# Cancer Research Secrets

by Keith Scott-Mumby
MD, MB ChB, HMD, PhD

Second Edition Sep 2015.

**Scott-Mumby Wellness is an imprint of Mother Whale Inc.**
PO Box 19452, Reno, Nevada, 89511, USA
Email: scottmumbywellness@gmail.com

ISBN-13: 978-0983878407

Library of Congress: this work is acknowledged by the Library of Congress, with dated receipt and is therefore fully protected. We are awaiting a registration number, which will be affixed to subsequent print runs.

Printed in USA by CreateSpace

# Are You Paying Attention?

Cancers figure among the leading causes of morbidity and mortality worldwide, with approximately 14 million new cases and 8.2 million cancer related deaths in 2012.

The number of new cases is expected to rise by about 70% over the next 2 decades.

Among men, the 5 most common sites of cancer diagnosed in 2012 were lung, prostate, colorectum, stomach, and liver cancer.

Among women the 5 most common sites diagnosed were breast, colorectum, lung, cervix, and stomach cancer.

**Around one third of cancer deaths are due to the 5 leading behavioural and dietary risks: high body mass index, low fruit and vegetable intake, lack of physical activity, tobacco use, alcohol use.** (my emphasis)

Tobacco use is the most important risk factor for cancer causing around 20% of global cancer deaths and around 70% of global lung cancer deaths.

Cancer causing viral infections such as HBV/HCV and HPV are responsible for up to 20% of cancer deaths in low- and middle-income countries.

More than 60% of world's total new annual cases occur in Africa, Asia and Central and South America. These regions account for 70% of the world's cancer deaths.

It is expected that annual cancer cases will rise from 14 million in 2012 to 22 million within the next 2 decades.

**Source:** World Health Organization website, accessed 21 Sep 2015, 1.00 pm PST.

# Important Disclaimer

# Contents

## 3. The Oxygen Connection .................75

## 4. Enzyme-Based Therapies.................87

## 5. Promising New Therapies .................97

## 6. Herbs Against Cancer ..................... 111

# Section 1

## The Politics
## Of Cancer

What you are NOT permitted to think in a society dogged by medical fascism! (beware the Gestapo tactics)

"Of course, it's in the interests of the cancer industry to keep everybody completely misinformed about cancer cures. They can't afford to let you learn the truth about how easy it is to cure cancer. Cancer cures are so commonplace now that you'd have to actually make a conscious effort not to see them."

**Mike Adams**
The Health Ranger

# 1.1 Is it cheating to win?

Welcome to the game of winning against cancer. It's a serious game and you don't want it to be like a crap shoot. You want the odds in your favor. That means you have to rig the game so that you win!

From the reaction of some of my medical colleagues, you would think they consider this to be worse than cheating at cards! Some of them have even been known to get angry at the patient who takes charge of his or her life and tries to influence the outcome of disease, as if it was a personal affront to them and their supposed skills.

But you need to be clear about one thing: the conventional treatment of cancer has been an unmitigated disaster. It is getting better and there are new "smart" therapies on the way. But cutting, burning and poisoning with chemo does as much, or more, to finish off the patient as the disease itself.

**170 Million Life Years Lost To Cancer in 2008**
Apparently, we lost approximately 170 million years of healthy life worldwide due to cancer in 2008.

That's pretty arresting. Ouch!

Researchers analyzed cancer registries from around the world and used a measure called disability-adjusted life-years (DALYs) to assess not only the impact of fatal cancer, but also the effects of disabilities among cancer survivors, such as breast loss due to breast cancer or infertility due to cervical cancer.

The researchers also determined that men in Eastern Europe had the largest cancer burden worldwide (3,146 age-adjusted DALYs lost per 100,000 men). Among women, the highest burden was in sub-Saharan Africa (2,749 age-adjusted DALYs lost per 100,000 women).

Colorectal, lung, breast and prostate cancers were the main contributors to total DALYs in most areas, accounting for 18 percent to 50 percent of total cancer burden.

Infection-related (viral-based) cancers such as liver, stomach and cervical cancers accounted for a larger part of overall DALYs in eastern Asia and sub-Saharan Africa (27 percent and 25 percent, respectively)

In addition, the study revealed that improved access to high-quality treatment has not improved survival for a number of common cancers associated with poor outcomes, especially lung, stomach, liver and pancreatic cancers.

Translation: conventional treatment doesn't work for most cancers (and is therefore not "high quality" care).

This study also shows quite starkly that cancer is emerging in poorer countries. As they adopt the much-desired Western lifestyle, they get our diseases too.

[The study was published online Oct. 15, 2012, in The Lancet]

**Immune System Disease**

Cancer is best seen as a failure of the immune system—we all develop cancer cells (all the time) but it's no problem for our immune systems to identify the rogue cells and destroy them. So, logically, how can poisoning the immune system with chemo help? Radiation too destroys immunity. That the main thing that later killed victims after Hiroshima and Nagasaki. Lowered immunity is recognized as one of the disastrous side-effects of radiation overdose!

So it's no surprise that, contrary to all the propaganda, we are NOT winning the war against cancer. That's just sales talk to raise more funds for cancer charities. Not that the money goes on research mind but it goes on huge unjustifiable salaries for officers of the trust; the ones who are putting out these misleading claims of success.

Whenever you hear of a new cancer "breakthrough" treatment in the press, you need to realize there is probably no breakthrough, nothing new even. It's just posturing by the Cancer Mafia, trying to raise the share value of this or that company. If you watch carefully for these orchestrated press releases, you will notice, as I have done many times over the years, that they are preceded by an onslaught on alternative therapies which they claim are proven worthless – or even dangerous. That's a joke when you consider the extreme dangers of chemo and radiation.

Having established the position that there is nothing you can do, no hope, alternative therapies won't save you, then BINGO! there is a sudden announcement of a new breakthrough drug or therapy that will save everyone.

I don't want to break your hopes but I do want to say that statistics for survival with cancer have not improved in 80 years, apart from a few very select cancers, such as childhood leukemias, chorion cancer and testicular cancer. Couple that with the fact that cancer is rising and you'll see we are NOT winning the war.

Well, I'm saying all that to make sure you understand that you have choices and you may want to turn against the orthodox approach and try something more holistic. This is just to say that you will not be harming your chances of survival, no matter what you are told.

However I do not suggest it is "wrong" to have chemo or radiation and many patients opt for that. I support that decision if that's what you want to do and, as we will see shortly, alternative medicine has a lot to offer you. It can protect you against the worst side effects. In over a decade I never had any patient who lost his or her hair!

All that said, let's take a look at what you can do. Here there is almost a feast of choices. What's great is you can try several different things at once and, again despite all the heavy-handed attacks and propaganda, none of it is incompatible with conventional therapies. One can help the other. Most of my successes were on patients who wanted to follow both pathways, some conventional therapy to maybe get started and then they took over with their own chosen treatment modalities.

I like to get a patient to the level where he or she has enough knowledge to make wise decisions and to manage their own condition. This empowers patients and it also lightens the physician's burden. Weekly appointments were often like a corporate business meeting, discussing strategies and voting on what action to take. My vote, incidentally, did not outweigh that of the patient. Not unless he or she was acting out of ignorance—and I would do everything in my power to provide the missing knowledge.

But you will see why conventional doctors may not be the place to get the right advice, from the next two sections...

# 1.2 We're All Battling Cancer!

This section heading might seem a bit of an exaggeration but some years ago cancer overtook heart disease as the number-one killer disease of the West. It's not just a question of an aging population, as we shall see, but cancer is p rimarily a disease of civilization. Elderly people among ethnic groups all around the world who have followed a natural traditional lifestyle simply do not get cancer: period.

Meanwhile, in the Western or "civilized" world, cancer has become a disaster. As I said, the incidence for both sexes is around 1:2 or fifty-fifty. That means either you, or someone who is very close to you, is going to contract the disease. While we might feel very sorry for the patient, let me assure you that it is no picnic being with someone you love while they suffer and eventually die, miserably and painfully. In some ways the survivors need more supportive care and sympathy than the victim. Once the patient is gone, it's over for them. But those left behind still have to pick up the pieces and live their lives as best they can, with the haunting memories of a stark reality that is often hard to bear. Even a belief in a higher presence to our lives does little to assuage the pain and grief of loss.

So once again let me invite you to join me in learning how this brute can be subdued. Here is a whole book crammed full of knowledge about how to overcome cancer. Make no mistake, it can be beaten. In some ways it is like a game—a very serious game—but there are rules. If you don't know the rules, you have very little chance of winning.

In the next few sections I am going to teach you the rules as I know them. I'll be sharing with you lots of tried and proven strategies that have been successfully used. Nothing in these pages is mere speculation.

With so much information available to you, you will be able to make wiser choices and certainly you will be in a position to influence the progress of your disease favourably. If you are learning for a friend or family member, make sure they learn too and become involved with their outcome. It's one of the oldest dictums in all of healing that you can't want recovery for a person more than they want it for themselves. It just doesn't work.

Bear in mind that not all the tactics I shall be sharing with you are therapies, as such. For example the report on understanding and monitoring your own tumor markers provides at least a dozen tools for beating cancer. Good nutrition is not just one answer but covers hundreds of different supplements and oral remedies, scattered throughout the book. The fact remains that there are over 500 different tips and wrinkles, theories, strategies and facts that you need to know and understand, in order to be truly DIET WISE.

# 1.3 Beware Phoney Stastitics

**The Lies We Face**

*The five year cancer survival statistics of the American Cancer Society are very misleading. They now count things that are not cancer, and, because we are able to diagnose at an earlier stage of the disease, patients falsely appear to live longer.*

*Our whole cancer research in the past 20 years has been a failure. More people over 30 are dying from cancer than ever before...More women with mild or benign diseases are being included in statistics and reported as being "cured". When government officials point to survival figures and say they are winning the war against cancer they are using those survival rates improperly."*

**Dr J. Bailer, New England Journal of Medicine**

**This is how the authorities work this "improvement" scam:**

1.  First of all you need to understand that official "survival" figures are based upon a five year period. To them, that's an achievement. Personally I don't think living for five years is satisfactory; I want to live for decades to come. But let's see how they play the game.

2.  Vigorous screening programs allow a certain number of cancers to be diagnosed earlier than normal. Because the patient shows up on the radar, maybe 12 months sooner, he or she appears to make it to the six-year mark and is therefore a success.

    But look at it this way: on the old system, you might have been diagnosed in the year 2000 and be dead by the year 2005. Therefore you would show up in the official five-year survival period (as a failure!) In the new system, you would be diagnosed in 1999, and therefore still alive at the end of 2004 (5 years) and apparently now, a survivor!

    However, you still die in 2005, the same year it was always going to happen. So therapy had no success whatsoever in your case, but you looked good. If there are tens of thousands like you, then officials can boast an improvement in overall statistics. But in fact, this is meaningless; just massaging of figures.

3.  The fraudulent claims don't stop there; they are adding in lots of harmless lesions, claiming these are cancerous or "pre-cancerous" (how do you like that word?) None of these lesions will cause any harm, they don't need treating and are best left alone (as we shall see in the next section). When these too don't kill the patient, this is claimed as a successful cure or "treatment".

You need to bear this in mind when you look at success stories about how we're winning against cancer. It's all just phoney posturing.

The truth is that chemotherapy and radiotherapy, also most surgery, is completely unjustifiable in terms of the results that are achieved. However this doesn't stop the medical establishment from continuing to push these treatments on unfortunate patients. They want their money and are not about to be deterred by the fact that they're giving deplorably bad, even dangerous, service.

You might think I am being unduly cynical with my colleagues. But consider the matter of radical mastectomy. It's now been over two decades since it was proven that this procedure added nothing whatever to a patient's life span or quality of life. It's just a hideous mutilation, serving no purpose, and yet surgeons all over the globe continue to assault women in this cruel and unnecessary way.

And while we are talking about cynicism, what about this story...

## Wrong Cell Lines Catastrophe in Cancer Research

It's me that used the word catastrophe for what I am going to reveal next; most doctors are talking of "a minor glitch". But then most doctors and scientists are gullible or frauds. The fact that 100 scientific papers and 11 US patents are invalidated by the discovery that trials were done on the wrong type of cells is very major indeed.

Know what's weird here? Hardly anybody is concerned. Doesn't that say volumes for the fact that they don't believe their own story anyway? I think it does.

If you had the "latest drug" for pancreatic cancer, that was "proven" to work, but in fact had been tested only on lung cells or ovarian cancer, wouldn't you worry... just a little?

Well, that's what patients are now facing. *It seems there has been a huge mix up and scientists supposedly doing research into cancer therapies have been testing out on any old cell line, not necessarily the one they claimed.* In other words all the science is fraudulent and should be re-done, even if not an intentional mistake.

The study which stirred all this up is a Dutch study (you'd never get this degree of honesty from an American study or researchers), showing that 3 of 13 human esophageal cancer cell lines widely used for worldwide research were actually cell lines from lung, colorectal and other malignancies.

Two of the contaminated or misidentified cell lines were involved in research published in more than 100 papers and in the issuance of 11 U.S. patents, which led to clinical trials in patients. Winand N.M. Dinjens, senior author of a short paper published online Jan. 14 in the *Journal of the National Cancer Institute* and head of molecular diagnostics in the department of pathology at the Josephine Nefkens Institute, University Medical Center Rotterdam in The Netherlands.

Predictably, "experts" are stating that the unintentional misidentification or contamination of the cell lines is not critical and is even a fairly common occurrence. Well, they would say that, wouldn't they, since they got egg all over their faces...

"From the scientific point of view, it's not a huge deal, but it's certainly something you're glad you found out," said Charles Saxe, scientific director of the Program in Cancer Cell Biology and Metastasis at the American Cancer Society in Atlanta [Yeah, I'll bet he was real glad]. "This probably doesn't surprise anybody. The surprise is probably that there were only three."

The unpleasant surprise for the rest of us, Mr. Saxe, is that you seem to play down mistakes of this order, yet belong to a lobby which wants to jail honest holistic practitioners for staking out part of your money-grabbing territory with something a little less twisted (Saxe works for the corrupt charity known as the American Cancer Society; most countries have a version of this "cancer charity" scam).

"The issue of misidentification/crosscontamination is not a new thing," said Robert H. Shoemaker, chief of the screening technologies branch at the U.S. National Cancer Institute and author of an editorial accompanying the study, who also did not deem the finding a huge catastrophe.

What? A kid in 2nd or 3rd grade who turned in such sloppy work would be punished by the teacher. If you got an assignment to write about European history and wrote instead about Japanese history, you'd get whalloped--- and expect to be, right?

Notice that my own concern here is not that this happened or that there was contamination: *it's that nobody in responsible positions seems to give a damn.*

It shows just what cynicism and phoney science is out there. It's not science: it's pre-packaging drugs for sale to an unsuspecting public.

SOURCE: Jan. 14, 2010, online *Journal of the National Cancer Institute*; comments from www.medicine.net

# 1.4 Do Doctors Create The Cancer Problem?

The fact is clear that in primitive societies, people don't die of cancer. This is supposed to be because they are healthier and eat properly. But who dares think the unthinkable: that the cause of the problem is doctors and when you don't have them, cancer is insignificant?

It's only when doctors using Western methods get involved that cancer actually becomes a problem at all. Then it's suddenly a serious and probably fatal condition.

But it may be time for a re-think. On Tuesday Dec 16th a major study was published which could change EVERYTHING doctors know and think about cancer.

If you've spent any time on my website you'll know I'm a fan of Dr. Ryke Geerde Hamer (http://www.alternative-doctor.com/cancer/hamers_page.htm or see section 14) who's radical cancer theory is that all cancers are Nature's healing response to something, typically a severe psychic trauma or some other threatening event.

This makes sense to me. I've never believed in the absurd attitude towards cancer that it's some kind of alien growth from another planet. It's YOU, I mean it's your own body tissue that has changed and started to do something else. It's not a package from outer space that landed in your body!

I believe that if we seek to understand the true purpose of cancer (and ALL diseases have a purpose, whether or not it's clear to us), we can solve this problem once and for all. Nature is not a fool and therefore, if she switches on a mechanism, she has a reason for it.

To assume Nature is stupid and misled is the most dangerous kind of arrogance I know, and not just physicians and surgeons, but most scientists are guilty of it.

In my profession, it's killing people.

But the question hangs: **is it because doctors are messing with it that cancer becomes so uncontrollable and dangerous?** Well, new evidence suggests that's very much the case.


# 1.4a Natural disappearance

Doctors and lay people have always known that some cases of cancer just go away without treatment. If Dr. Hamer is right, this is what should happen. The cancer manifests as a healing mechanism, the problem is resolved and the cancer heals and disappears!

*Voila!* As the French say.

How often this happens we have no way of knowing, because doctors get on the case and mess things up. I can infer from less-doctored societies, like the Eskimos and natural-born Indians, that if there is little or no doctoring, that the low rates of cancer are due to the fact that doctors are not getting involved.

The cancers are there allright, but they go away! Nature takes her course; the "disease" resolves.

Now a new study had shed a great deal of light on what I'm talking about here. This is not some miraculous "spontaneous remission"; this is *what is supposed to happen* and does happen, when doctors leave matters alone.

Cancers heal themselves! And it's NOT a rare thing at all.

The study, from Norway, was published in *The Archives of Internal Medicine* (Dec 2008), and it suggests that even invasive breast cancers may sometimes go away without treatment and in larger numbers than anyone ever believed.

Maybe doctors should re-consider what they do? If the spontaneous remission hypothesis is credible, it should cause a major re-evaluation in the approach to breast cancer research and treatment; in fact all cancers.

But predictably, the old guard entrenched against any new discoveries, reacted with fury: "Their simplification of a complicated issue is both overreaching and alarming," said Robert A. Smith, director of breast cancer screening at the American Cancer Society.

He's paid a lot of money to keep cancer cures from the public (by which I mean if a cure is ever found, he's out of his job, per the terms of the Society charter).

But many doctors have responded as I would wish and have started to re-think things. Robert M. Kaplan, the chairman of the department of health services at the School of Public Health at the University of California, Los Angeles, has already suggested that it could eventually be possible for some women to opt for so-called watchful waiting, monitoring a tumor in their breast to see whether it grows. "People have never thought that way about breast cancer," Kaplan told the New York Times.

The study was conducted by Dr. H. Gilbert Welch, a researcher at the VA Outcomes Group in White River Junction, Vt., and Dartmouth Medical School; Dr. Per-Henrik Zahl of the Norwegian Institute of Public Health; and Dr. Jan Maehlen of Ulleval University Hospital in Oslo. It compared two groups of Norwegian women ages 50 to 64 in two consecutive six-year periods.

One group of 109,784 women was followed from 1992 to 1997. Mammography screening in Norway was initiated in 1996. In 1996 and 1997, all were offered mammograms, and nearly every woman accepted.

The second group of 119,472 women was followed from 1996 to 2001. All were offered regular mammograms, and nearly all accepted.

It might be expected that the two groups would have roughly the same number of breast cancers, either detected at the end or found along the way. Instead, the researchers report, the women who had regular routine screenings had 22 percent more cancers. For every 100,000 women who were screened regularly, 1,909 were diagnosed with invasive breast cancer over six years, compared with 1,564 women who did not have regular screening.

Of course the old guard is quick to point out that the findings do not mean that the mammograms caused breast cancer! That's false: evidence shows that there is a significant increase in the risk. The "guidelines" are no more than a smokescreen for profiteering, not science.

John Gofman, M.D., Ph.D. – a nuclear physicist and a medical doctor, and one of the leading experts in the world on the dangers of radiation – presents compelling evidence in his book, *Radiation from Medical Procedures in the Pathogenesis of Cancer and Ischemic Heart Disease,* that over 50 percent of the death-rate from cancer is in fact induced by x-rays.

The routine practice of taking four films of each breast annually results in approx-imately 1 rad (radiation absorbed dose) exposure, which is about 1,000 times greater than that from a chest x-ray (remember, mass screening with chest x-rays was stopped, because it caused more cancer than it detected!)

Dr. Epstein, M.D., professor emeritus of Environmental and Occupational Medicine at the University of Illinois School of Public Health, and author of an amazing book *"The Politics of Cancer Revisited"* has described the guidelines as a sham.

According to him "They were conscious, chosen, politically expedient acts by a small group of people for the sake of their own power, prestige and financial gain, resulting in suffering and death for millions of women. They fit the classification of 'crimes against humanity.'"

It remains that, one way or the other, the die-hards have got to face the fact they are killing women. Either the mammograms cause cancer, in which case they should stop, or there is spontaneous disappearance of many cancers, which is be-ing thwarted by medical intervention.

They can't lie their way out of it in both directions at once!

"Intellectually bankrupt, fiscally wasteful and therapeutically useless", said Dr. James Watson, Nobel Laureate when asked about cancer research and the National Cancer Program.

The problem, as always, is money and greed. Doctors want to make money out of patients who don't need any medical care, as well as the ones who are sick. Dropping the present approach would mean their revenues would suffer (smaller mortgages, less marble in the villa!)

The fact remains that many actions are carried out in the US that other countries don't do. Here there is the insistence in biopsying every lump. That means women with no real cancer are being subjected to unnecessary procedures and run the risk of being inadvertently diagnosed as having cancer, being subjected to chemo and dying as a result.

In fact I have good evidence that women are being falsely (fraudulently) diagnosed as histologically positive, to help attract more revenues through costly and protracted chemo and radiotherapy. In any other sphere that's murder; indeed, in medicine it's murder, but is not being picked up.

These are hot claims, so let me steer back towards the main point I'm making, which is that doctors may "cause" a lot of cancer and unnecessary deaths, by refusing to allow that this disease will resolve naturally.

After all, in simple societies—like traditional Eskimos, the Hunzas in the Himalayas and Amazon Indians—the disease is virtually unknown. I recently also published an article, quoting research into the Victorian diet, showing that even with less doctoring they had far, far fewer cancer deaths.

Actually, it was almost unknown at that time. A physician at one of London's main hospitals (Charing Cross) told his medical students that lung cancer was "One of the rare forms of a rare disease. You may probably pass the rest of your student's life without seeing another example of it".

Don't get caught by the phoney propaganda argument we are living longer than ever, so more cancer is showing up. In my piece I quoted extensive research showing we are NOT living significantly longer than our mid-Victorian counterparts (once past the first 5 years, our survival rates are pretty similar to those of 1850).

In any case, there is more to this; not only were cancers rarer but Victorians seemed to withstand the disease better than our modern citizen. It was not feared nearly so much, for this reason. Take breast cancer: the average survival time was 4 years, with a maximum time of 18 years. But this was almost all due to stage 3 and 4 (late) cancers.

If Victorian physicians had had our modern sophistication in diagnostic equipment, they would have picked up stage 1 and 2, so dramatically extending average post-diagnosis survival times. The average may well then have shot up to 10 years and maximum to 40- 50 years!

Let's go back to the Norwegian study that is so exciting and controversial:

The study's design was not perfect, but researchers say the ideal study is not feasible. It would entail screening women, randomly assigning them to have their screen-detected cancers treated or not, and following them to see how many untreated cancers went away on their own.

But, they said, they were astonished by the results.

"I think everybody is surprised by this finding," said the journal editors. They spent a weekend reading and re-reading the paper (see, not every doctor is a crook or a sham). "Our initial reaction was, 'This is pretty weird' but the more we looked at it, the more we were persuaded."

Dr. Barnett Kramer, director of the *Office of Disease Prevention at the National Institutes of Health*, had a similar reaction. "People who are familiar with the broad range of behaviors of a variety of cancers know spontaneous regression is possible," he said. "But what is shocking is that it can occur so frequently."

Although the researchers cannot completely rule out other explanations, they went to a lot of trouble to show these other interpretations are not valid.

A leading alternative explanation for the results is that the women having regular scans used hormone therapy for menopause and the other women did not. But the researchers calculated that hormone use could account for no more than 3 percent of the effect.

Maybe mammography was more sensitive in the second six-year period, able to pick up more tumors. But, the authors report, mammography's sensitivity did not appear to have changed.

Or perhaps the screened women had a higher cancer risk to begin with. But, the investigators say, the groups were remarkably similar in their risk factors.

Die-hard Dr. Smith of the American Cancer Society, predictably, said the study was flawed and the interpretation incorrect. Among other things, he said, one round of screening in the first group of women would never find all the cancers that regular screening had found in the second group. The reason, he said, is that mammography is not perfect, and cancers that are missed on one round of screening will be detected on another.

But the study authors debunked this nonsense. Chief author Dr. Welch said that he and his colleagues considered that possibility, too. And, he said, their analysis found subsequent mammograms could not make up the difference.

The fact remains that now doctors must seriously worry themselves that they are blunderingly wrong by rushing to treatment:

I like the comments of Dr. Laura Esserman, professor of surgery and radiology at the University of California, San Francisco:

> "I am a breast cancer surgeon; I run a breast cancer program," she said. "I treat women every day, and I promise you it's a problem. Every time you tell a person they have cancer, their whole life runs before their eyes.

> "What if I could say, 'It's not a real cancer, it will go away, don't worry about it,' " she added. "That's such a different message. Imagine how you would feel."

Now that WOULD be progress!

Well, I hope this article has brought you some hope. The main thing we have to fear with cancer is fear and confusion. All this will vanish when we understand it properly. Meantime, it's a wake up call but not a death knell: you just have to get your health in order.

As I said, cancer is not some package from outer space dropped inside your body. The tumor is YOU. If you make the right changes, those tissues will go back to being healthy and normal.

Your diet, lifestyle and state of mind are absolutely critical. Do not allow shallow-thinking, ignorant doctors to tell you otherwise.

[MAIN REFERENCE: November 25, 2008, on pg. A19 of the New York Times]

# 1.5 The "Arrow Of Cancer"

The hero scientist who defeats cancer will likely never exist. Cancer is an intricate, potentially lethal collaboration of genes gone awry, of growth inhibitors gone missing, of hormones and epigenomes changing, and rogue cells breaking free.

**Dr. Garry Gordon**

Garry is right up to a point. But there's a missing sentence: **Nature will cure anything, if you only remove the barriers to healing!** Check this out:

Call it the "arrow of cancer". It's been likened to the arrow of time, it was supposed to point in one direction. Cancers starts, grows and just worsens relentlessly. That's what they said. The "Norway Study" I just referred to on page 9 changes all that.

Now an article in The New York Times (Oct. 26, 2009) featuring interviews on the same theme with recognized cancer experts, has called a whole doctrine into question (that cancer is relentless and early detection saves lives). It also raises the other BIG question that noone is still talking about (except me): do doctors cause cancer deaths by getting involved in a natural process that will often heal, if just left alone?

A review of more than two decades of screening for breast and prostate cancers, published in the Journal of the America Medical Association (Oct 2009) has shown simply that screening appears to be finding many small tumors that would not be a problem if they were left alone, undiscovered by screening. They were destined to stop growing on their own or shrink, or even, at least in the case of some breast cancers, disappear altogether.

No oncologist will tell you that.

[JAMA. 2009;302(15):1685-1692. doi:10.1001/jama.2009.1498]

Dr. Barnett Kramer, associate director for disease prevention at the National Institutes of Health, questioned the old idea that cancer is an automatic linear process.

"A cell acquired a mutation, and little by little it acquired more and more mutations. Mutations are not supposed to revert spontaneously."

That's the current model, Dr. Kramer said, "an arrow that moves in one direction." But now, he added, it is becoming increasingly clear that cancers require more than mutations to progress. They need the cooperation of surrounding cells and even, he said, "the whole organism, the person," whose immune system or hormone levels, for example, can squelch or fuel a tumor.

And remarkably, even some of the skeptics have changed their minds and decided that, contrary as it seems to everything they once thought, cancers can disappear on their own. They may not be happy about it but what can an honest physician think?

Dr. Robert M. Kaplan, the chairman of the department of health services at the School of Public Health at the University of California, Los Angeles, thinks, "The weight of the evidence suggests that there is reason to believe..." that cancer is rigged to heal itself in many cases.

Disappearing tumors are well known in testicular cancer. Dr. Jonathan Epstein at Johns Hopkins says it does not happen often, but it definitely happens. A young man may have a lump in his testicle, but when doctors remove the organ all they find is a big scar. The tumor that was there is gone. Or, they see a large scar and a tiny tumor because more than 95 percent of the tumor had dis*app*eared on its own by the time the testicle was removed.

There is more and more evidence that cancers can go backward or stop, and researchers are being forced to reassess their notions of what cancer is and how it develops.

Of course, doctors are quick to point out patients should not avoid treatment because of such occasional occurrences. That's the party line.

"Biologically, it is a rare phenomenon to have an advanced cancer go into remission," said Dr. Martin Gleave, a professor of urology at the University of British Columbia. **But how does he know? Since doctors always get involved, there is no true measure of how cancers on the whole progress if left** alone. What I pointed out eleswhere in my writing is that cancer in Victorian times was not feared as it is today. The real fear element seems to be something that has been manufactured by modern science; critics would say deliberately.

What we do know is that the vast majority of us have cancers already circulating in our bodies. There are more as we get older. By middle age or beyond we are riddled with cancer cells, according to Thea Tlsty, a professor of pathology at the University of California, San Francisco.

She is referring to the discovery made in autopsy studies of people who died of other causes, with no idea that they had cancer cells or precancerous cells loose in their bodies. They did not have large tumors or symptoms of cancer.

"The really interesting question," Dr. Tlsty said, "is not so much why do we get cancer as why don't we get cancer?" I like this lady (pronounced Tulsty, I think).

You know, maybe cancer is a healing process, not a disease process! Why not? It is proper to think of ALL disease as a healing process. Diarrhea is trying to get rid of toxins, so is eczema and lumps and cysts. There a whole model here in which cancer is vibrant new tissue, trying respond to some biological trigger. But then it goes wrong...

This possibility is backed up by the simple observation that the earlier a cell is in its path toward an aggressive cancer, the more likely it is to reverse course. So, for example, cells that are early precursors of cervical cancer are likely to revert. One study found that 60 percent of precancerous cervical cells, found with Pap tests, revert to normal within a year; 90 percent revert within three years.

Do you ever get told that? No, never. You get told you are in grave danger and you need treatment right away to have even a chance of beating the cancer!

Probably this early detection of cancers, that will go away if left untreated, is the reason that we are finding huge numbers of early cancers without a corresponding decline in late stage cancers.

If, as the story goes, every one of those early cancers were destined to turn into an advanced cancer, then the total number of cancers should be the same after screening is introduced, but the increase in early cancers should be balanced by a decrease in advanced cancers—and therefore a drop in deaths.

That has not happened with screening for breast and prostate cancer, for example. So the hypothesis is that many early cancers go nowhere. And, as with breast cancer, there is indirect evidence that some actually disappear.

Prostate cancers are among the "safest" to have. Many stop growing or grow only very slowly, even after a fast start.

When men have small tumors with cells that do not look terribly deranged, doctors at Johns Hopkins offer them an option of "active surveillance."

Almost no one agrees to such a plan. "Most men want it out," Dr. Jonathan Epstein at Johns Hopkins said. But, following those men who do chose not to be treated, the investigators discovered that only about 20 percent to 30 percent of those small tumors actually progressed at all.

In Canada, researchers have been doing a similar study with small kidney cancers, among those that are reported to regress occasionally, even when far advanced. As many as 6 percent who received no treatment, or a placebo, had tumors that shrank or remained stable. The same thing happened in those who received the therapy, leading the researchers to conclude that the treatment did not actually improve outcomes.

So the message is encouraging. Do NOT get railroaded into hasty choices. The only reason an oncologist would do that is he's ignorant, or greedy (he wants your money), or both (most likely).

As my good friend Dr. Garry Gordon likes to say: Early detection should not be used as a means to shuttle people into surgery, radiation, and chemotherapy. Mainstream treatment for cancer is usually a waste of time and money, yet amazingly no one in academia ever mentions how easy it is to bring PSA into safe ranges and keep it there for life.

With early detection, the net has become so fine that we are pulling in small fish as well as big fish. What oncologists need to start doing is to identify the small fish can be let go. Time to start slinging some back in the sea!

I'm not telling you not to get screening tests. It could help detect early risks. But never swallow the junk science that says: we have found markers, therefore you have cancer, therefore you are in danger unless you start our treatments right away. Keep in mind that standard treatments seem to have been shown to have the potential to waken a sleepy cancer and turn it into an avenging giant!

# 1.6 Inflammation Is The Big Worry

That brings me to an another important topic and a very special and easy way you can "solve" the cancer puzzle.

We know the hallmarks of cancer, the properties that endow the cells with mischief, such as self-sufficient growth, resistance to anti-growth and pro-death signals (apoptosis), activated oncogenes or dysfunctional tumor suppressors, but these alone it has emerged are not sufficient for the development of cancer.

There needs to be a shift in the surrounding cells, which are not necessarily cancerous themselves, but create a growth-friendly environment for the tumor to flourish.

Specifically, there needs to be inflammation for cancers to flourish! [Yale J Biol Med. 2006 Dec; 79(3-4): 123–130. Published online 2007 Oct.]

That's good news, because inflammation is relatively easy to quench and should follow naturally from a healthy diet and lifestyle.

**Mechanics**

Here may be a good point to lay down some basic principles.

There are six fundamental properties or, if you like hallmarks, of cancerous cells:

self-sufficient proliferation

insensitivity to anti-proliferative signals

evasion of apoptosis (programmed cell death)

unlimited replicative potential

the maintenance of vascularization (for food supply)

and, for malignancy, local tissue invasion and eventually metastasis

However the adoption of any or all of these characteristics will not lead to successful tumor growth.

Research over the last two decades has solidified the concept that tumor development and malignancy is the result of processes involving both the cancer cells themselves and non-cancer cells around them, many of which compose a hetero-geneous multicellular mass.

Cancer we know is an "outgrowth" of normal healthy tissue that has gone off in a different direction and regulation of growth and multiplication has been lost. There are four essential phases in this outgrowth process.

These are: 1) Predisposition, 2) Precipitation and 3) Prolongation and 4) Progres-sion. What I call **The Four Ps**.

Without all stages in place, the cancer either won't grow or won't survive long. The single word "carcinogenesis" does not really cover all this.

> **Predisposition** means genomic changes within the "cancer cell," such as point mutations, gene deletion and amplification, and chromosomal rear-rangements leading to irreversible cellular changes and the potential for ab-normal growth.

> **Precipitation** means certain cells break through and go "rogue". These will then start to clone. In other words, tumor suppressor genes have failed. The cells are now imbued with certain dangerous propensities.

> **Prolongation** needs encompassing survival factors. It has become clear that surrounding cells need to "enable" the tumor. Inflammation is important in this stage. It means that the immune system has lost the battle, at least for the time being.

> **Progress** is the stage where the cancer propagates, grows and eventually spreads. Again, support from the surrounding tissues is necessary, if the can-cer is to spread. For examples vascular tissue needs to proliferate, to bring more food to the rapidly growing object, a process called "angiogenesis". A go-it-alone tumor wouldn't last long, without adequate food.

# The Role Of Inflammation

An association between inflammation and cancer has been long known. For exam-ple continuously abraded wounds (rubbing, as in asbestosis and mesothelioma), localized toxins (pipe smoking or tobacco chewing leading to oral cancers), infec-tions (papilloma virus and hepatitis B and C).

There are also a number of specific infections, associated with specific cancers: Burkitt's lymphoma; Kaposi's sarcoma (AIDS); gastric cancer secondary to *Hel-icobacter pylori*; and colon cancer because of long-standing inflammatory bowel disease precipitated by the intestinal microflora. Or in the case of ulcerative colitis, which is notoriously pro-cancerous, inflammation of a non-infectious kind.

Even if there is no direct evidence of infection or irritation, where is always a sig-nificant leucocyte infiltration and often wound repair responses observable at sites which eventually become cancerous.

All of these cases are situations where the immune system's inflammatory re-sponses are in over-drive, trying to overcome the local tissue insult. There is leu-cocyte infiltration at the site of any chronic irritation. We are already very clear that cancer follows any immune dysfunction. A flustered, over-worked immune system is not doing its job.

Conversely, there are reverse clues; further evidence for the role of inflammation has come from the use of non-steroidal anti-inflammatory drugs (NSAIDs) in the prevention of spontaneous tumor formation in people with familial adenomatous polyposis (FAP). http://www.ncbi.nlm.nih.gov/pmc/articles/PMC1994795/]

Joining the dots and interpreting the picture which emerges is not very difficult: *cancers and inflammation are related by epidemiology, histopathology, inflammatory profiles, and the efficacy of anti-inflammatory drugs in prophylaxis.*

Chronic inflammatory states associated with infection and irritation are well-proven to foster genomic lesions in cells. One way this occurs is the production of free radicals such as reactive oxygen intermediates (ROI), hydroxyl radical (OH) and superoxide (O2) and reactive nitrogen intermediates (RNI), nitric oxide (NO) and peroxynitrite (ONOO-). These can damage DNA and increase the risk of genetic mutations. [http://www.ncbi.nlm.nih.gov/pmc/articles/PMC1994795/]

Moreover, in the face of massive cell death, as occurs in infection or non-infectious tissue injury, lost cells must be repopulated by the expansion of other cells, often undifferentiated precursor cells such as tissue stem cells. There is a risk of these turning wild, in their enthusiastic growth.

It is important to remember that a competent and not-overstressed immune system is quite capable of picking off cancer cells and neutralizing them. We therefore need to protect and enhance our immune systems. That includes lowering inflammation in the tissues as drastically as possible.

No effort in this direction is wasted.

# 1.6a 10 Tips To Reducing Inflammation

1.  Immediately begin a search for non-inflammatory foods and eliminate them. Ignore ALL the advice you read about what are supposed to be "allergenic foods" and "anti-inflammatory foods". Foods that cause inflammatory reactions are NOT the same for everybody. We are all unique.

    The way to identify your highly inflammatory foods is to follow the detailed self-help plan I gave you in my book Diet Wise (www.DietWiseBook.com) and is also managed for you in detail, with over 50 instructional videos, at my membership site: www.dietwiseacademy.com The membership is very modest and you only pay once.

    At the very least you will avoid all manufactured foods, with their added sweeteners, hidden trans-fats and other texturings, flavorings and chemicals that you body definitely does not want.

2.  Take adequate omega-3s. These are among nature's finest anti-inflammatory substances. 3 grams a day.

3.  Avoid all sugar in foods and keep your glucose metrics in a good range (fasting insulin, HbA1C, etc.) If you already have type II diabetes, you already have

roaring inflammation going on in your body and you must work extra hard to get it down.

4. Flood your body with molecular hydrogen (H2). This has nothing to do with hydrogen ions (which create acidity). Molecular hydrogen is one of the best selective antioxidants known, that knocks out the very dangerous hydroxyl radical, without harming the oxidative signalling pathways. [get Activ-H2, from Purative: www.purative.com]

5. Eat plenty of fresh fruit and veggies and enjoy juices and smoothies, but this is subject to what you find in 1.

6. Sleeping soundly is vital and you must address any sleep-deficit disorder. This is one of the most powerful ways I know of reducing inflammation. (section 1.6)

7. Losing weight is essential if you are obese or significantly overweight. You must understand that belly fat particularly is highly inflammatory.

8. Anti-Inflammatory Herbs (these are just a sample):

   - **Boswellia (Boswellia serrata)**. Also known as Indian frankincense, Boswellia serrata has long been recognized in Ayurvedic medicine for its anti-inflammatory benefits. Today scientists studying extracts of boswellia report that it can switch off key cell signalers and pro-inflammatory mediators known as cytokines in the inflammatory cascade.

   - **Ginger (Zingiber officinalis)**. Ginger has been valued for centuries the world over for its medicinal qualities, including its analgesic, anti-inflammatory, anti-nausea, and sugar-moderating effects in the body.

   - **Turmeric (Curcuma longa)**, has been used for centuries in Indian Ayurvedic medicine as an anti-inflammatory agent. Also known as cucurmin, it is a mild COX-2 inhibitor, but works differently from the prescription-strength drugs (they can increase your risk of myocardial infarction or stroke). Like Boswellia and ginger, curcumin seems to inhibit the production of prostaglandins and helps inflammation-regulating genes through its effects on cell-signaling.

9. Mild exercise is also known to lower inflammation. Heavy exercize is bad for you; it releases lots of free radicals. Avoid cardio and do only 20 – 40 minute *walks*.

10. Massage and aromatherapy are also believed to help.

**Less popular advice—but important none the less—would be to stop smoking, calm down (avoid stress, which is also highly inflammatory) and get rid of all unnecessary chemicals in your home, including cosmetics and cleaners.**

Start a "fresh" life!

# 1.6b The Microbiome and Inflammation

Finally, let's not forget the role of our intestinal flora; the so-called microbiome. Its becoming more and more obvious that the microbiome influences many disease. It probably, in truth, will cause death when sufficiently out of balance.

I have already written extensively of the effect of the human microbiome on health and disease, in my classic book "*Fire In The Belly*". Vast number of pathological process, even a number of psychiatric conditions, start in the gut; a result of that metabolic "fire" (inflammation).

Here's is more information, to make clear how important our gut health is in the matter of developing cancer.

Dr. David Johnson, professor of medicine and chief of gastroenterology at Eastern Virginia Medical School in Norfolk, Virginia, recently edited a book on the human microbiome's role in health and disease, and shared with subscribers at Medscape. com what he had learned.

It is well known that the gut serves as the largest immune system in the body. A study of special germ-free mice has shown that the gut can be humanized with human gut flora and has demonstrated that switching from a plant-based to a Western-based high-fat and high-sugar diet causes distinct shifts in the microbiome. Such shifts can occur very rapidly (within one day).

[Turnbaugh PJ, Ridaura VK, Faith JJ, Rey FE, Knight R, Gordon JI. The effect of diet on the human gut microbiome: a metagenomic analysis in humanized gnotobiotic mice. *Sci Transl Med*. 2009;1:6ra14]

The question is then, how much of a role bacterial flora play in systemic diseases, rather than simply in the day-to-day processing of the food groups that we eat.

## Gastrointestinal Cancers

The majority of our microbiome's diversity resides in the colon. Already a study has linked certain pathogenic bacteria with the development of colorectal cancer. The current thought is that selected microbiomes can mediate a chronic inflammatory environment, which contributes to the progression of colorectal cancer.

For example, the incidence of cancer in rural native Africans is lower compared with African Americans, something that has been attributed to a higher amount of indigestible polysaccharides in the diet of the former. Undigested polysaccharides passing into the gut, primarily as dietary fiber, are metabolized by the microbiome into short-chain fatty acids. These are then converted into acetate, propionate, and butyrate. These in turn down regulate the pro-inflammatory cytokines and induce differentiation of T cells into regulatory T cells (the ones which turn off inflammation).

There is a sharp drop in inflammatory mediators in the colon. This underlines the importance of fiber for colon cancer prevention. [ Louis P, Hold GL, Flint HJ. The gut microbiota, bacterial metabolites and colorectal cancer. Nat Rev Microbiol. 2014;12:661-672]

Conversely, a high-fat diet has been shown to promote small-bowel cancers. Researchers were able to demonstrate an acceleration to small-bowel cancer in specially-bred mice. Importantly, the researchers could decrease the cancer risk in these mice by deliberately modying the microbiome (in this case through the use of antibiotics).

## Breast Cancer

But it's not just bowel cancer. Diet and microbiome are also postulated to influence the course of breast cancer.

One of the most powerful inflammatory substances in a woman's body is estrogen. However, the microbiome is capable reducing circulating levels of this estrogen (because it is excreted from the liver, via the bile, into the intestine, where it may or may not be re-absorbed). Once again, evidence shows that breast cancer risk may be diminished with a high-fiber, low-fat diet.[ Shapira I, Sultan K, Lee A, Taioli E. Evolving concepts: how diet and the intestinal microbiome act as modulators of breast malignancy. ISRN Oncol. 2013:2013;693920]

## Inflammatory Bowel Disease

There has been a growing focus on the impact that dietary influences can have on inflammatory bowel disease, although the causal relationship remains somewhat unclear.

Mice deficient in Interleukin-10, an anti-inflammatory cytokine, have been shown to develop spontaneous inflammatory colitis. This colitis is prevented, however, when the mice are reared in a germ-free environment, which eliminates the role of the gut microbiome.

When these mice are then re-exposed to specific gut flora, they can experience a flare up of colitis, suggesting the important role the microbiome plays. It's probably worth adding that when these mice were fed a high-fat diet, it was possible to induce small intestinal inflammation.

It all adds up. Keep your bowel flora sweet and healthy. Maybe Old Man Kellog was right when he famously said, "Death begins in the colon"! Eating right is over 100 times more important than swallowing probiotics. You have just read that changes can take place in as little as a day.

There's one more thing you can do. It appears, as a result of research, that taking the supplement tryptophan can also help. Tryptophan is metabolized by gut *Lactobacillus*, the resulting metabolite altering the microbiome in ways that enhance the mucosal inflammatory protection.

[ Zelante T, Iannitti RG, Cunha C, et al. Tryptophan catabolites from microbiota engage aryl hydrocarbon receptor and balance mucosal reactivity via interleukin-22. Immunity. 2013;39:372-385]

I've been banging on about the importance of this gut flora thing for decades. Now at least science is backing me up, instead of arguing the point!

## 1.6c Add the Inflammasome Theory

Now we have new levels of understanding, thanks to the inflammasome model.

Inflammasomes are small molecular complexes that activate the inflammation process. They were discovered in 2002, by Prof. Jürg Tschopp and his team working at the University of Lausanne in Switzerland. According to this theory, the effect of inflammasomes is to produce inflammation as part of your body's immune system response.

It's a necessary mechanism but with inherent dangers, as I have said. Inflammation is a healthy response of the body to the early stages of fractures, wounds, toxins and numerous pathological microbes. Without this "acute" inflammation, your body wouldn't heal, because no white blood cells from your immune system could move in and fight off the foreign bodies attacking you.

But once it becomes chronic and non-resolving, inflammation is a danger, especially to potential cancer cases. Inflammation contributes to the cancer burden and is an important trigger. Inflammasomes also cause the low-level inflammatory responses you can't see but go on for years and slowly kill you with cancer and the other chronic diseases.

Inflammasome triggers are all around us. In fact, they attack every day. These include: bacteria and viruses, chemical pollutants, such as Bisphenol A (BPA), stress, excess weight, cigarette smoke (active and passive) and, of course, reactive oxygen species (free radicals).

The exact mechanism and pathways of the inflammasome response is very complex and need not be explained here.

**But the good news is that oxygen quenches inflammasomes.** For example, a 2015 study published in *Molecular Medicine Reports* showed that inflammation after spinal cord injuries in rats was benefitted by oxygen.

[Liang, F., Li, C., Gao, C., Li, Z., Yang, J., Liu, X., Wang, Y."Effects of hyperbaric oxygen therapy on NACHT domain-leucine-rich-repeat- and pyrin domain-containing protein 3 inflammasome expression in rats following spinal cord injury". *Molecular Medicine Reports* 11.6 (2015): 4650-4656]

See the oxygen section 3 for details on the administration of therapeutic oxygen.

# 1.7 Whether To Opt For Chemotherapy Or Just Go Natural?

Before we go any further, let's address that vexed question of whether to opt for chemo or radiotherapy, or go "natural" and just do an alternative program

This is one of the most important questions for some patients and they agonize over the choice before them. It is made so much more difficult by the dread that a wrong decision could lead to fatal consequences. You see, everyone knows that it is not really as straightforward as the oncologists like to claim.

There is no question that the older conventional therapies you will encounter are pretty toxic. They are supposed to be: the idea is to kill the tumor but just stop short of killing the patient. Unfortunately, it can be a dangerous and narrow line between the two. Once your body defences are damaged, then you are in a worse position than before because, in the end, your immune system is going to be the only thing that's saves you.

Obviously, all cases are different, so we can only talk in general principles. But having been told you have cancer is a time of great fear and uncertainty; all the more reason then to keep our thoughts clear and balanced. The first big relief is that you can do both types of therapy in conjunction!

Talk about hedging your bets! It is possible to view holistic therapies as a stand-alone treatment of cancer, leukaemia etc. But why not see them as an adjunct to conventional therapy? Hit it both ways?

You have the right to choose whichever treatment you like, without hostility or ridicule from supposed members of the holistic community; it's your health, after all. Sometimes it isn't clear where your best chance lies. I would only ask you to be cautious in evaluating the data presented to you.

It's shocking to realize that many of the scientific studies quoted by oncologists, supposedly supporting the conventional approach, have actually been faked. Even articles in prestigious journals are known to have been fraudulent and yet were still published. I give you an example in section 4.4 (Gemcitabine+Gonzalez), of a study which was faked but nevertheless published in the *Journal of Clinical Oncology*. The official *US Office of the Human Research Protection* has made it clear on their website that this trial was deliberately manipulated against a holistic therapy.

This may change but that could take years. There are signs of orthodox medicine digging itself out of the primitive "kill-'em-all" cut, burn and poison mode it has fallen into.

Modern chemical treatments for tumors are becoming quite specifically targeted and not so dangerous as old-time chemo and radio therapy. Modern substances can be created which release their deadly load only on certain chosen tissues: a sort of "smart bomb" for chemo. It might be wise to give these new methods consideration, as they come onto the market.

But what you want then is to give your body every possible aid in resisting the damaging chemicals or radiation, so that only the tumor gets hit, not your valuable defence tissues. The big danger of powerful and sophisticated conventional therapy, as I have explained, is that it harms your defences almost as much as it does the tumor.

Doctors and drug manufacturers alike persist in seeing the body merely as the battle ground, not as one of the key friendly combatants. Yet the body is capable of exerting enormous influence on your behalf, against cancer (or viruses, bacteria, parasites etc). It is stupid to ignore this important biological resource or risk harming it in any way.

Let me tell you how important your own body tissues are: did you know (very few doctors know this) that a cancer tumor is typically composed of about 50% your own immune white blood cells, in there, fighting for you against the bad cells? Shrinking the size of the tumor sounds great; but it may mean mostly the loss of white defensive cells and not cancer cells.

Yet shrinkage of the tumor, regardless of what this may mean, is the only criterion that is used to judge the worth of a chemo drug. Increased survival time is not even considered as a measure of the drug's efficacy. Yet time is the only thing that matters to the cancer victim!

Protecting your defence mechanisms is probably the most critical reason I would encourage patients to adopt alternative and holistic remedies, like vitamins and herbs. You can, to a degree, measure how well you are doing so by how much you can reduce the ugly side-effects of chemo. For example, very few of my patients ever lost their hair because of chemo, even on the Rubicin family of drugs.

Chemo is intended to hit at rapidly dividing cells, which is what cancer cells are. Unfortunately, hair cells also rapidly replace themselves and the lining of the gut and bone marrow cells too. So the common side effects of this treatment are hair loss, nausea and stomach upset, and dangerous lowering of both red and white blood cells.

Good nutrients, like vitamins and detox supplements, which I'll explain in due course, can be very helpful in removing these unpleasant side effects. Yet here the exasperating ignorance of orthodox doctors becomes evident, when you hear stories of patients being told not to take vitamins because "it will help the cancer".

First off, there is no evidence of any kind whatsoever that vitamins and minerals can do this - it's opinionated prejudice of the first order, which could cost you your life (well, there appears to be one tiny sub-set of lung cancer patients, in one study, where the patients continued to smoke—Duh! I wouldn't worry about that small group)

Secondly, it shows remarkable ignorance of basic life biology: cancer cells are malformed rogue cells that do not behave as normal cells do and for whom vitamins and minerals are probably about as useful as daylight is to a vampire! Cancer cells, for example, don't like oxygen; whereas normal cells thrive on it!

In fact a rpublished paper in April 2007—which was a review of randomized controlled trials evaluating the effects of concurrent use of antioxidants and chemotherapy—antioxidant use during chemotherapy was not found to decrease the effectiveness of chemotherapy, as I said, and in fact, was associated with increased survival time, increased tumor responses, and fewer toxicities.

The authors of the study searched various medical databases and identified 845 articles, out of which 19 randomized, controlled clinical trials met their inclusion criteria. Antioxidants used in the studies included glutathione, melatonin, vitamin A, antioxidant mixtures, vitamin C , N-acetylcysteine, vitamin E, and ellagic acid. Analysis of the results of these studies found no sign of decreased efficacy of chemotherapy as a result of antioxidant supplementation, as has been argued by some.

On the contrary, increased survival times, increased tumor responses, and fewer toxicities were found among persons taking antioxidants along with chemotherapy as compared to those on chemotherapy alone. The authors point out that lack of adequate statistical power was a consistent limitation and conclude, "Large, well-designed studies of antioxidant supplementation concurrent with chemotherapy are warranted."

How absolutely true and how much better than attacking nutritional therapy. Unfortunately, the ignorance persists out there. The chances of your oncologist having read this review are very small. As soon as he or she sees the word antioxidant he or she will turn the page to something more interesting, something more in keeping with their rigid prejudices.

There is no question then, that if you want to help yourself, you are going to have to get informed on the issues.

But now a serious word of warning: be just as suspicious of claims by practitioners in the alternative field as you are about patronizing advice from doctors. There are many dangerously well-intentioned therapists out there, who make all kinds of claims they can help you. Some of it is nothing more than dogma with zeal and that kind of ignorance is no better (just as deadly) as advice from the misguided oncologist. They too are after your money, remember, and may want to exploit you for cash, even when they have no real ability to help.

Hopefully, this book from a doctor who is not trying to recruit you as a patient or sell you any products, will enable you to make more informed decisions on what your choices are, without any commercial bias whatever.

# 1.8 The One Approach Myth

One of the absurd follies of conventional medicine is that there is only one "proper" treatment (the one they make lotsa money on, of course!)

Common sense says you would do several things at once. Gamblers call this "mini-max"; it's something I talk about a lot in my writings. You do what you can in order to minimize the negative and whatever you can to maximize the chances of a positive.

It's not about drawing a royal flush every time. It's about the fact that **if you win 51% of the time, consistently, you'll eventually break the house!**

Gamblers are not fools; they do this because they know it works. It can work for you too. If you tip the odds even slightly in your favor, eventually you will repel the cancer.

Yet time and again the oncologist will say "Don't take vitamins" (without testing if you are deficient), "Stress isn't the cause of cancer" (it's probably the 1 cause), "Diet is irrelevant, eat what you like" (they would probably say that to anyone with any condition because they don't understand that all disease stems from faulty nutrition, one way or another).

They also argue venomously against taking any kind of alternative remedy.

Of course, not all doctors are motivated by greed; but vanity and fear comes into it. They are frightened of the possibility that their cutting, burning and poisoning may turn out to be the wrong strategy. It will show them up as dangerous and incompetent (statistics already do that).

You can take it from me (or any source of common sense), that adding several healing modalities will all help you overcome your cancer. By that I mean both the possibility of increased survival and also a great improvement in the quality of your time with us.

I never argue with patients that they should not opt for chemo or radiation. It's their own choice. But later I'll talk about ways to use alternative modalities to block the dreadful toxic effects of chemo. This big improvement in quality of life is a very important contribution to real health care and should not be overlooked or denied.

Just to emphasize my point about the two approaches working synergistically, I'd like to report to you a very significant study which shows that fasting alongside may improve cancer response to chemotherapy. Fasting seems to help protect healthy cells and help them become as much as 5 times more resistant to chemo than the cancer cells.

It's only an animal study but is nevertheless significant, because it backs up everything we alternative doctors have said is critical about diet and cancer. Stressful foods help the cancer; a good diet holds it back. Fasting has been shown to be beneficial for humans with cancer.

Nowadays, with our much increased knowledge of epigenetics, we also understand that we can switch off bad genes, incvluding cancer genes, by changes in diet and lifestyle. Indeed, it emerges this is rather easy to do. In the next section check out some cool ways to increase your sensitivity to chemo (in other words, it will work better).

# 1.8a Making Cells More Sensitive To Chemo

If you choose the chemotherapy route, don't let anyone scoff at you. People do survive with chemotherapy. It doesn't seem to do much good, according to the figures. But you might be among the lucky ones.

It is not my purpose to tell you are foolish to choose that path. It's your call! But do remember that chemotherapy agents are known to sometimes actually cause cell DNA mutations. In other words they can actually lead to cancerous changes. Paradoxical, I know. This may be the reason cells can develop "chemo resistance". They quickly develop new strains, which are not affected by the current drug.

> Children who are "successfully" treated for Hodgkin's disease are 18 times more likely later to develop secondary malignant tumors. Girls face a 35% chance of developing breast cancer by the time they are 40 - which is 75 times greater than the average. The risk of leukemia increased markedly four years after the ending of successful treatment, and reached a plateau after 14 years, but the risk of developing solid tumors remained high and approached 30% at 30 years.

(SOURCE: New Eng J Med, March 21, 1996)

Here are some natural things you can do, to maybe improve the effectiveness of chemotherapy.

It's been found that inducing temporary starvation increases the cells' resistance to stress, which may allow doctors to use higher doses of current cancer chemotherapy treatments to make them more effective.

In the study, published in the March 31 2008 *Proceedings of the National Academy of Sciences*, researchers studied the effects of starvation on cancerous and normal cells. First, they induced a starvation-related response in yeast cells, which made them 1,000 times more protected than untreated cells.

Then, they tested the effects of fasting on human and cancer cells in a test tube and in mice. The results showed starvation produced between a twofold and five-fold difference in stress resistance between the normal, starvation-treated cells and normal cells.

In tests with live mice, of 28 mice starved for 48-60 hours before chemotherapy, only 1 died (less than 4%). Of 37 mice that were not starved prior to treatment, 20 mice died from chemotherapy toxicity (over 50%). [Raffaghello, L. Proceedings of the National Academy of Sciences, online early edition March 31, 2008. News release, University of Southern California.]

It would explain why fasting, juicing and extreme diets could be beneficial; as well as starving the patient, the cancer is weakened.

Why is this important? Well, there's nothing wrong with chemo, at least in principle. It's just that it kills good cells at about the same rate as bad cells. It's VERY toxic. But if we could increase what is called the therapeutic margin (the difference between the dose which cures and the dose which kills), then all of a sudden it's a completely different game against cancer.

We don't yet understand what fasting works so well. Researchers believe genetic cues prompt starved healthy cells to go into a hibernation-like mode that produces extreme resistance to stress (chemo is stress). But cancerous cells don't obey those cues and remain stuck in growth mode.

I doubt this and it does not explain why even just modifying the diet helps so much. I think the explanation lies in removing stressor foods (intolerance, allergies, junk chemicals and other poisons). This is why my *Diet Wise* book is so valuable for cancer victims. It enables them to produce a well-tolerated personal program that provides adequate nutrition.

It's needed because patients cannot stay on a fast; but they can stay on my program for months or years!

http://www.dietwisebook.com

# 1.8b Other Ways To Enhance Chemotherapy

## Fish Oils

Eicosapentaenoic acid (EPA) concentrated from fish oil was shown to sensitize colon cancer cells to Mitomycin C, a chemotherapy agent [Tsai et al. 1997]. It should be noted that fish oil also suppresses the formation of prostaglandin E2, an inflammatory hormone-like substance involved in cancer cell propagation.

In fact omega-3 essential fatty acids have long been known to quench inflammation. Inflammation is bad for cancer patients. Stay cool!

In a group of dogs with lymphoma were randomized to receive either a diet supplemented with arginine and fish oil or just soybean oil. Dogs on the fish oil and arginine diet had a significantly longer disease-free survival time than dogs on the soybean oil (Ogilvie et al. 2000).

## Caffeine

Caffeine, we are slowly realizing, is an extremely healthful substance, despite the unpleasantness of its jag effect.

Recently, the use of caffeine in combination with chemotherapy has been shown to enhance the cytotoxicity of chemotherapy drugs. Caffeine occurs naturally in green tea and has been shown to potentiate the anticancer effects of tea polyphenols, such as epigallocatechin gallate (EGCG). When mice were fed caffeine as sole source of drinking fluid for 18-23 weeks (they must have been pretty jumpy), it inhibited the formation and decreased the size of both nonmalignant tumors and malignant tumors.

In cancer, p53 gene mutation is one of the most common genetic alterations observed. It may not be causative but is fully involved. Caffeine has been shown to help the destruction of p53 defective cells.

This unique ability of caffeine is the basis of many anticancer therapies, aimed at damaging tumor DNA and destroying the replicating cancer cells. Caffeine uncouples tumor cell-cycle progression by interfering with the replication and repair of DNA

[Blasina et al. 1999; Ribeiro et al. 1999; Jiang et al. 2000; Valenzuela et al. 2000]

## L-Theanine

I introduced L-theanine into my amazing "Doctor's Chocolate", so I know it's good and has many healthful properties. In fact so good companies have been buying it up in bulk and have driven the price through the roof.

Now it appears, L-theanine has been shown to enhance Adriamycin concentration in tumors 2.7-fold and reduce tumor weight 62% over controls, whereas Adriamycin by itself did not reduce tumor weight. [Sugiyama T and Sadzuka Y, Enhancing effects of green tea components on the antitumor activity of Adriamycin against M5076 ovarian sarcoma, *Cancer Letters* 1998; 133(1): 19-26]

Additionally, L-theanine was shown to reverse tumor resistance to certain chemotherapeutic drugs by forcing more of the drug to stay inside the tumor. It does not, however, increase the amount of drug in normal tissue, which sets it apart from other drugs designed to overcome multidrug resistance.

In 1999 researchers performed a study testing the use of L-theanine in conjunction with a drug similar to doxorubicin known as idarubicin. The use of idarubicin has been tried in drug-resistant leukemia cells, but it caused toxic bone marrow suppression.

But when coupled with L-theanine, the idarubicin worked well at one quarter of the standard dose (meaning it was enhanced at least four-fold). In larger doses, L-theanine blocked the toxic bone marrow effect of idarubicin. Leukocyte loss was reduced from 57% to 37%. [Sadzuka Y, et al., Improvement of idarubicin induced antitumor activity and bone marrow suppression by theanine, a component of tea, *Cancer Letters* 2000;158(2): 119-24]

## The LEF Protocol

If you really want to go the chemo route, the Life Extension Foundation recommends the following protocol. I can't improve on it:

1. Decide on an appropriate chemotherapy regimen and plan to increase its efficacy, as outlined in the previous sections. Chemosensitivity and immunohistochemistry tumor cell tests can help you and your physician make a more informed decision.

2. Be certain your physician understands the importance of guarding against hypoxia. This means keeping your hematocrit and hemoglobin in the upper ranges of normal. Since chemotherapy often induces anemia, the drug Procrit along with supplemental iron is often required.

3. Based on tumor type, consider asking your physician to prescribe a COX-2 inhibiting drug, such as Lodine.

4. Based on findings from the immunohistochemistry test, if your tumor expresses the K-Ras oncogene, consider high-dose statin drug therapy such as lovastatin (80 mg a day).

5. The following supplements might help block growth signals used by cancer cells to escape eradication by chemotherapy. These supplements have also displayed antiangiogenesis properties. Some of these supplements may be best initiated 3 weeks after cessation of chemotherapy if one believes that antioxidants will protect cancer cells from the effects of chemotherapy drug(s):

   • Soy Extract (40% isoflavones), five 675-mg capsules taken 4 times a day. The only soy extract providing this high potency of soy isoflavones is a product called Ultra Soy. Note that isoflavones from soy have antioxidant properties.

   • Curcumin, 900 mg, with 5 mg of Bioperine (an alkaloid from Piper nigrum), 3 capsules 2-4 times a day taken two hours away from medications. Super Curcumin with Bioperine is a formulated product that contains this recommended dosage. Warning: Use caution when combining curcumin with other chemotherapy drugs. Do not take curcumin with the chemotherapy drugs Irinotecan, Camptosar, or CPT-11. Watch for NSAID-like side effects such as gastric ulceration because curcumin is a COX-2 inhibitor. Do not take curcumin if you have a biliary tract obstruction. Also note that curcumin is a potent antioxidant.

- Green tea extract, two-three 725-mg capsules with meals. Each capsule should be standardized to provide a minimum of 200 mg of epigallocatechin gallate (EGCG). It is the EGCG fraction of green tea that has shown the most active anticancer effects. These are available in a decaffeinated form for persons who are sensitive to caffeine or who want to take the less stimulating decaffeinated green tea extract capsules in the evening dose. Note that green tea is a potent antioxidant.

6. To possibly enhance the efficacy of certain chemotherapy drugs:

- Fish oil, 7-11 capsules of Super Omega-3 EPA/DHA w/Sesame Lignans & Olive Fruit Extract throughout the day.

- L-theanine, five 100 mg capsules twice a day.

7. The following natural supplements may reduce side effects and healthy tissue damage caused by chemotherapy. All of these supplements except shark liver oil are potent antioxidants:

- Vitamin E, 400 IU a day of vitamin E succinate (dry powder natural vitamin E).

- Vitamin C, 4000-12,000 mg throughout the day.

- Coenzyme Q10, 200-300 mg daily in a softgel capsule for maximum absorption. (Refer to cautions about CoQ10 and chemotherapy.)

- Melatonin, 3-50 mg at bedtime. Dose may be reduced after chemotherapy ends if too much morning drowsiness occurs. After several months, most cancer patients take 3-20 mg of melatonin at bedtime.

- Se-methylselenocysteine (SeMSC), 200-400 mcg daily.

- Whey protein concentrate isolate, 30-60 grams, in divided doses, daily. Note: Cancer patients undergoing chemotherapy should consider taking whey protein concentrate at least 10 days before beginning therapy and during therapy and then continuing with the whey protein for at least 30 days after completion of the therapy.

- Shark liver oil, 200 mg alkyglycerols, 5 capsules daily for 30 days.

- Digestive enzyme capsules may reduce the gas and bloating associated with high soy intake.

8. Ask your oncologist to consider prescribing immune-enhancing drugs suggested in this protocol, such as Leukine and alpha interferon or IL-2 (along with a retinoid drug).

Cancer patients may want to refer to the other protocols suggested by the Life Extension Foundation. You visit their website at www.lef.org or www.lefcancer.org.

# 1.9 Doctors Must STOP Giving Out Death Sentences

It's great to be smarty Aleck and pronounce when a patient is going to die. It gives you immense power and prestige, doesn't it?

Well, it didn't for me when I was an interne (hospital "house" doctor in the UK terminology, actually about one grade up from interne). Yet doctors go on doing it and I can't think of any other reason. Or actually, I can: cruelty or stupidity are the other two obvious reasons.

Stupidity I put there because the average doctor cannot seem to get it into his or her head and work schema that Nature heals, that patients recover and that disease has a healing purpose.

Why else would doctors go on telling cancer patients "You have 6 months to live" (or weeks or whatever)?

Don't they see it's going to be a self-fulfilling prophecy in most cases? A patient under the duress of feeling sick and frightened is told by this powerful authority figure, "You are going to die soon"; what do you think will happen?

Right! The patient's subconscious will take this pronouncement on board and make it come true. That way the doctor looks good – he or she got it right. But it doesn't come under the functions of a doctor as I understand them.

If a doctor ever says such words to you, translate them as follows: "I don't know what I'm talking about and I don't know what I'm doing. I suggest you find a natural healer and follow a spiritual and lifestyle path to a cure."

The fact is that every disease you can name, of every severity, has been survived by others before you. People sick unto death and not expected to last the day have got up and walked out of hospital; terminal cancer patients, whose bodies were riddled with secondaries, have recovered and the tumors gone away (and stayed away for the rest of their lives); people who were paralyzed have walked again (done a few of those myself) and even genetically-determined conditions have disappeared, no matter the DNA message.

Doctors must stop pronouncing on patients what becomes a death sentence by impact. Don't let 'em scare or bully you!

It usually needs little more than a change of mind, a determination by the patient, the will to survive, and the natural healing process kicks in. Mostly, I have noticed, the patients who survive have a slight scorn or even contempt for the doctors who failed them. That's probably why they won't agree to the death sentence.

The fact is, whatever you are facing, there is a path back to health. You may have been living where this path is very hidden and overgrown with weeds. But it's there. It's ALWAYS there; God makes sure of that. You only have to find your path!

**Here's a Cheerful Story!**

I recently ran across a patient who had been told "You have six months to live". Well, that was twenty years ago; she was fine and still in good health, having beaten her cancer with the kind of methods I'm sharing with you in this book.

But... here's the kicker... *the doctor himself died more than ten years ago!*

Just ignore these pompous fools.

# 1.9a Immoderate Language

And while we are visiting the topic of doctor's immoderate language, beware a subtle killer in what they tell you.

Doctor's love to say "We fixed it. It's gone. You're blood work is fine. There is no trace of the cancer". While this is probably the most wonderful news a patient can get, you must beware of this reckless language.

Patients, quite naturally, really *want* to believe this is true. They so much want it they let go of logic and reason.

The point is that *if nothing whatever has been done to deal with the cause of the problem, then it has not been conquered at all.*

If you had rats in your property, is it enough to just set traps and kill the rats? Shouldn't you figure out how they are getting in and block up the access? Get a cat or more and bigger cats (immune system)?

One of the main things in conventional medicine that kills patients is complacency. In a sense this is more dangerous than the effects of chemo and radiation.

You see, the cancer is the SYMPTOM, not the disease. The real disease is the person's life.

It's all part of the differing philosophies between conventional and holistic therapy. It applies to all diseases, not just to cancer. The conventional doctor thinks of symptoms and results. That's the "problem". A holistic doctor thinks of *causes*. Where is this coming from? **What caused the disease to come about?**

My experience of conventional doctors is that they never try to fix causes, only the results. They speak in terms of "treating" the cancer, without ever getting to grips with why the patient has got it in the first place (they seem to think cancer is no different to getting a bad throw in a cosmic crap shoot, instead of being the result of preventable health causes that need to be fixed).

So while it's wonderful to be given the "all clear", remember it's coming from doctors as ignorant of health as you are (maybe more so).

If you don't deal with the real problem (why you got cancer in the first place) it will very likely come back. The door is still wide open to all the rats and they will try to come back!

And while I am sounding off here, let me also warn you against the same smugness in alternative practitioners. It's especially easy to when you have a good result from holistic therapies.

But the same warning applies: you must get the real cause of the problem as, for example, there is *always* an element of emotional toxicity that you need to eradicate.

I lost a wonderful patient who set up the local Gerson support group. She had overcome breast cancer, using the Gerson method. So when the disease came back a second time, she naturally had great faith in it and went through the program again.

But this time she was a little more nervous and came to me for IV infusions. It went well; we beat the disease a second time.

Throughout her visits I begged her to get to work on emotional issues. Apart from my knowing they are always there, the fact that she had a recurrence was a clear signal (to me) that something was not resolved.

But no; she thanked me for my help and went away, believing she was OK. Or if it recurred, she thought, there was always the Gerson method again. This was very blind but, being very keen on Gerson, she could not see the truth which is that it had actually failed her. It hadn't dealt with the core issues in her life.

It makes me angry when Charlotte Gerson has the effrontery to stand in front of an audience and say that emotional issues are of no consequence to a cancer patient. She is of course protecting her father's position (and also looking after her own financial empire). But this is the kind of ignorance among alternative practitioners that I deplore

The next time I saw this patient was over a year later. She came to see me short of breath. I ordered an immediate chest x-ray and, sure enough, she was riddled with lung secondaries. I was unable to work with her this time because this was only days before my passage to a new life in Sri Lanka, with my lovely new wife.

The patient, by the way, had been seeing a chiropractor for months, who kept assuring her that it was just a spinal mal-adjustment and could be easily fixed (a chiro who thinks that, in a cancer patient with those symptoms, should lose her license).

# 1.9b Half Of Cancer Cases Die Of Something Else

This is welcome news in a couple of ways. If the conventional analysts and doctors are faking cancer stats and their claimed recoveries (as many of us suspect), then it shows up in this fact: *half of all people with cancer will die of something else!* Betcha didn't know that!

Secondly, even if the stats are real, it means cancer is less to be feared than many people think.

I think the third interpretation... that we are winning the war against cancer, is the least likely to be true!

## What are the facts?

Officially (this is the USA), there are now 12 million cancer survivors… up from 3 million in 1971 and 9.8 million in 2001. Other territories will have proportionately similar figures.

Two-thirds of them have survived cancer for at least five years, according to Yi Ning, MD, ScD, of the Virginia Commonwealth University Massey Cancer Center in Richmond. He and his colleagues examined data on 1,807 cancer survivors who participated in the 1988-1994 and 1999-2004 *National Health and Nutrition Examination Surveys* (NHANES).

The most common forms of cancer among the survivors were breast, prostate, lung, and colorectal. Fifty-one percent died from cancer and 49% died from other causes. Let's call that UN-cancer death!

## Died Of What?

Heart disease was the number one killer, responsible for over two-thirds of the UN-cancer deaths. Chronic lung diseases like emphysema claimed 15%; Alzheimer's disease and diabetes were each responsible for 4% of UN-cancer deaths.

The study also showed that that the longer people lived after their initial cancer diagnosis, the more likely they were to die from another disease. In the first five years of diagnosis, 33% of survivors died from a condition other than cancer compared with 63% after 20 years.

Also, people diagnosed with cancer at older ages were more likely to die from diseases other than cancer, Ning says.

## So Are Cases Really Cured?

I have to say this, but yes. You'd think, to read articles and comments in the holistic field, that chemo and radiation therapy is a dismal 100% failure.

That's not true, really. The 12 million survivors are mainly from the conventional route. There is no evidence that more people survive using holistic methods (there are just NO figures, so please don't write to me and tell me I am idiot). All we can say is that the quality of life is generally far better using a holistic approach.

Of course, once orthodox therapy has done its job and treatment discontinued, then the quality of life issue is irrelevant.

## But What About Recurrence?

One is left with the question: does chemo etc. set you up for a recurrence? Figures say many cancers recur. You know that.

But what we lack is stats to tell us how often the cancers come back, after holistic therapy. And there are NO figures again, so again… don't write and tell me I am idiot.

People on my list like me to tell the truth and not propagandize for holistic therapies. I'm just telling it like it is.

Orthodox or holistic is a personal choice and everyone is entitled to make their own decision. I'm disgusted at the number of "holistic" people who sneer at those who choose conventional therapy.

I put "holistic" in quotes because it is not nice to judge and stupid to believe only you are right, neither action of which is in any way in accord with Mother Nature and holism.

Lots of people die choosing the holistic route; some after seeing celebrated cancer heroes. So don't be naïve.

### Take Home

I think the message is very clear. Survival of cancer requires general health measures that will protect you against ANY disease process. That starts and ends with diet; includes detoxing; oxygen is a great idea; it requires elimination of toxic emotions; and not smoking, taking exercise and generally being moderate in all things.

Adequate restful sleep is another major linch-pin that is often not mentioned. Exhaustion is not a good state to be when fighting any potentially killer disease.

We should all be doing these things. In which case we are unlikely to get cancer and will probably survive it if we do!

[SOURCE: American Association for Cancer Research
Meeting 2012, Chicago, March 31-April 4, 2012]

# 1.10 This Is The Age Of "Personalized Oncology"

The latest buzzword in cancer is "personalized oncology." The phrase originated mid-decade, especially in relation to nanotechnology. John Niederhuber, MD, director of the National Cancer Institute, endorsed personalized oncology in his *Cancer Bulletin* editorial of August 19, 2008, where he wrote about the dawn of a new era of "personalized cancer medicine," with "specific, targeted therapeutic solutions."

This reflects a general development in treatments that has been stylized as "personalized medicine".

### Consider the following proposition:

Every human being on planet Earth is 5ft 9inches tall, weighs 150 pounds, blonde hair, blue eyes, male, and with dark skin, right? No? You mean we're all different? Not according to the medical profession. Doctors and the drug industry regard everyone as being the same. We're all supposed to be "average", whatever that means. The joke is that *nobody is average*. I'll say that again: nobody is average, not one single human being.

Take height. The average height for a white man is 75 inches at age 25 years. But less than 0.1% of the population measures 75 inches. Many are close, say between 74 and 76 inches; many more measure between 70 inches and 80 inches; and so on. But very few are right on 75 inches!

Height of course is only one genetic trait: add hair color, gender, eye color and skin, making just 5 traits and virtually nobody is close to average. Investigate a lot of traits and... just forget it.

So why do doctors and the drug industry persist in believing the same medicine at the same dose is right for everyone? We are not all the same and to treat us as such is bad medicine. But it is also very bad science.

In fact even the sluggardly FDA has embraced this concept. An FDA position paper published as long ago as March 2005, took a stand in supporting personalized medicine. They even hinted that it would soon become considered malpractice, if doctors did not establish what each individual's tolerance and type was, and amend treatment accordingly.

No sign of that happening yet. But we are getting closer, as gene testing (genomics) gains ground.

Meantime, personalized medicine has developed a face in oncology. Not before time. This is the future and, if you are facing cancer, be sure you work with an oncologist who understand and practices personalized oncology!

It's all about our genomes. There are countless tiny variations in our DNA that make us all unique. There is no real "human genome"; there are an infinite number of human genomes.

Unfortunately, this is an area of skill and commitment. At this time, it is doubtful if the "Cancer Mmafia" are committed to personalized oncology, since current procedures put profits before patients and convenience before scientific credibility. But change will only come if patients demand it.

Again, I must repeat my caveat that medicine is better practiced elsewhere in the world than the USA and with more integrity and less focus on profit.


# The Past Is Outdated

Treatment still chosen based on predetermined protocols for particular stages of the disease, usually according to universally-defined tumors rather than individual characteristics. These protocols are chosen based on empirical evidence derived from previous clinical trials. A particular drug or combination of drugs is favored because, on average, it performs somewhat better than another combination. Or at least it does in the rather shaky and propped up scientific trials that are carried out.

Let me remind you here of the philosophy of the pharmaceutical industry, which is that "scientific studies" are concerned only with creating some credibility for an expensive drug and not about efficacy at all.

In reality, current therapy isn't about science in the true meaning of the word, but is about *consensus*. The vast majority of oncologists suggest treatment protocols which are merely the standardized recommendations of the National Comprehensive Cancer Network (NCCN), or some other "authority", rather than individualizing the choice of drugs based on the characteristics of the individual in their office.

Nowadays, patients are demanding better. Blogging at Medscape.com, oncologist and pathologist Cary A. Presant, MD explains the public relations dilemma that doctors now face:

> "The first implication of personalizing oncology is that the way in which we communicate with patients has to change. Because patients are seeing personalized cancer care as a recurring emphasized theme in newspapers and television, *it is important for each oncologist to assure patients that their treatment plans are optimized for personalized therapy."*

In other words, oncologists need to reassure their patients that they are indeed getting "the best and most up-to-date care...." But unfortunately, Dr. Presant does not address the question of whether this in fact is true. Otherwise, he's advocating that doctors just lie to people, to continue getting their business!

Make up your own mind. Don't be bullied and browbeaten. Threaten a malpractice suit and a complaint to the licensing authority, even before treatment, making it clear you will do so automatically, if you don't get "personalized oncology"

At the minimum, the following should happen:

Surgeons must be informed that fresh tumor tissue removed during biopsies or operations needs to be preserved for microarray DNA testing and for chemotherapy sensitivity or drug induced apoptosis. The drug(s) chosen for therapy must show activity against the patient's OWN tumor, not some laboratory line.

However, this regimen (entirely scientific and sound) has been around since the 1980s, supported by doctors like me, yet has been resisted tooth-and-nail by the cancer establishment. They hate all that extra work and expense and would rather give their patient standardized treatments, fully knowing that it will kill a significant number of those people they are pretending to help

I repeat, *standardized chemotherapy does not work.* Required doses differ. That's one of the reasons it's so toxic. The lucky patients who get the right dose (for them) will recover and sing its praises. The others die of the cancer or die of the therapy.

# 1.11 Cancer Means A Career Shift

I've said it before and it bears repeating: *cancer is a wake up call but it is not a death knell.* It tells you loud and clear that something is wrong with your life and lifestyle and that has now reduced your health and vitality to ruinous levels. You must listen to the message from Mother Nature and take appropriate action.

If you heed the warnings and put matter right you will probably be safe. Many people have had cause to bless the fact that they got cancer: it alerted them to the fact that their life was wildly off track and that they must do something effective to put matters right—or pay the ultimate price.

I'm going to be telling you what your treatment alternatives are. You'll be surprised how many different actions you can take that will raise your chances of beating the disease successfully. In fact I'd like to encourage you that, in the early stages at least, cancer isn't that difficult to conquer at all.

Yes, I did say conquering cancer. You can survive this affliction and it never return. There are many success stories that prove this. Unfortunately, the prevailing attitude in the medical profession is that of ignorance and disinformation. Doctors seem to have a very negative view of cancer survival, despite all the propaganda. In some territories it is even illegal to talk of cancer cures.

But my years of experience allow me to assure you that if you approach the disease properly and tackle its causes at root, then that cancer isn't going to come back. There is more likelihood of someone else getting the disease—who hasn't taken the proper steps to put their health issues right—than someone who has already beaten off cancer. You just need to take effective action and correct the obvious problems that led to the disease.

Now by "effective action" I do not mean leave it to the oncologist. The single biggest mistake that you can make if you are diagnosed with cancer is to leave it to the experts to save your life. Conventional doctors are pretty useless at dealing with this disease. Despite all the propaganda, the survival rate for cancer treated solely by conventional means is largely unchanged over the last 50 years.

Only a few breakthroughs, which I'll be discussing with you, have shown any real promise (like anti-cancer vaccinations) and, hey, you know what? These are the methods that work along with Nature and her wisdom. So they are not so much a breakthrough as a "back to basics" approach.

I repeat: To beat cancer you must take charge of your own health. You need to become the executive manager or chief-of-staff for your own case. Don't be panicked by threats that you will die horribly and quickly if you do not opt for surgery, chemo or radiation: doctors who treat you in this way are a disgrace to the profession and should lose their right to practice. Remember their motivation is primarily to make money from your plight; platitudes and assurances are really only to disguise the financial nature of their interests.

I am on record in several places as saying that if I were a really cynical doctor and wanted only money, I would choose to be an oncologist. I would get to face people at the moment of maximum terror when they have just been told the news they most dread; I could work on their fears, stoke up the panic some more, and then demand anything up to half a million dollars for helping them to survive, knowing the law backed my claim exclusively and criminalized anyone who tried to move in on my patch and started offering an effective cure for just a few cents on the dollar!

Fortunately, I am not a cynical doctor.

At the same time, I am not saying that you must necessarily abandon the conventional approach. The final choice must be yours and not some oncologist panting for the cash for a down payment on his or her Tuscan villa. Unfortunately, in some territories (such as here in California), it is illegal for a doctor to offer any other therapy than conventional chemo or radiation. That's "freedom" for you.

Notwithstanding the political failings of these crazy bureaucracies, there is thankfully no law that says you must abide by what the oncologist recommends. For the time being, at least, even Californians have the right to opt out of the mainstream approach (some of us are concerned that even this small freedom will eventually be taken away).

## Update

Since I wrote the above, a number of years ago, I am somewhat disturbed to have to tell you there there increasing incidents of the huge might of the law being used to browbeat patients. In the USA, "Land of The Free", you can now be accused of murder or attempted murder, if you deny anyone the dubious "benefits" of the "proper" cancer treatment.

Take the sad story of a Massachusetts woman who withheld at-home chemotherapy medications from her autistic, cancer-stricken son and was convicted of attempted murder.

Kristen LaBrie also was found guilty of child endangerment and assault and battery for failing to give her son, Jeremy Fraser, at least five months of cancer medications after the boy was diagnosed with non-Hodgkins lymphoma in 2006. He died in 2009 at age 9.

LaBrie, 38, told the jury she stopped giving him the medications because she couldn't bear to see how sick the side effects made him.

Jeremy's oncologist, Dr. Alison Friedmann of Massachusetts General Hospital, had testified that she told LaBrie her son's cancer had a cure rate of 85 percent to 90 percent under a two-year, five-phase treatment plan that included some hospital stays, regular visits to the hospital clinic to receive chemotherapy treatments and at-home administration of several cancer medications.

Friedmann said the boy's cancer went into remission after months of treatment. But in early 2008, Friedmann said she discovered that the cancer had returned in the form of leukemia and that LaBrie had not filled at least five months of prescriptions she was supposed to give him.

LaBrie said she told her son's doctor two or three times that she was afraid that "he just had had it."

I think what's "had it" is the idea of a compassionate medical system! It an industry!

# Section 2
## The Three Pillars
## Of Cancer Healing

But today in the United States, and this shows you where fascism REALLY exists, ANY doctor in the United States who cures cancer using alternative methods will be destroyed. You cannot name me a doctor doing well with cancer using alternative therapies that is not under attack. And I KNOW these people; I've interviewed them.

**Gary Null**
(1994)

# 2.0 First pillar - Nutrition

The argument about diet was settled long ago. **There isn't an argument.** Only the die-hard fools don't get it.

Diet is everything. In fact some people beat cancer on this one trick of cards!

The World Cancer Research Fund, the UK's leading independent cancer research foundation, states very plainly that 40% of cancers are diet-based. I know it is far higher. The truth will emerge gradually. I have been proved right over all my major predictions in the last 38 years.

It is important to remember that cancer is a degenerative disease of modern times.

It was unknown among hunter-gatherer and pastoral peoples living in remote parts of the world, such as the Himalayas, the Arctic and equatorial Africa, when these were first visited by explorers and missionaries. One of the first medical teams to study the Hunza, remote recesses of the Himalayan Mountains, between West Pakistan, India and China, was headed by world-renown British surgeon Dr Robert McCarrison (the McCarrison Society is named after him).

Writing in the AMA Journal Jan 7, 1922 he reported: "The Hunza has no known incidence of cancer." McCarrison went on to remark about apricots: "They have an abundant crop of apricots. These they dry in the sun and use largely in their food". This led in the 1970s to the laetrile frenzy.

Trying to pick on an extract of apricot as "the" cause of the Hunza longevity is just plain stupid, and shows just as little understanding of Nature, as drug companies trying to extract "the active ingredient" in a herb! But that's what the laetrile lobby got started with and it is nonsense.

I have never seen a successful trial of the value of amygdalin (Laetrile) that specifically excluded other change modalities, which of course would have to be done for any meaningful "proof" that laetrile works. While it is combined with diet (as is usually the case) then the diet may be the real cause of recovery and not the laetrile at all. See section 10.4.

The Eskimos are another people that have been observed by medical teams for many decades and were found to be totally free of cancer. Alaska's most famous doctor Joseph H. Romig, in an intwerview with Dr Preston A. Price claimed that, "In his [Dr. Romig's] 36 years of contact with these people he had never seen a single case of malignant disease among the truly primitive Eskimos, although it frequently occurred when they were modernized".

[reported in Nutrition and Physical Degeneration. London and New York]

An interesting point to note is that when an Eskimo leaves his traditional way of life and begins to rely on a western/modern diet he becomes even more cancer prone than the average American.

The Indians of North America are another people who are remarkably free from cancer. The AMA went as far as conducting a special study in an effort to discover why there was little to no cancer amongst the Hopi and Navajo Indians. The February 5, 1949 issue of the journal of the American Medical Association declared that they found 36 cases of malignant cancer from a population of 30,000. In the same population of white persons there would have been about 1,800 current cases.

In 1843, a French surgeon, Stanislas Tanchou, MD, formulated a doctrine that the incidence of cancer increases in direct proportion to the "civilization" of a nation and its people.

This theory was embraced by John Le Conte, MD (1818-1891), first president of the University of California, and his enthusiasm led medical missionaries, ship surgeons, anthropologists and others to undertake an avid search for cancer among the Alaskan Eskimo (Inuit), northern Athapaskans of Canada and the native peoples of Labrador.

The result was always the same: **for 75 years, not a single case of cancer was documented among the tens of thousands of such people studied by competent medical examiners.** The Harvard-trained anthropologist, Vilhjalmur Stefannson, for instance, lived for 11 years among the Eskimo and never saw a case. In later life, he wrote a book on the topic, *Cancer: A Disease of Civilization?*

Similar stories are told about the indigenous peoples of Africa and Asia. Albert Schweitzer, MD, the famous Nobel laureate, testified: "On my arrival in Gabon, in 1913, I was astonished to encounter no case of cancer... The absence of cancer seemed to me due to the difference in nutrition..."

Is this beginning to add up to a pattern for you?

Indigenous people of regions across the globe seem protected so long as they eat the diet that their ancestors ate for millennia. But once they adopt Western dietary habits, cancer appears and then rapidly grows to being a major killer, if not the number one.

# 2.1 Notable Anti-Cancer Diets

Couple this with the fact that the main effective regimens against cancer (once contracted) are dietary. Most famous is the Max Gerson diet. It has its successes. However it is a formidable diet to follow, practically a career move in its own right, including juicing and coffee enemas several times a day. My belief is that it singles out very determined people and only those with an intense desire to stay alive at all costs will put up with it! This makes it hard to evaluate properly.

Less demanding is the Budwig diet, named after Johanna Budwig. She advocates lots of good fresh food, which is great. But the keynote of her plan is flaxseed oil (omega-3s, of course – back to the Eskimos), which is taken with quark or cottage cheese (very unnatural and nothing to do with the basic hunter-gatherer diet). She has lots of success stories too.

**I suggest that all those who find it necessary to add other protocols or to add supplements to it have not even given the Budwig Protocol half a chance. They just don't look beyond the flaxoil/quark part. There is much more to it than that. It is a scientifically well thought out, all natural ap-**

**proach to health, that has a tremendous rate of success and track record... and it costs next to nothing. I think that if it were very expensive and much money could be made on it, it would be much more popular because it would be pushed by business. But as it stands, it doesn't lend itself to that. So you have to take it at practically no cost or go for some other high priced methods.**

*I'll tell you a bit more about the science behind the success of Johanna Budwig's diet after you have read the section on oxygen pathways (section 3.2. Sunlight and magic electrons)*

Dr William C. Kelley also deserves a big place in the history of anti-cancer diets. Kelley cured himself of virulent pancreatic cancer, using a mainly dietary approach. He had a questionnaire-based analysis of metabolic types, which led to customized dietary recommendations. Kelley developed ten basic diets with 95 variations. These ranged from pure vegetarian to exclusively meat. The diets forbade processed foods, pesticide residues, milk, soy beans, peanuts, food concentrates, white sugar, and white rice. It allowed almonds, low protein grains and nuts, yogurt, "organic" raw vegetable and fruit juices, salads, and whole grain cereals.

You can find Kelley's complete first edition book *One Answer to Cancer* on my website, http://alternative-doctor.com/drkelley [Kelley gave John Scudamore and me permission to publish his first edition free on the web before he finally passed on—38 years after cancer of the pancreas tried to claim him!]

All this should make it clear that the number one factor in controlling and beating cancer is to follow a safe diet. Here's where I differ from some of the experts. There is no universal safe diet. Even the famed vegetarian diet or avoiding red meat is no guarantee. Everyone is different. My approach is to work with each individual and have them figure out their own safe eating plan.

If I should develop cancer, I will do exactly what I tell you to do in my own book *Diet Wise*, which is to work out which foods are stressing your immune system and remove them from your diet. Eat fresh food, salads and smoothies (not much raw), organic if you can and include lots of brightly colored foods. Get rid of any food which reacts to a proper food challenge test—for you they are poison. What is surprising it that whole foods, including fruit, beans and vegetables, can be stressor foods. Each one has to be verified as safe.

In over a decade I never lost a patient to cancer at my office. It was not till years after I quit England they started going down one by one.

It's quite hard work to approach it this way but not as nearly hard as the Gerson diet and certainly not as tough as losing to cancer.

I am not giving details of these three key diets (Gerson, Budwig, Kelley), because they are readily available on the Web. To find out how to carry out my own immune regulator diet, you just need copy of my book "Diet Wise" and do what it says!

**http://www.dietwisebook.com**

# 2.2 Fasting and Near-Fasting

## 2.2a Rudolph Breuss And The Severe Fast

Another herbal naturopath to "cure" cancer was the Austrian, Rudolph Breuss. He healed cases of cancer of the larynx, intestines, breast, kidney, leukemia, abdominal, uterine, hodgkin's, during the 1970's.

Breuss maintained that cancer, whenever it occurs in the body, feeds and grows from protein. He therefore deduced that if one fasted for what has now been confirmed as an ideal period of 42 days, during which various herbal teas and juices are taken to detoxify, cleanse and eliminate, the cancer would starve, be absorbed and subsequently pass out of the body one way or another. Radical thinking that flew in the face of the accepted medical wisdom, but is now used all over the world and known as the Breuss Total Cancer Treatment.

Raw fruit and vegetable juices have always been used and recommended in natural medicine as part of the healing system for many ailments and chronic complaints. Raw juices contain antioxidants and living enzymes that science has identified as an imperative part of everyone's diet if they wish to stay healthy and maintain a defense against all the toxins of today's environment.

It is against this backdrop that Rudolf Breuss developed his Total Cancer Treatment, utilising the therapeutic properties of vegetable juices and herbal teas that have been implicated in the cure of many types of cancer.

The Breuss Tea mix and a specific mixture of organically grown carrot, beetroot, celery, Chinese radish and potato worked wonders on his patients. His mixture provided, in liquid form, all of the minerals and vitamins required by the body during the 42 day fast, whilst the body's own resources are used in dealing with the diseased tissue.

The same blend of the Breuss Vegetable Juice is used in all manners of diseases, taken for a lesser period of time or with food, depending on the severity of the condition. Breuss's book outlines cures for a variety of ailments - serious and those not so serious.

## 2.2b Fasting Helps Chemo Side-Effects

Fasting is prescribed in the Bible and is considered a path to physical and spiritual purity. There are books, articles and Web sites that advocate fasting, some of them even for cancer patients. But many oncologists understandably become alarmed when their patients suggest fasting. After all, cancer is a disease sometimes characterized by unintended weight loss (cachexia). Doctors may feel that fasting will only worsen the situation. But what is the actual science of fasting and its relationship to cancer treatment?

Recently Dr. Valter D. Longo, Fernando M. Safdie and colleagues at the University of Southern California (USC) Andrus Gerontology Center and Department of Biological Sciences, have shown that a 48-hour fast protects normal cells in mice, but not cancer cells, against high-dose chemotherapy.

They also described 10 patients who voluntarily fasted prior to and/or following chemotherapy. None of these reported side effects caused by fasting other than lightheadedness and, of course, hunger. However, most patients reported less fatigue, weakness or gastrointestinal side effects from chemotherapy if they also fasted before and/or after receiving the drugs.

Nor did fasting decrease the effectiveness of the chemotherapy. These USC scientists therefore suggest that fasting, in combination with chemo, is "feasible, safe, and has the potential to ameliorate side effects." They also recommend consulting one's physician before undertaking a fast, and I totally agree. There are certainly individuals with cancer who should not fast. But fasting should be feasible for other patients, is cost-free and, at least in this preliminary report, effective at reducing the side effects of chemotherapy.

There's also the possibility that fasting increases the cancer's vulnerability to chemo (section 2.2).

Resource: http://www.ncbi.nlm.nih.gov/pmc/articles/PMC2815756/?tool=pubmed

# 2.2c The Johanna Brandt Grape Cure

The Brandt grape cure is named for its chief proponent, Johanna Brandt, a South African naturopathic doctor, who published her protocol in a book *The Grape Cure* (1928). The book details Brandt's experiences after she was diagnosed with stomach cancer in 1916. She claimed that fasting and eating only grapes actually kept her cancer in check!

It's true there are several potentially anti-cancerous substances in grapes, like beta carotene, ellagic acid, lycopene, quercetin and selenium (depends on the ground supply)

But I don't think it's due to any magic about grapes. I think it's just a full exclusion program, of the kind I recommend in all my writings.

Scott-Mumby rule: It's what you stop eating that does the most good, not what you eat instead!

### 2.2c.i The Brandt Protocol (from Brandt's own notes)

1. To prepare the system for the change of diet, the better practice is to fast for two or three days, drinking plenty of pure, cold water and taking an enema of a quart of lukewarm water daily with the strained juice of one lemon therein (skip the lemon juice; this is housewife's stuff. There are no taste buds to amuse up your bum! Moreover, citrus foods are common allergens - KSM)

   During the fast the body will cleanse. This is, of course, a complete exclusion program, which accords entirely with my hypo-allergenic approach to cancer nutrition.

A good point Brandt makes is that becoming very, very hungry will make grapes taste wonderful, when you get to your first one!

2. Breaking the fast. The patient drinks one or two glasses of pure, cold water the first thing in the morning.

3. Half an hour later the patient has his first meal of grapes. Wash them well. (Chew the skins and seeds thoroughly and swallow only a few of them as food and roughage.)

4. Time. Starting at 8 a.m. and having a grape meal every two hours till 8 p.m., this would give seven meals daily. This is kept up for a week or two, even a month or two, in chronic cases of long standing. Not longer under any circumstances.

5. Variety. Any good variety may be used - purple, green, red, white or blue. Hothouse grapes are better than none, and the seedless varieties are excellent. The monotony of the diet may be varied by using many varieties. Different varieties contain different elements so it is advisable to use as many kinds as one can get. Some like them acid, others like them sweet.

The best time is when the grape season is at its height.

6. Quantity. This varies according to the condition, digestion and occupation of the patient. It is well to begin with a small quantity of one, two or three ounces per meal, gradually increasing this to double the quantity.

In time about a half pound may safely be taken at a meal. To make this point quite clear, a minimum quantity of one pound should be used daily, while the maximum should not exceed four pounds. Patients taking larger quantities at a meal should allow at least three hours for digestion and should not take all the skins. Invariably, the best results have been effected when grapes have been taken in small quantities.

7. Enjoyment. A loathing for grapes may indicate the presence of much poison in the system, Brandt says, and the need of another short fast. Go back to just water, until the symptoms clear.

(Well from my experience, I should point out that this is often a "detox" effect. There are "withdrawal" symptoms and the simplest answer is just keep going.

When the last of the allergy-addictive food residues leave the bowel, these "detox" symptom clear up like magic. This usually happens on the morning of the 5th day - KSM)

Brandt continues: We hear of over-zealous relatives forcing grapes down the throats of unfortunate patients. This is a great mistake (always remember that grapes are nourishing and maintain life in the body while the cleansing process is going on). Loss of strength is due to the presence of poisons in the system. The patient continues to weaken under the grape diet and under the complete fast, until the poison has been expelled. Then, without a change of diet (and in case of a complete fast, without any food whatsoever), the patient returns to strength and in some cases even puts on weight.

It is a well-known fact with scientists and physiologists that a person can go from 90 to 115 days without any food and live, and that he can go without water 12 days and live.

The outcome stages are given here, described in Brandt's own flowery words

## 2.2c.ii Four Stages

There are four stages in a complete treatment and these stages must be followed closely; heavy foods must not be eaten until the completion of the four stages.

At the conclusion of the exclusive diet, the patient is in much the same condition as a typhoid patient when the fever subsides! Extreme care must be taken to prevent him from eating heavy foods.

### First Stage

*(a) In every case reactions are different.*

It is, therefore, impossible to say beforehand how long it will be necessary to use grapes only. But this may be stated definitely - the cleansing of the alimentary canal takes time, and until this has been accomplished, the real relief does not begin. It is safe to say that the first seven to ten days on grapes only would be required to clear the stomach and bowels of their ancient accumulations. And it is during this period that distressing symptoms often appear. Nature works thoroughly. She does not build on a rotten foundation. The purification of every part of the body must be complete before new tissue can be built.

Note: I think this is the only explanation of the excessive loss of weight under the grape diet.

This question is of so much importance that we refer to it in detail under the treatment of cancer elsewhere.

If we could remove every trace of fear from the mind of the patient, the correct procedure would be to continue the exclusive grape diet until he stops losing weight. By watching the symptoms - the temperature, the excretions, eruptions, etc., we know when the work of purification is complete. When this point has been reached - and it may last from two weeks to two months - it is advisable to go on to the

### Second Stage

*(b) The gradual introduction of other fresh fruits, tomatoes and sour milk or cottage cheese.*

We do not expect anyone to live on grapes forever. The grape contains many of the most valuable elements necessary for life, but it does not contain everything. To live on grapes indefinitely would be to rob the system of some of the elements essential to life. When we are sure, therefore, that the grape has done its work by breaking up the unhealthy tissue and purifying the blood, the careful introduction of other bodybuilding foods is the next step.

Grapes still form the main food and are always taken as the first meal in the morning and at 8 p.m. But now, during the day, some other fresh fruit may be used instead of grapes. An endless variety presents itself - a slice of melon, an orange, a grapefruit, an apple, a luscious pear, the scarlet strawberry, the golden apricot -

one fruit more appetizing than the other. Let the patient choose. Only one kind of fruit to be taken at a meal but something different every day.

After a few days a glass of sour milk or buttermilk, yogurt, or cottage cheese may be taken instead of grapes for supper. Patients who dislike milk should take a ripe, finely-mashed banana, or some other nourishing fruit.

(Don't do milk or cheese! Dairy allergy is about the commonest imflammatory food effect there is. Milk contributes to cancer, I and several other experienced doctors agree. Start with fish or exotic foods you don't normally eat, like persimmons, kiwis etc. - KSM)

After a week or ten days, every other meal may consist of different varieties of fruit, or sour milk, taking them, for example, in the following order:

8:00 A.M. Grapes.
10:00 A.M. Pear, banana or peaches.
12:00 Noon Grapes.
2:00 P.M. Sour milk, buttermilk, or cottage cheese.
4:00 P.M. Grapes.
6:00 P.M. Orange, grapefruit, plums or apricots.
8:00 P.M. Grapes.

At this point some patients crave for something savory. The sweet fruits begin to pall. There may even be a positive aversion to grapes, in which case they should be omitted altogether and the other foods taken every three hours.

One or two sliced tomatoes with pure olive oil and a little lemon juice may safely be included in this diet. The tomato is more of a fruit than a vegetable, containing many valuable properties, and it forms an indispensable part of the diet in the second stage of the treatment. Third Stage

*(c) The raw diet.*

This includes every food that can be eaten uncooked - raw vegetables, salads, fruits, nuts, raisins, dates, figs and other dried fruits, butter, cottage cheese, sour milk, yogurt and buttermilk, honey and olive oil.

Begin the day as usual with cold water and grapes or some other fruit for breakfast, but instead of sour milk or fruit for lunch, have a substantial salad of raw vegetables. Reduce the number of meals, as raw vegetables require longer to digest.

It is surprising to some people to find that nearly all the vegetables can be used raw - young green peas and string beans, celery tomatoes, cucumbers,) lettuce, sprigs of cauliflowers, squash, shredded cabbage leaves, grated carrots, turnips, beets and parsnips, finely chopped onion and spinach.

(sprouted is even better, taste great raw, and I don't know why she missed this point - KSM)

After the light fruit diet, it is wise not to start out too soon with a large variety of vegetables. Choose two or three of the above-named as a foundation for your salad and mix them with lemon juice and olive oil. Try different varieties the following day and watch the combinations of flavors. Salad-making is a supreme art.

Above all things, this noonday meal should be made palatable. Patients who have been used to animal food crave for something stimulating. There can be no objection to adding one or two savory ingredients to this salad - some finely-chopped nuts, grated cheese, sour cream, or a good homemade mayonnaise made of eggs, lemon juice and olive oil. In some cases a finely-chopped hard boiled egg may be included in the salad.

### Time to Digest
Give this meal more time to digest than is required for raw fruits, especially if nuts, dates, raisins or other dried fruits have been added to it.

The supper should consist of sour milk or fruit, or a highly nourishing and digestible dish may be made of ripe bananas mashed, with sour cream.

### The Raw Diet
Sufficient stress cannot be laid upon importance of the raw diet. If we could only educate the people to this fact it would help to eradicate disease.

The raw foods digest more easily than the cooked and pass through the system far more rapidly. The result is that they have no time to decompose in the alimentary canal. There is no undue fermentation and no fear of toxic poisoning.

Therefore patients are strongly advised to abstain from every form of cooked food during the full period of treatment.

Thus far the course then consists of the three stages as outlined above and if followed the highest results are obtained.

When it is difficult to convince people that they derive more nourishment from uncooked foods, we reluctantly consent to the introduction of one cooked meal a day, but do not recommend it.

### Fourth Stage
*(d) The mixed diet.*

With this innovation, there is sometimes a recurrence of the old trouble, and the patient, sadder and wiser for the experience, is glad to go back to the raw diet. But if the disease has not been very deep-seated and the cure is complete, the following regimen is recommended: - Three Meals a Day

(1) A fruit breakfast, one kind only.
(2) A cooked dinner.
(3) A salad supper.

For breakfast eat plentifully of any of the juicy fruits that may be in season. Make a strict habit of this and observe it for the rest of your life if you want to be healthy.

The No Breakfast Plan does not apply to fruit at all. It was and is, a splendid rule for people who have been systematically overeating, and especially those who are in the habit of indulging in heavy dinners and late suppers. But when the supper is taken not later than 7 P.M. and consists of raw salad or fruit, the stomach of one who has been on a proper grape diet is free from acidity and accumulations.

In such cases, the fruit breakfast is better than the fast, in that it supplies the body with cleansing and building material.

One can, moreover, do a hard morning's work on a fruit breakfast.

Be sure to connect this program in your mind with the section that shows how fasting helps increase chemo-sensitivity too (section 38). Even if you don't do chemo, it's clear that fasting helps weaken the cancer cells, as Rudolph Breuss too noticed.

# 2.3 How Do Polyphenols Prevent Cancer?

Polyphenols are antioxidant compounds found in the skin and seeds of grapes. When wine is made from these grapes, the alcohol produced by the fermentation process dissolves the polyphenols contained in the skin and seeds. Red wine contains more polyphenols than white wine because the making of white wine requires the removal of the skins after the grapes are crushed. The phenols in red wine include catechin, gallic acid, and epicatechin.

However, white wine has plenty of polyphenols, and champagne, which contains such active polyphenols as tyrosol and caffeic acid, may turn out to be the best antioxidant of all.

Antioxidants are substances that protect cells from oxidative damage caused by molecules called free radicals. These free radicals can damage important parts of cells, including proteins, membranes, and DNA. This sort of damage has been implicated in the development of cancer. Research on the antioxidants found in red wine has shown that they may help inhibit the development of certain cancers.

Resveratrol is a type of polyphenol and is actually produced by the plant in response to an invading fungus, stress, injury, infection, or ultraviolet irradiation. In other words, protection. Red wine contains high levels of resveratrol, as do grapes, raspberries, peanuts, pistachios, blueberries, cranberries, and even cocoa and dark chocolate.

Resveratrol has been shown to reduce tumor incidence in animals by affecting one or more stages of cancer development. It has been shown to inhibit growth of many types of cancer cells in culture. Evidence also exists that it can reduce inflammation. That's good for cancer too.

Remember, although consumption of large amounts of alcoholic beverages may increase the risk of some cancers, there is growing evidence that the health benefits of red wine are related to its nonalcoholic components.

[http://www.cancer.gov/cancertopics/factsheet/prevention/
redwine; recovered: 2/16/10: 11.00 am PST]

Resveratrol is like several anti-cancer drugs rolled into one. Resveratrol works in so many ways to block cancer, researchers can't find a cancer-promotion pathway it doesn't inhibit. It is virtually non-toxic since, after oral ingestion, it is quickly metabolized by the liver, attached to a detoxification molecule called glucuronate, which renders it harmless, though biologically inactive, at least for a time.

At the site of tumors cells there is an unzipping enzyme (glucuronidase) that uncouples resveratrol from glucuronate. This is nature's "smart bomb" drug delivery system, releasing resveratrol right on target, inside the tumor.

So maybe the observation that heavy drinking can stem cancer has some scientific merit. This is not what you will hear from the "bread and butter" thinkers.

[Cancer Letters 231: 113–22, 2006; Oncogene 23: 6702–11, 2004; Toxicology Letters 161: 1–9, 2006; World Journal Gastroenterology 12: 5628–34, 2006; Investigative Ophthalmology Visual Science 47: 3708–16, 2006; Cancer Detection Prevention 30: 217-23, 2006; Molecular Cancer Therapy 4: 554–61, 2005; Journal Biological Chemistry 278: 41482–90, 2003]

# 2.4 Wine Is Good Against Some Cancers

We know that wine helps with heart disease. But a little wine may be a very good thing for cancer too.

Researchers at the Yale School of Public Health studied more than 500 women with non-Hodgkin's lymphoma, a cancer of the lymphatic system.

At the time of their diagnosis, the women were asked a battery of questions regarding alcohol: whether they drank, what they drank, how much they drank, and for how long they had been drinking. Then they were followed for 8 to 12 years.

Among the findings, it was noted that:

- About three-fourths of women who drank at least 12 glasses of wine over their lifetime were alive five years after diagnosis, compared with two-thirds of those who never drank wine.

- 35% of never-drinkers relapsed within five years vs. 30% of wine drinkers.

- The longer a woman drank, the lower the chance she would suffer a relapse or die within five years of diagnosis.

- Patients who had been drinking wine for at least 25 years prior to diagnosis were 26% less likely to relapse or develop a secondary cancer and 33% less likely to die over the five-year period, compared with non-wine drinkers.

The protective effects of wine were strongest among women with diffuse large B-cell lymphoma, the most common type of non-Hodgkin's lymphoma. Women with this type of cancer who drank more than 6 glasses of wine a day were about 60% less likely to relapse or die within five years, compared with non-wine drinkers.

Note that 6 glasses of wine a day (for a woman especially) is considered heavy drinking. So on the face of it (careful!) heavy drinking of wine could be a protective.

Beer and liquor consumption did not appear to affect lymphoma risk.

**And this from the US's National Cancer Institute site:**
Red wine is a rich source of biologically active phytochemicals, chemicals found in plants. Particular compounds called polyphenols found in red wine—such as catechins and resveratrol—are thought to have antioxidant or anticancer properties.

Please know that I NEVER recommend beers and spirits. Only wine seems to have any protective effect and is a healthful food for many, that goes back many centuries. One big surprise is that champagne has a powerful anti-oxidant (tyrosol), which is much more potent than the anti-oxidant effects of blueberries and resveratrol!

Always drink moderately and only with food.

# 2.5 The Question of Supplements

People sometimes ask (maybe without voicing the question): "Will vitamins and minerals save me?"

The answer is NO. It would be like closing the stable door after the horse has bolted. But they are great in prevention. Vitamin D, for example, is a well-proven anti-cancer vitamin.

Nevertheless, there is every reason to supplement your diet with good nutrients, including simple prorietary multi-vitamin and mineral formulas. As part of a good health regimen, nutrient supplements are vital for health. Just be realistic about what to expect.

Rather than me parading the value of numerous individual vitamins and minerals, let me just say that I expect you to get plenty of everything. A good fresh food diet will help too, with bags of antioxidants.

All this is in accordance with my "Cancer Rule 1:

**every good health measure is an anti-cancer measure.**

Supplementing is a vast subject, all on its own.  So I will just mention a few specifics here, to get your started and to press home my point.

Good supplements will protect you from the dire effects of chemo and radiation.

# 2.6 Positive Evidence For The Value Of Supplements

Not much gets published these days that isn't bought-and-paid-for lies by the Pharmaceutical industry and the Cancer Mafia. However, as I keep pointing out, there are good, caring, honest researchers out there. Their voice is suppressed by the giant propaganda machine. But then it's up to doctors like me to make sure that what they say gets heard.

It's my pleasure to report yet another (of very many) studies that show nutritional supplements have powerful and far-reaching benefits for determined cancer survivors.

Dr Bob Lister, co-author of a study by British and Danish researchers, said the results from taking supplements were similar to the survival gains from new drugs and in some cases better. *But the important difference was there were no side effects reported by patients taking vitamins.*

> Dr Lister, chairman of the Institute of Brain Chemistry and Human Nutrition at London Metropolitan University, said: "People with cancer are constantly asking what can we do, not necessarily to beat the cancer but to have a better quality of life whatever the length of survival.
>
> "Most importantly, taking these supplements is extremely safe, and there were no adverse reactions among the patients."

The study followed patients suffering from breast, lung, brain, colon and other forms of cancer in Denmark between 1990 and 1999 who continued taking conventional cancer medication.

During the nine-year period, the patients were treated with coenzyme Q10 – a vitamin-like compound-essential for producing energy made naturally in the body – and six other antioxidants including vitamins A, C and E, selenium, folic acid, and beta carotene (which were not given to lung cancer patients for safety reasons).

The patients were predicted to live for an average of 12 months, but 76 per cent lived an average of 17 months longer. That's an extra 30% life.

The doses of the supplements, supplied by manufacturers Pharma Nord, were large but were within recommended safety limits, said Dr Lister.

In addition, patients received small amounts of other nutrients including fish oil and B vitamins.

The findings are published in the *Journal of International Medical Research* (February 2010).

The study was paid for by Pharma-Nord, a very fine Scandinavian holistic health company which manufactures good products. I dealt with them for years during my hegemony in the UK.

[http://www.dailymail.co.uk/health/article-1251286/
Cocktail-vitamins-cancer-patients-extra-years.html]

And yet another study which neatly proves the point: the daily use of multivitamins may reduce the incidence of cancer in men, according to the results of a very large randomized trial. The study was on male doctors as patients, which could be important.

After about 11 years, multivitamin use resulted in a modest but statistically significant reduction — specifically, an 8% reduction in total cancer incidence.

In fact, if you remove prostate cancer cases from this study, the remaining cancers showed a MASSIVE 12% reduction in total cancers which was "significant", said lead author John Michael Gaziano, MD, MPH. He was speaking at a press briefing ahead of a presentation at the Annual American Association for Cancer Research (AACR) *Frontiers in Cancer Prevention Research* meeting.

Significant means it's scientifically proven, not a hoax or anomaly.

That's 1 in 10 lives saved!! Chemo and other pharmaceuticals cannot come close to that.

This study was a large-scale, randomized, double-blind, placebo-controlled trial that included 14,641 male US physicians who were 50 years or older when the study began. The cohort included 1,312 men with a history of cancer. The multivitamin study began in 1997, with treatment and follow-up that continued through June 1, 2011.

In other words, it was really good science. But when reporting it, the medical press keep factoring in the word "modest" gain, which is a bit different to Big Pharma lies and exaggerations. Also, they quickly limited it by saying this benefit only applies to men over 50... As if!

# 2.7 Antioxidants Reduce Cancer By Two Thirds

Finally, here's a refreshing study that shows without question that antioxidants will not harm you and will even reduce the incidence of deadly pancreatic cancer by *two thirds*.

In this latest study, researchers led by Dr. Andrew Hart of the University of East Anglia tracked the long-term health of more than 23,500 people, aged 40 to 74, who entered the study between 1993 and 1997. Each participant kept a food diary that detailed the types, amount and method of preparation for every food they ate for seven days.

After 10 years, 49 participants (55 percent of whom were male) had been diagnosed with pancreatic cancer. By 2010, the number of participants diagnosed with pancreatic cancer increased to 86 (44 percent were men).

On average, patients survived six months after diagnosis.

The researchers found that people with the highest dietary intake of selenium were half as likely to develop pancreatic cancer as those with the lowest intake. Those who consumed the highest dietary intake of all three antioxidants -- selenium and vitamins C and E -- were 67 percent less likely to develop pancreatic cancer compared to those with the lowest intake.

That's down two thirds.

Need I say more?

The study was published online July 23, 2012, in the journal *Gut*.

# 2.8 Vitamin D A Truly Vital  Anti-Cancer Nutrient

A study published in the Journal of the National Cancer Institute in 2006 showed that even small rises in vitamin D levels in the blood produced a dramatic lowering of cancer risk.  For 6 years nearly 50,000 men were followed, while taking an average of 1500 IU daily. The results showed a 17% reduction in the incidence of cancer, almost 30% reduction in overall cancer mortality and a massive 45% reduction in deaths for bowel cancer.

Another study in the same year, involving more than 120,000 women participating in two studies at Harvard University and Saint George's Hospital Medical School In London, showed that women with high levels of vitamin D were 50% less likely to get breast cancer; even those with moderately raised vitamin D levels had a measurable 10% lower risk. Yet another study showed that women who spent a lot of time in the sunshine – which is what creates vitamin D – had between 25% and 45% less cancers than the average woman.

You'd think the medical profession would jump at these findings and recommend everyone take vitamin D. But I'm afraid that's sadly not the case. In fact, although studies make it clear that 1000 to 1500 IU is required to protect men and women from cancer, official government figures still insist that 200 IU is enough. This advice is not merely bad - it's criminal, given the level of scientific knowledge on this topic that says different.

# 2.9 Apatone®
## (vitamins C and K3 combined)

You know, I keep saying that some of my orthodox colleagues are coming round to our way of thinking (I dissociate myself from silly, petulant "holistic" writers, who think everything is evil about conventional cancer treatment).

As I like to point out: there are some great doctors out there, trying hard. Not everyone is corrupted by Big Pharma. Some good techniques are emerging, with great promise and sound science.

I'm talking now about a novel combination of vitamin C and vitamin K3 called Apatone®. It selectively targets tumors by entering cancer cells as readily as glucose. It then suppresses certain inflammatory reactions that cancer cells use to escape destruction by chemotherapy agents.

When administered prior to chemo, vitamin K3 appears to decrease the tumor resistance to chemo drugs. It has helped prostate cancer patients, who were getting no help from chemo, to start making progress knocking out the cancer.

Coupling it with vitamin C is a smart move. According to *Science Daily*, "This non-toxic approach weakens and kills cancers in a novel way." In fact quite a few studies published since 2008 have shown vitamins K2 and K3 to be intriguing agents in both cancer prevention and treatment.

Apatone was discovered by Dr. Henryk Taper from the Catholic University of Leuven in Brussels, Belgium and was developed by Dr. James Jamison and Dr. Jack Summers, both of Summa Health System, and Dr. Jacques Gilloteaux, now with the American University of the Caribbean in St. Maarten. Their groundbreaking discovery found that moderate doses of Apatone eliminate many types of cancer cells, including prostate, bladder, renal and ovarian.

"This strategy targets cancer cells by their inflammatory response," explains Dr. Jamison. "It's a different approach than most other anti-tumor drugs, which target dividing cells or the development of blood vessels within the tumor. Since normal cells use sugars or fats for energy and cancer cells rely on glucose, the real key here is that Apatone resembles glucose. As Apatone preferentially accumulates in cancer cells, it also supplies quinone that weakens and can destroy the cancer cell from within.

"The bottom line is: Apatone selectively targets and kills tumor cells using non-toxic biochemistry that protects surrounding healthy tissue."

In a March 2008 study, Apatone® significantly slowed prostate cancer and lowered PSA levels; 16 out of 17 patients responded positively (no chemo agent can equal that!) Moreover, of the 15 patients who continued to take it, only one death occurred after 14 months of treatment. The doses were: 5,000 mg of vitamin C and 50 mg of vitamin K3.

The doctors concluded that Apatone showed promise in delaying biochemical progression in this group of end stage prostate cancer patients.

[*ScienceDaily*, 9 Oct 2007. www.sciencedaily.com/
releases/2007/10/071005143631.htm]

Well, the real key here is that Apatone resembles glucose! We all know how precious glucose is to cancer cells. They need it to burn for energy. That's Otto Warburg's glycolysis theory. So it is preferentially taken into cancer cells, where it accumulates. It also supplies quinone that weakens and can destroy the cancer cell from within.

The bottom line is: Apatone selectively targets and kills tumor cells using non-toxic biochemistry that protects surrounding healthy tissue.

You can ask your oncologist for Apatone. But for home therapy it has no value: it needs to be taken IV. However, you need nobody's permission to take lots of vitamin C (10 – 20 grams a day or more) and vitamins K2 and K3 (try to get 50 – 100 mg if you can get it and can afford it). Double these doses if you are obese. Note that vitamin K1 is worthless in this context.

Additional clinical trials are planned for intravenous administration of Apatone in patients who have failed chemotherapy. Apatone has been granted orphan drug status by the FDA to treat advanced bladder cancer.

# 2.10 Potassium

This is a surprise cancer need. Most doctors would assume automatically that the body has enough (if supplies go too low, the heart stops). But in fact this is far from the case. Max Gerson MD was made famous for his "diet" but I think his contribution to the understanding of the need for huge doses of potassium are, if anything, the major factor in the success of his program (meaning almost any old good diet will work; there are very many that do, so his diet may not be the really critical factor in his program—just thinking out loud here...)

Gerson carefully researched and established that the toxins from cancer reduce potassium levels. That's made worse by the toxins from the destructive breakdown of cancer tumors, caused by chemo and radiation, which also dramatically lower potassium levels.

[ Physiol.Chem.Phys.1978; 10(5):465-468]

So logically, potassium supplementation is paramount. Freeman Cope, M.D., wrote in Physiological Chemistry and Physics in 1978, "The high potassium, low sodium diet of the Gerson therapy has been observed experimentally to cure many cases of advanced cancer in man, but the reason was not clear. Recent studies from the laboratory of Ling indicate that high potassium, low sodium environments can partially return damaged cell proteins to their normal undamaged configuration.

# 2.11 Iodine

Lack of iodine is now endemic in the US and the Western world. Iodine is added to salt but so much propaganda about avoiding salt has resulted in civilized nations being chronically deficient in iodine.

That coupled with the fact that iodine in bread is now replaced by bromine, a competitive antagonist of iodine, has caused a health problem of vast proportions. Iodine deficiency has many consequences, including thyroid troubles and cancer susceptibility.

Iodine enhances oxygen metabolism and that has significant consequences, as we shall see later.

Make sure you get enough and read the book *Iodine: Why You Need It, Why You Can't Live Without It* by Dr. David Brownstein.

# 2.12 Shark's Cartilage and Angiogenesis

**While we are on the subject of nutrients, let's look at a couple of other examples:**
Like healthy tissue, tumors need a steady blood supply. By creating their own "network" of blood vessels, tumors develop an independent and reliable source of nutrients and oxygen, which "feed" the tumor. Without new blood vessels, tumors cannot grow beyond the size of a pea. *Angiogenesis* is a word that means new growth of blood supply.

In fact tumors are very sneaky and secrete hormone-like substances called growth factors, especially one known as vascular endothelial growth factor, or VEGF. This attaches to nearby cells and triggers new blood vessels to sprout toward the tumor. These blood vessels provide the tumor with a steady blood supply and nutrients. Without VEGF, new blood vessels are unable to grow and support the tumor. The tumor dies.

Anti-angiogenic agents (blocking VEGF) are thought to work by stopping the growth of new blood vessels. This process "starves" the tumors of the blood and nutrients necessary for growth. These types of treatments are called angiogenesis inhibitors. Of course the majority are just complicated and expensive drugs.

But did you know that shark cartilage has exactly the same action—at a fraction of the cost? No, of course you were not told. It's bad news for sharks! In fact liquid bovine (beef) cartilage appears to give similar results. That's easier on the environment and actually tastes better.

# 2.13 Supernutrient Vitamin C

The cancer-curative properties of vitamin C is its most controversial benefit by far. Oncologists hate it and regular media splurges try to discredit it and even claim it causes cancer, based on a very miserable inadequate study showing if you drenched chromosomes in vitamin C in a test tube there were minor changes which *might* (they said) indicate a cancer risk.

Having used it IV for over 2 decades with cancer patients I can attest with certainty to its beneficial effects.

One good study showed a cytotoxic effect (like chemo) against cancer cells at around 3 grams per 100 mls in blood. That's way below any possible toxic effect in humans. In fact there is no such thing as a toxic effect from vitamin C. None ever recorded, even at doses over 300- 400 grams IV. It really is remarkable.

[Please note a study in 2008 which showed that vitamin C in the presence of fats in the stomach created more nitrosamines. We know nitrosamines are carcinogenic. It's a paradox because vitamin C, without fats, normally lowers nitrosamine levels in the stomach. So the culprit is really the fats. Unfortunately, this study did not fully reveal what type of fats].

**Most objective studies show vitamin C significantly decreases cancer of the mouth, esophagus, stomach, colon, rectum and lung.**

One prospective study of 870 men over a period of 25 years found that those who consumed more than 83 mg of vitamin C daily had a striking 64% reduction in lung cancer compared with those who consumed less than 63 mg per day. That's a 2/3rds reduction: pretty hard to argue with.

Although most large prospective studies found no association between breast cancer and vitamin C intake, two recent studies found dietary vitamin C intake to be inversely (which is good) associated with breast cancer risk in certain subgroups.

In the Nurses' Health Study, premenopausal women with a family history of breast cancer who consumed an average of 205 mg/day of vitamin C from foods had a 63% lower risk of breast cancer than those who consumed an average of 70 mg/day.

In the Swedish Mammography Cohort, women who were overweight and consumed an average of 110 mg/day of vitamin C had a 39% lower risk of breast cancer compared to overweight women who consumed an average of 31 mg/day.

# Quality of Life

In the 1970's and 1980's pioneer vitamin C researcher Linus Pauling and his medical collaborator, Dr. Ewan Cameron, former Chief of Surgery at Vale of Leven Hospital in Scotland, published several studies in the 1970s on the beneficial response of cancer patients to large doses of supplemental vitamin C as an adjunct treatment to conventional cancer therapies (10 grams/day intravenously for 10 days followed by at least 10 grams/day orally indefinitely).

They found repeatedly that benefits ranged from an increased sense of well-being and an increased survival time for terminal patients to rare complete regressions of malignancies.

However, two randomized placebo-controlled studies carried out by Drs. Edward Creagan and Charles Moertel of the Mayo Clinic and published in 1979 and 1985 found no differences in outcome between terminal cancer patients receiving 10 grams of vitamin C/day orally or placebo. But the difference is clear: *the Mayo studies used oral vitamin C, Cameron and Pauling used IV*. The intravenous route will result in far higher blood levels of ascorbate; we know that, it's proven science.

In studies like this, with faulty technique, it's hard to avoid suspicion that the researchers were trying to avoid getting a beneficial effect.

The National Cancer Institute website is more to be trusted, I think, and contains several pages of evauation of usage of vitamin C (ascorbate) in cancer therapy, and I quote:

Studies have demonstrated tumor growth inhibition after treatment with pharmacological ascorbate in animal models of pancreatic cancer, liver cancer, prostate cancer, sarcoma, mesothelioma, and ovarian cancer.

The effects of high-dose ascorbic acid in combination with standard treatments on tumors have been investigated. In a mouse model of pancreatic cancer, the combination of gemcitabine (30 or 60 mg /kg every 4 days) and ascorbate (4 g /kg daily) resulted in greater decreases in tumor volume and weight, compared with gemcitabine treatment alone. According to a study reported in 2012, ascorbate enhanced the cancer cell–killing effects of photodynamic therapy in mice injected with breast cancer cells. A study of mouse models of ovarian cancer found that ascorbate enhanced the tumor inhibitory effect of carboplatin and paclitaxel, first-line chemotherapy used in ovarian cancer.

Yet all you ever hear is vitamin C is "proven" to interfere with chemo, which is not the case.


# Vitamin C Latest

This is hot: well, 2015!

Researchers Jihye Yun from John Hopkins University, Baltimore and Lewis Cantley of Weill Cornell Medicine, New York City along with Cantley's lab and his collaborators noticed that large volumes of vitamin C could indeed eliminate cultured colon cancer cells in mice with FRAF or KRAS mutations.

Thing is, more than half of human colorectal cancers (CRCs) carry either KRAS or BRAF mutations, and are often refractory to approved targeted therapies, so this is excellent news, both for the patients and for the credibility of vitamin C cancer therapy.

If these findings also apply to humans, researchers have possibly found a means of treating a large number of tumors that have not seen any effective drug till now. Channing Der from the University of North Carolina, a molecular biologist, stated that the present study could be the answer to the one question that everybody is striving to find. He added that the study is gratifying for the small number of researchers who were pursuing Ascorbic acid or Vitamin C as a cancer drug.

A Vitamin C researcher from National Institute of Diabetes and Digestive Diseases stated that he is encouraged and may be, people will start paying attention.

[Science| DOI: 10.1126/science.aad7397]

No KRAS-targeted therapeutics have emerged despite decades of effort and hundreds of millions of dollars [spent] by both industry and academia," said Cancer geneticist Bert Vogelstein of Johns Hopkins University.

Others caution that the effects seen in mice may not hold up in humans. But because high dose vitamin C is already known to be safe, says cancer researcher Vuk Stambolic of the University of Toronto in Canada, oncologists "can quickly move forward in the clinic."

One drawback is that patients will have to come into a clinic for vitamin C infusions, ideally every few days for months, because vitamin C seems to take that long to kill cancer cells, Levine notes. But Cantley says it may be possible to make an oral formulation that reaches high doses in the blood—which may be one way to get companies interested in sponsoring trials.


## Detox

It would be remiss not to share one of the important benefits of vitamin C which a few of us discovered in the 1980s, even though no direct scientific research has been done in this field.

We became keenly aware that significant doses of vitamin C were beneficial in cases of chemical overload. By the late 70s we were encountering more and more patients with "chemical allergy" syndrome.

Some individuals are super-sensitive to ambient chemicals. This is partly a genetic thing, as we shall see later. They simply didn't have the right enzymes, or not enough, to adequately detoxify so-called xenobiotic (unnatural) chemicals. The result was much suffering and incapacity.

But large doses of vitamin C would prove helpful. How big a dose? We used a crude strategy called "fill and flush"; the patient would take increasing doses in 2 gram increments (a teaspoon is 4- 5 gms). Eventually, the side effect of diarrhea would manifest and we told the patient to take just less than that as their personal level. So, 10 grms = diarrhea; dose = 8 grams.

It was all rather crude by modern standards but it got results and, as I have already said, there are no known toxic effects of vitamin C, even at levels exceeding typical oral doses by 10- 20 times.

The result was that chemically-sensitive patients could get through their working hours, endure traffic fumes and aircraft travel, without being sick for days afterwards.

For cancer patients, most of the toxins arise internally, either generated by the cancer or (sometimes) in massive amounts when the cancer was overthrown and began to break up, releasing a lot of poisons.

That's probably why vitamin C makes a cancer patient feel a lot better.


## Vitamin C: Attacks Never Go Away

Have you ever wondered WHY there is such a frenzy to discredit vitamin C?

They tried again in 2008. A study published in *Cancer Research* (2008; 68:8031-8038) warned that high doses of vitamin C could harm cancer patients by making chemotherapy drugs ineffective. This was based on research on "vitamin C" given to mice or cultured cells treated with common anti-cancer chemotherapy agents. Apparently their "vitamin C" hampered those drugs' anti-tumor effects.

Why do I keep putting "vitamin C" in quotes. Because they did not use vitamin C (ascorbic acid) but a totally different (but related) substance known as dehydroascorbic acid. It's not used therapeutically. It's useless and was clearly chosen deliberately, to obscure the results.

What's more, in the experiments with laboratory rodents, the mice were given excessive and probably toxic doses of dehydroascorbic acid. In other words, it's a straight fix.

Of course the media picked this up; the media are bought and paid for by the establishment and Big Pharma. Clearly they had their instructions to run another trashing campaign against natural therapies. If you saw it, don't let it put you off.

We know that REAL vitamin C selectively kills cancer cells, while leaving healthy cells untouched. Countless tests and trials shown that natural vitamin C (even when it's manufactured in a laboratory) is non-toxic and can be safely administered in HUGE doses of over 100 grams a day, IV.

It also has a protective effect against the toxicity of chemo and radiation and enhances the quality of life right to the last.

# IV administration of vitamin C

Today, we highly recommend IV vitamin C at doses around 50 grams, for cancer.* Tests show it is cytotoxic to cancer cells at this level, without harming normal, healthy cells.

Most of us using this method took the chance to provide a whole bunch of other good nutrient stuff, some complex homeopathics maybe (section 8.6) and adjuvant therapy like DMSO (section 10.9).

Each patient's program was personalized. Everyone is different. But with this kind of therapeutic regime I was not only able to keep patients alive who might have died, but they were extraordinarily healthy.

One of my boasts is that none of my patients lost their hair or had unpleasant side effects, over a 10-year period. That's how good it was at protecting the patient, while at the same time giving cancer cells a deadly cocktail!

If you cannot find a physician willing to do IVs for you, then be sure to take liposomal vitamin C: 1 gram of liposomal vitamin C is equivalent to 10 grams orally and without the side effects.

*Daily if the patient is very sick, dropping to twice a week and then weekly.

# 2.14 Second Pillar of Healing - Cleaning up your emotions

The first reference I know to emotions and cancer comes from the great Roman doctor – Galen: "Cancer does not strike happy people" (well, actually, he said cancer was caused by an excess of black bile = melancholy!) The dogma of black bile as the source of cancer reigned for over 1500 years after Galen wrote his treatise.

Surprisingly, he was right! Nowadays we don't think of the four "humors" (black bile, yellow bile, blood and phlegm) but certainly negative emotional humors and cancer go hand in hand.

A defining study was carried out by Stanford psychiatrist David Spiegel, who set out to examine just to what extent the mental state of a patient influenced the survival outcome of 86 women with advanced breast cancer (advanced is a euphemism for close to death). Spiegel, like most doctors, did not believe that attitude had any effect on the disease at all.

But he was shocked to find that, after reviewing the results at the 10-year mark, that the women who had weekly support psychotherapy lived *twice as long* as those who did not. That's far better than any chemotherapy or other conventional treatment. Yet doctors never mention it.

Other research has only confirmed this important principle. For example a carefully conducted study carried out at Yale in 1987 found that breast cancer spread fastest among women who had "repressed personalities" (meaning feelings of hopelessness and the inability to express anger, fear, and other negative emotions).

However this re-examination of emotional issues mustn't be used as a ridiculous guilt trip. The aforementioned David Spiegel tells how he was telephone by a woman in great distress. She had gone to a "cancer support group" because of her desperately sick child. There the members had stared accusatively at her and told her she needed to realize first of all that "every child with cancer is an unloved child". This kind of abusive and judgmental nonsense, which so often circulates at so-called support groups, is clearly worse than unhelpful. It's wicked and false.

So it's not true that "any" support therapy is going to be helpful. Just choose wisely.

## 2.14a The Iron Rule of Dr Hamer

Controversial Dr Ryke Geerde Hamer from Germany claims to have documented over 40,000 cancer cases in which he has proof that before the onset of the disease the patient underwent a major psychic trauma in the previous 3 years. Hamer calls it his "Iron Rule" of cancer.

Recently I learned that my one-time sweetheart from medical school days went down with breast cancer exactly 3 years after her husband drowned suddenly. Believe me, Hamer is on the right lines. I have reported Hamer's work on the website at:

http://www.alternative-doctor.com/cancer/hamers_page.htm.

I only disagree that the trauama may be much earlier, for example childhood abuse. But there is always some kind of psychic trauma at work or "stress". What Hamer doesn't mention—and I am telling you is crucial—is that the stress may only *surface* shortly before the diagnosis.

Hamer's model is that all cancers are a healing response: for example loss of a child will set up cell proliferation in the breast, to prepare for new offspring and lactation.

Naturally, Hamer was attacked. Physicians in his home town of Tübingen, near Stuttgart, tried to have him barred. Courts eventually came the rescue of Hamer and demanded his opponents looks at his mass of evidence. They never did.

Recently Hamer had to serve a jail sentence in France for practicing unlicensed medicine, after giving advice to a person. This is despite the fact that France and Germany are in a common alliance (the EU) and what is licensed in one state is automatically licensed throughout the union. All Hamer had done was give somebody advice in an airport (a set-up stooge).

In mocking style, his opponents introduced the term "Hamersche Herde" (Hamer's comical seats) for certain lesions which show up on the brain. These can be photographed with a computed-tomography (CT) and look like the concentric rings on a target, or like a picture of a surface of water into which a stone has been dropped. Hamer considers these to be the sign of intense overactivity and stress in the brain, as a result of the psychic trauma.

Radiologists mistake these rings as a defect in the equipment. An "effective blow for ignorance", a term I got from the late Lawrence Dickey MD and I have adopted myself latterly, since Lawrence's death.

Nothing will stop the march of truth however. The Spanish have already embraced Hamer and call his work "La Medicina Sagrada" (sacred medicine). He has a huge and loyal following there. The torrents of recoveries are testimony to his work.

Hamer himself tells a good story in an interview with "Amici di Dirk" Verlag, Cologne in 1992. I reproduce it here for you all to understand the popularity of this work:

"…After a lecture I gave in Vienna in May 1991, a doctor handed me a CT brain scan of a patient and asked me to disclose the person's organic state and to which conflict it belonged. There were twenty colleagues present, including some radiologists and CT specialists. Of the three scan levels, I had only the brain level in front of me. From these brain CT scans I was able to diagnose a fresh bleeding bladder carcinoma in the healing phase, an old prostate carcinoma, diabetes, an old lung carcinoma and a sensoric paralysis of a specific area in the body and, of course, the corresponding conflicts. The doctor stood up and congratulated me. "Five diagnoses and five hits. That's exactly what the patient has, and you were even able to differentiate what he has now and what he had before. Fantastic!" One of the radiologists told me " I'm convinced of your method. How could you have guessed the fresh bleeding bladder carcinoma? I could find nothing in the CT scan but now that you have shown us the relay, I can follow the findings."

The important point, of course, is that if you reverse the psychic trauma, recovery will take place. Cancer is the result of thoughts. First comes the thought, then the illness.

The cure therefore must come from the thoughts and the energy that created them. Please bear that in mind.

# 2.14b The Journey

Psychic healing and recovery is not always an easy path. But you've got help from writer's like Brandon Bayes and her "Journey". She discovered she had a uterine tumor the size of a basketball and that an operation was essential. She resisted conventional treatment and her doctor gave her one month to make a difference. After a lifetime of teaching and following a healthy lifestyle Brandon was not going to give in without a fight.

Brandon used every moment of her waking hours to focus on her problem. She new that the body cells have amazing regenerative powers. Six weeks later and with no surgical intervention the doctors found no trace of the tumor.

Today, Brandon is healthy and vivacious. She teaches "The Journey" to other people, showing individuals how to overcome issues and illnesses that prevent them from living fully.

Yet, however much I appreciate her work and "The Journey", I cannot help but extrapolate from knowledge and the scientific proofs already quoted in section 1.4, which is that *cancer often heals spontaneously*.

If that is correct, Brandon is hardly in possession of specialist insight; she was just lucky enough to stay out of the hands of doctors for long enough for natural healing to take place!

## The Healing Path

Marc Ian Barasch is another writer you should read. His book *The Healing Path: A Soul Approach to Illness* (Penguin) is one of the best books ever written about the mind-body connection.

When Marc was thirty-five years old, he had a series of vivid and startlingly detailed dreams about cancer. Though he had no physical symptoms, he went to see a doctor, insisted on medical tests, and was diagnosed with thyroid cancer. At the time, Marc was the editor of *New Age Journal* and they fired him because it was bad for the magazine image if he got sick. Nice people! Marc always thought himself "quite knowledgeable about the realms of healing." But he found it was one thing to read and study and write about disease, and quite another thing to experience it.

In February 1985, he had conventional surgery. It was pronounced a success, although sorting through the spiritual, psychological, and social implications of the illness, the treatment, and its aftermath would take many years. Barasch explains the path he took and the book is highly informative and will help you understand what you are undertaking.

## 2.14b Bernie Siegel

Then comes Bernie Siegal and his healing book *Love, Medicine And Miracles*. You must read this. Segal was a general and pediatric surgeon. In 1978 he originated Exceptional Cancer Patients, a specific form of individual and group therapy utilizing patients' drawings, dreams, images and feelings. His work is based on "carefrontation," a safe, loving therapeutic confrontation, which facilitates personal lifestyle changes, personal empowerment and healing of the individual's life. The physical, spiritual and psychological benefits which followed led to his desire to make everyone aware of his or her healing potential. According to Bernie, exceptional behavior is what we are all capable of.

# 2.14c Bert Hellinger's "Family Constellations"

Bert Hellinger's highly original and moving work, centering around what he calls family constellations, has a lot to offer the cancer sufferer. If you can find a good practitioner, you should not pass up an opportunity to investigate where your cancer came from and why it happened.

The revelations which come about from engaging in Hellinger's work can be deeply insightful and, importantly, very healing.

### Family Constellations

The key modality in this work, as I said, is the Family Constellation, which is used to investigate the patterns operating in a client's family system. A family system consists of the client, plus his or her:

- children
- spouse
- siblings
- parents
- siblings of parents
- grandparents
- siblings of the grandparents
- former partners of the parents and grandparent

Also, anyone who suffered so that the family might gain in some way becomes connected to the system. For instance, if a family business took great advantage of its employees, there would be an unconscious need to resolve this injustice by those in following generations.

So, for example, a woman's breast cancer might be rooted in a loss of connection to her mother or to her mother's mother. Or perhaps a hidden desire to follow another family member who died of cancer.

## Practitioners Skills

The outcome you get depends on just how good the practitioner is. I personally attended a demonstration, with Bert himself in control, and it was a very profound and moving experience. The subject was a cancer survivor.

I could feel the emotional dynamic in the room and, as individuals were moved around and "placed" where Bert wanted them, we could see the destructive picture emerging.

It was quite remarkable that, as the person representing a suicide from an earlier generation approached their "correct" spot in the room, most of us literally burst into tears. It was uncontrollable, the room was so charged with emotional energy, that did not belong only to the role actors: we all shared it.

# 2.14e My Own Supernoetics™ Piloting

**Transformational Mind Dynamics™** (TMD) is a term for an entirely new kind of mental cleansing and energizing. It does not concentrate on actual thoughts (which are non-material) so much as the energy, emotion and dynamics involved in a situation.

These are discharged fully, using an immersion technique we call "repeat and tell."

Moreover, we do not take the view that a person's troubles are theirs alone. In line with Virginia Satyr's *Conjoint Family Therapy* and Hellinger's *Family Constellations*, rather we recognize that persons around the target individual contribute greatly to the mental imprint formed at the time of any significant event.

In TMD practice, we have our willing client take up the viewpoint of others, starting with the main antagonist or opposition, and have the client discharge the *other person's* emotion and energies. What did the rapist feel at the moment he was carrying out the brutal assault? What in God's name was she thinking of when she walked out the door? Why did Mom always talk to me that way?

The strange thing is, we seem to know! If you occupy the viewpoint of the domineering husband, the inept boss at work, the chump who stole your first girlfriend, and find *his emotions*, *his effort* and what *disastrous thought computation he was struggling with*, suddenly you are released and cleansed from something you didn't even think belonged to you! It's wonderful to behold.

By having the client see the events of their lives through the eyes of others and with the others' feelings, we gain a far deeper insight into the meaning of what we jokingly call life.

It builds compassion. It builds wisdom. We grow immensely in stature as we finally learn tolerance and forgiveness. We come at last to understand, as John Dunne said so beautifully, in his famous poem *No Man Is An Island*: "Never send to know for whom the bell tolls; it tolls for thee..." It's your funeral, as well as the dead guy's burial. We are all in this together!

But this isn't just poetic whimsy. Surprisingly, as I revealed in my book *Medicine Beyond*, there is science to back this idea. Advanced physics proves that we radiate outwards energetic effects into space, which can travel many miles and influence others around. Indeed, they could not help being influenced and becoming, in turn, a part of the event's dynamics.

To find out more about this wonderful new therapy, go here and read more:

**http://alternative-doctor.com/supernoeticspiloting**

# 2.15 Third Pillar - Chemical Detox Is Vital

It would take a textbook to talk about personal pollution and the dire negative health effects of the environment we are living in. Even eskimo mothers now have chemical toxins in their milk. Little babies in remote climes cannot avoid what I have christened the "Chemical Blizzard".

I get asked a lot about "organic food". Well, what does that mean when the very sky rains chemicals and pollution on all your nice clean "organic" crops? Not a lot.

We are faced with so-called "brown aerosol" pollution. This is mostly made up of miniscule particles. Aerosols consist of sulfates, nitrates, black carbon, hundreds of organic compounds, and fly ash. When sunlight is absorbed and scattered by aerosols, it creates a brown colored haze, hence the name. Satellite data reveal thick, polluted haze layers scattered all over the globe, from populated regions to the once-pristine Alps, the Himalayas, and the Pacific and Atlantic Oceans.

One of the main sources of this pollution today is China! Ironically, because of prevailing winds, Chinese atmospheric pollution is raining down on North America. Streams of yellowish dust have been seen streaming across the Pacific since 1998. Mercury emitted by power plants and factories in China, Korea and other parts of Asia wafts over to the USA and settles into the nation's lakes and streams, where it contributes to pollution that makes fish unsafe to eat. Solid particles from Asian primitive oil and coal burning is now a source of solid sooty deposits high in the pristine mountains anywhere you go in the US. Birds are being poisoned as far inland as Payson Arizona, where the trees are thick-crusted with Chinese effluvia.

What has all this to do with cancer?

If you follow Sam Epstein's writings, everything. Dr. Sam Epstein is a Professor of Occupational Health and Environmental Medicine at the University of Illinois School of Public Health and he is recognized as perhaps the world's most influential critic of official cancer policy. Dr Epstein provides copious evidence that chemical pollution is one of the major causes for the soaring cancer rates.

Epstein's book *The Politics of Cancer* (now TPC Revisited) documents a great many disturbing facts, including the shocking truth that cancer charities are actively opposing progress in alternative treatments, because of corruption. He also attacks the "white collar crime" of lying and cover-up, to divert attention from the way Big Business is killing everyone with its dirty fall-out.

"As recently as 1986, the NCI (National Cancer Institute) promised annual cancer mortality rates would be halved by the year 2000. The establishment now belatedly admits that cancer rates are increasing sharply. However, with the enthusiastic support of the chemical industry, these are ascribed exclusively to smoking, dietary fat itself (ignoring the tenuous evidence relating this to colon, breast and other cancers) and "mysterious" causes.

"Meanwhile it discounts substantial evidence incriminating and wide range of chemical and radioactive carcinogens permeating the environment, air, water, food, and the workplace... Non mysterious causes of breast cancer, which the establishment ignores, let alone investigates, include carcinogenic contaminants in dietary fat, particularly pesticides; PCBs; and estrogen (with extensive and unregulated use as growth promoting animals food additives)."

[The Politics of Cancer revisited, East Ridge Press, NY, USA 1998, p. 355]

As Sam points out boldly, you are not going to get the truth from official sources. Something is causing the soaring cancer rates and anyone intelligent can quickly spot that increased levels of personal and environmental carcinogens are one of the main cause of the problem. The establishment, so closely tied to the huge chemical industry lobby, is simply not going to support your interests over those of Big Business.

So, it's vital we all take control and reduce our personal pollution load where possible.

It's playing Russian Roulette to use after-shave, cosmetics, gels, hair-set, paints, household cleaners, solvents, herbicides, insecticides and other pesticides in the torrents that we do. Did you know that women absorb about half a kilo of cosmetics every year – through their skin? Add what is in the air to what's in our food and in the water and we have a big problem. Our liver and major de-tox systems try to keep pace with this lethal tide of chemicals but we are not winning.

These chemicals accumulate and do not decay, since they are such strange substances, Nature doesn't have a means of getting rid of them (xenobiotics). All we can do is reduce the load, keep clean and do everything possible to help the detox mechanisms. Unfortunately they too are poisoned, as the rest of us, when this tide of chemicals rises too high; that which protects us one of the first things to be damaged.

The immune system gets hurt too.

Today, as I teach, one of the number one aspects of what we call "nutrition" is merely supplementation to help our detox pathways. Magnesium, for instance, is involved in over 300 pathways, including the all-important Phase I detox. Glutathione is another powerful tool, an anti-oxidant. But it gets used up every time it walks off with a toxic molecule and we need to take phenomenal amounts. Unfortunately, glutathione by mouth doesn't work. But you can take lashings of the precursors that help create glutathione inside your cells: alpha-lipoic acid (200 mgm), N-acetyl cysteine or NAC (500 mgm) and s-adenosyl methionine (SAMe) 100 mgm.

We also need B6, zinc and B3, molybdenum and more. That's just to cope with the additional oxidative stress of our poisonous world.

Not really what you think of as nutrition is it? But because these beneficial supplements are taken by mouth, what else can you call it?

For more information, I can do no better than recommend Sherry Rogers' book *Detoxify or Die*. Another cracking read is by my old friend Dr Doris Rapp: *Our Toxic Word: a Wake Up Call*. You'll be sadder but I lot wiser when you have read them.


# 2.15a Heavy Metals are Carcinogenic

And before we leave the subject of toxic overload, I must mention what we call heavy metals. A number of metals are known to be carcinogenic. These are:

- arsenic and arsenic compounds,
- beryllium and beryllium compounds,
- cadmium and cadmium compounds,
- nickel compounds and
- hexavalent chromium (remember the movie "Erin Brockovich"?).

The usual target is the lung, though arsenic has a unique association with skin cancers that has been recognized for many years.

You should know that in the US there is a heavy burden of arsenic poisoning carried to humans via chickens. Roxarsone is a very common arsenic-based additive used in chicken feed, used to promote growth, kill parasites and improve the color of chicken meat. It is normally benign, but under certain conditions that can occur within live chickens or on farm land, the compound converts into more toxic forms of inorganic arsenic. Arsenic has been linked to bladder, lung, skin, kidney and colon cancers, and low-level exposure can lead to partial paralysis and diabetes.

Even if you don't eat chicken, don't think you are safe: chicken manure is used as fertilizer on vegetable farms and this contains arsenic which then contaminates the vegetables. Arsenic is everywhere.

You'll be surprised at some of the other sources of arsenic contamination. According to Consumer Reports Magazine popular rice products including white rice, brown rice, organic rice baby cereal, and rice breakfast cereals, were all found to contain arsenic, some at levels that well exceeded safety limits (the EPA recommends 5 parts per billion or ppb maximum).

You can reduce arsenic levels in rice by cooking with plenty of water and then rinsing it off (forget the cook's trick of measuring out the exact quantity of water to make rice, just drain through a sieve or colander when it's cooked).

Cadmium is also widespread: it is found in grains like wheat and leafy vegetables, which readily absorb cadmium from the soil. Cadmium may also contaminate fish. It is a constituent of alloys, pigments, batteries and metal coatings. Cadmium is also found in cigarette fumes and fumes from vehicles. There are many other places you might meet cadmium, even without knowing it.

Avoidance is very difficult, as I have explained. Even babies are being born with heavy metal poisoning in the womb. They didn't eat anything!

Yet if you have cancer, or want to prevent it, you must try to get rid of these dangerous metals from your body.

The known scientific method is called Chelation. Some very simple substances have Chelation possibilities: cilantro (coriander) for example. Apple pectin and seaweed, such as kelp.

Better is the green algae called chlorella. That's really quite successful. Chlorella is one of the most scientifically researched supplements in human history. There are thousands of research papers on chlorella from medical institutions, scientific journals and universities. NASA has decided it will be one of the first foods grown on the space station when it is completed. There is not a single report of toxicity to humans taking chlorella, though if you have too much iron on board—a disease called hemochromatosis—you should know that chlorella contains lots of iron.

Alpha lipoic acid, already mentioned as a glutathione precursor, also has chelation properties. That's useful at doses of 100- 200 mgms.

Beyond these simple compounds you will need to see someone who is licensed to carry out office chelation. Unfortunately, that is fraught with medico-legal problems. Chelation agents are much more controversial. The simplest is EDTA, which is added to food so it's pretty safe. Others include succinate, DMPS and DMSA. You can read about these widely on the web.

# 2.15b Update: TACT Trial

Fortunately, we have seen a diminution of attacks on chelation and doctors who practice it. That's as a direct result of a now-notorious clinical trial known as TACT (Trial to Assess Chelation Therapy). It was the first large-scale, multicenter study designed to determine the safety and efficacy of EDTA chelation therapy. It was co-sponsored by The National Institutes of Health's National Heart, Lung, and Blood Institute (NHLBI) and the National Center for Complementary and Alternative Medicine (NCCAM), and the results were presented at the American Heart Association Scientific Sessions in November 2012.

Orthodox doctors did everything in their to stop this trial. They even described the trial as "unethical" because there was no rationale for the use of chelation therapy. When that didn't work, they tried to discredit the results; when that failed, they have tried to ignore it and pretend it wasn't *really* a success.

The trial, which was aimed at vascular and heart problems, was an unqualified success, with diabetic patients in particular gaining great benefits; so much so that one of the trial's lead doctors, L. Terry Chappell MD, has posted on his own website, "I believe that ALL diabetics should take chelation, starting about age 30…"

Dr L. Terry Chappell also says this:

"I cannot wait to share with our patients and friends what TACT and previous studies mean to current medical science and to those who could benefit from them…

"Our experience is that chelation can reduce your chances for blindness, kidney failure, amputation and other vascular complications of diabetes.

"I believe that chelation is the most powerful prevention intervention that we have. Everyone should take it to improve his or her chances for living a disease-free life. Scientific evidence is accumulating to back me up...

"Chelation is not just a treatment that is slowly emerging into the spotlight. It is a movement against the forces that are resisting change, especially from powerful economic interests..."

[http://www.healthcelebration.com/#!what-you-dont-know/c2296]

The Science-Based Medicine website, a humbug for orthodoxy, says different and sarcastically remarks: Chelationists seem to have got exactly what they'd hoped for from the TACT: a free pass to peddle their favorite, lucrative 'remedy'... That's rich! Chelation costs about one tenth of conventional cardiac and vascular interventions, not to mention the cost of all the necessary amputations of their approach!

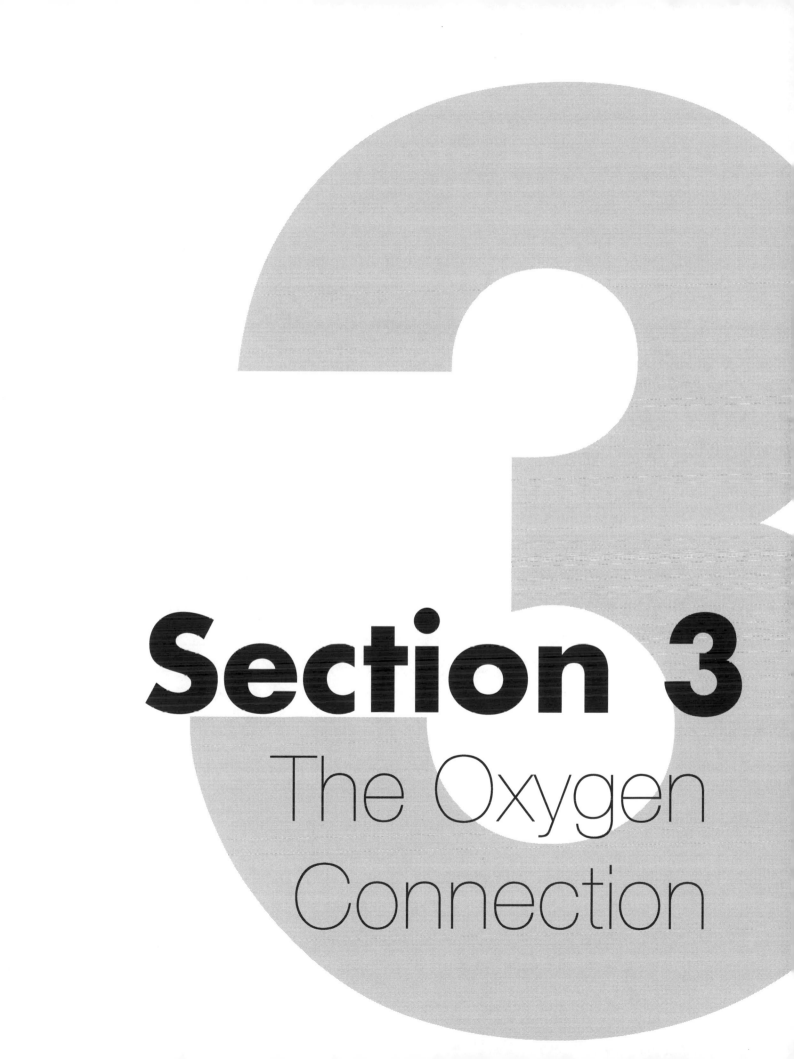

# Section 3

## The Oxygen Connection

We KNOW the answer to cancer...Yet the authorities, in the form of the law of the land (UK), will not allow this book (The Good News On Cancer) to be promoted to lay persons.....it is not permitted that they can even be told where to find information that might help them. That has got to be democracy with a very small d...... One eminent publisher...backed out as he feared he could be jailed for infringing the Cancer Act by offering the book to the public. Another...was deliberately pressured by an unnamed group after his medical reader (an M.D.), having checked the manuscript, leaked its contents to a confidential authority.

**Dr Richards & Frank Hourigan**

# 3.0 Cancer Doesn't Like Oxygen

I'm going to start with a little scientific and slightly technical background to a whole range of very useful therapies. It concerns the fact that cancer cells are not like any other cells—in a number of respects— but particularly in how they metabolize and create energy for living and multiplication.

Ordinary cells use a pathway that is rich in oxygen, called the Kreb's cycle. It is highly effective and is what breathes life into us humans. But cancer cells don't like oxygen. They use an alternative pathway, called glycolysis. That's just a fancy ancient Greek word for breakdown of glucose to release energy—but cancer cells do it with little or no oxygen. In fact cancer cells don't like oxygen at all—they cannot flourish in its presence.

All this was discovered over 70 years ago by a German doctor called Otto Warburg. He made a significant number of discoveries and was awarded the Nobel prize in 1931. He showed that cancer cells cannot use oxygen in the same way as normal cells and use anaerobic metabolism instead (which means without oxygen). Remarkably, his work was then ignored for the next 60 years. Only recently have scientific studies re-discovered what he said and proved he was right. Warburg's theories have even been extended.

He looked for an efficient way to supply the extra oxygen. Warburg understood that essential fats and oils were crucial in some way. He experimented with butyric acid, which is a saturated fatty acid. This was an unfortunate choice, which left him with frustration and failure. Butyric acid lacks what we now know are special pi electrons. I'll explain more about the significance of that in the following section. Suffice it to say that Warburg was unsuccessful in his search.

It was Johanna Budwig who gave us the breakthrough that we needed. In a sense, she made Warburg's prediction come true (see section 3.2).

Meantime, let's look mainly at oxygen therapies.

We know that the anaerobic pathway yields much less energy for every glucose molecule (2 ATP "energy molecules", instead of 36). So cancer cells have a higher than normal hunger for sugar. That means if you eat sugar and sweet foods, you are playing right to the cancer. You must get all sugar, honey and sweeteners out of your diet. *Sugar is deadly if you have cancer.*

In the meantime, many physicians got started treating cancer by flooding the body with extra oxygen: and it worked! It worked then and it works now. So one of the most important things you can do it to increase free oxygen in your body.

That can be done a number of ways. You may have heard of hyperbaric oxygen? That's a mechanism for increasing the air pressure of oxygen and so forcing more into the blood and tissues. However this one is not used so much for cancer; there's better.

Other approaches are to use oxygen flooding, peroxide and ozone. The latter two substances are super-charged with oxygen and deliver a high-impact yield. Needless to say, you do need to go to someone who knows what they are doing—and I don't just mean some alternative practitioner who *says* they know what they are doing. Both substances could be dangerous if misused though not, I hasten to say, as dangerous as chemotherapy.

Peroxide or ozone can be delivered either by an intravenous line or, I think much safer, removing some blood, oxygenating it and then returning that to the body.

Other routes of administration may sound strange but are perfectly valid scientifically and probably far safer. Ozone or peroxide can both be given rectally. This avoids the coughing reflex that patients sometimes get when administering ozone intravenously.

It is also possible to give just plain oxygen, oxygen flooding, from a cylinder, via the rectum, the vagina in women or even tubes in the ears. All that matters is that the oxygen gets into the body, where it will make the cancer cells sicken and die.

The best part of doing intravenous therapies and using other injectable healing substances is the chance to look at the patient's venous blood. I used to find it quite easy to recognize the difference in color: venous blood is normally dark purple, wine color—but when venous blood turns bright scarlet, you know the patient is receiving plenty of extra oxygen.

Treatments vary from several times a day if the patient is in dire straits, to twice weekly and then weekly, as recovery continues.

You may hear criticism of these therapies. There have been claims it is dangerous and one doctor, I know, was charged with murder because a cancer patient died while having peroxide treatment. In fact the patient died of his cancer (obviously) but that inconvenient truth doesn't stop the bigots of orthodoxy from attacking anything they hate.

You will notice that no doctor gets charged with murder for administering deadly chemical cocktails and brutal radiation, or performing mutilating surgery. They always blame the cancer and say the patient died of that "despite everything we could do to save the patient".

But when a patient dies during alternative therapy, it's said to be the treatment that killed him or her, not the tumor.

My advice is don't be afraid of oxygen therapy. It is used widely in Europe and with good results. But just choose wisely and beware of who you trust to give it. It may be sensible to find a doctor who is member of the International Oxidative Medicine Association (IOMA). But remember there is no exam; it's just a group of practitioners sharing the same interests.

# 3.1 The Reverse Warburg Twist

Hold on... It could be possible that Otto Warburg got it wrong; at least got the right answer for the wrong reasons. A fascinating new theory overturns everything we thought we knew about the biology of cancer.

As you have read, Nobel Laureate Otto Warburg suggested that cancer cells produce the bulk of their energy by breaking down glucose in the absence of oxygen, a process called *glycolysis*. The Warburg effect, as it is called, is now widely accepted in orthodox cancer research.

But it's WRONG, according to Michael Lisanti at the Kimmel Cancer Center in Philadelphia, Pennsylvania. He has a completely different model, which puts a whole new light on how cancer cells feed and grow.

Cancer, as we all know, is made up of rogue cells, where the DNA has gone frighteningly wrong and lets cells off the leash of restraint. They multiply out of control and often cannot be stopped: the immune system works hard against them but with certain cancers, they grow too fast, even for a competent immune system.

The missing part of the mechanism says Dr. Lisanti, with good evidence to back up his new theory, is that cancer cells release a lot of hydrogen peroxide, which hammers nearby support cells in the tissues called fibroblasts. These decay and lose their vital mitochondria.

Without their mitochondria, fibroblasts cannot now metabolize properly using oxygen. They switch to glycolysis, which we thought was being used by cancer cells. Not so, says Lisanti. According to him, "It's the Warburg effect, but in the wrong place." Lisanti calls is the Reverse Warburg Effect. He believes the reason Warburg got it wrong is because he looked at cancer cells in isolation, rather than in co-culture with fibroblasts.

So Warburg wasn't exactly wrong but this new idea takes things forwards several paces. It's a revolution, if true. But is it?

Surprisingly, there is an astonishing amount of evidence to suggest that it is.

This form of "metabolic coupling" is already known to exist and mirrors the way in which the epithelial cells that make up the skin and the surface of the body's organs produce hydrogen peroxide during wound healing. In doing so they rally immune cells to repair the damage - but in cancer the signal is never turned off. Cancer is "a wound that doesn't heal", because it keeps on producing hydrogen peroxide.

When Lisanti and his team cultured breast cancer cells alongside fibroblasts for five days, *they spotted the cancer cells releasing hydrogen peroxide on day two. By day five, most free radicals generated by the hydrogen peroxide were found inside the fibroblasts* [Cell Cycle, DOI: 10.4161/cc.9.16.12553].

Also, the team found a reduction in mitochondrial activity in fibroblasts, consistent with the cells self-destructing. There was also an increase in glucose uptake by the fibroblasts - a sign of glycolysis [Cell Cycle, DOI: 10.4161/cc.10.15.16585).

In a further experiment, they found that treating cancer cells with catalase, an enzyme that destroys hydrogen peroxide, triggered a five-fold increase in cancer cell death, possibly by preserving the fibroblasts and cutting off the cancer cells' fuel supply.

The theory looks pretty solid.

## Why Chemo Is Bad

This new theory would explain why chemo often makes things worse.

Lisanti makes the point that his own father was saved from colon cancer by timely and effective chemo (yes, it does happen). But he admits it's a fine line between success and damaging the body. If by chance the chemo is too much, it may be *damaging fibroblasts*.

That would help the cancer cells, by feeding them with more "victims". In certain circumstances, chemo or radiation therapy could be adding to the problem (as well as hurting the patient).

It would also reinforce my frequently voiced objection, that at least 50% of a tumor consists of healthy cells, including fibroblasts. So gauging the success of a treatment by tumor shrinkage is very foolish indeed. It could be just lining up "food" for the cancer cells. Yet that's what orthodoxy does and is the required proof of effectiveness for a drug to be officially approved.

# 3.2 Sunlight And Magic Electrons (pi-electrons)

In section 3.0 you read about 1931 Nobel Laureate Otto Warburg's major contribution to discovering the real cause of cancer. In fact he famously said "There is no disease whose cause is better known".

It's time to go deeper into this mechanism and in doing so we uncover one of the most wonderful of all natural anti-cancer remedies.

First, a little science, as the cosmetic ads say!

Warburg had learned that the delivery of oxygen to the tissues was critical for health. Cancer cells thrive in low oxygen environments. Adding oxygen, as you probably know, is called "oxidation". It can be bad, as in rusting of metal, or good, as in allowing our cells to burn food fuels and thus create energy.

In fact it is both good AND bad for our bodies. We need oxygen and respiration to live; we wouldn't last 10 minutes without it. But also active oxygen around the tissues can cause damage. Oxygen can reach a souped-up stage we call a super-oxide or "free radical", which can be very destructive. That's why we take antioxidants, of course.

But again, there is benefit in the bad. You see, our immune cells deliberately create free radicals from oxygen, to "zap" or destroy bacteria and other pathogens, including cancer cells (that's how dangerous free radicals are). Antioxidants are then needed promptly, on the spot, to quickly mop up the damaging weapons just created, before they damage us! It's all very paradoxical and scientists are not nearly humble enough in the face of these natural mysteries.

There is, however, one other important definition of oxidation you need to know. Oxidation is taking electrons. The opposite process, reduction, is giving electrons. So good oxidation sources need to have readily available electrons. Movement of electrons, especially across cell membranes, is crucial to oxygen enrichment—and therefore for fighting cancer.

Otto Warburg knew this and sought for dietary oils which were known to be electron friendly. He chose butyric acid to study. This was a mistake which cost him heavily. He was not able to create the effect that he predicted.

Now we know why and in a few paragraphs, you'll know too. It was just one of those unlucky turnings for Warburg. If he had chosen differently, everything since his Nobel Prize discovery would have been different.

Electrons can vary in their state of activity. As they jump up and down different orbits in the atom, they gain or lose energy. Indeed, this is the entire definition of quantum physics. The energy given off when an electron falls to a lower orbit is in the form of a little packet of energy called a quantum (plural quanta). The fact that electrons are in either one orbit or the other, and no transition or in-betweens, was what was so shocking and radical about quantum physics. It violated all other physics processes up to that point.

Think of it like the moon being suddenly instantly a million miles further away, then next night it was instantly back where it was, no time to travel between the two locations.

Now I can tell you what a quantum jump really is: an instant re-location, with no process by which it happens. It just does. It scared physicists to death and some still can't hack it. Einstein himself famously couldn't believe in the weird new order of quantum physics.

Well, now you understand where quantum physics came from and you've got the proper definition of a quantum jump! (no extra charge).

# 3.3 Quantum biology?

At first it was thought that quantum physics had no relevance to biology and living systems. Now we rather think that's what is exciting and different about living systems: they are quantum by very nature, strange and semi-mystical!

Erwin Schroedinger, one of the founder-fathers of quantum physics, wrote a classic book called *What Is Life?* In it he was among the first to point out that life had strange quantum properties. But mainstream biology is still fighting this (and, of course, the medical profession).

So, that was not a needless diversion. Warburg's oxygen theory and the amazing cancer cure it spawned is based soundly in quantum physics. See, we receive streams of highly charged photons from the sun (a photon is a *quantum* of light). These interact with electrons here on Earth and can boost their energy, causing them to flip to higher states of energy and higher orbits. They can then release this energy later, for the benefit of living organisms.

This is important in biology, since ultimately all life energy comes from the Sun, as you know. Plants harness sunlight and turn it into food. Animals then eat the plants and the energy is passed on. Fortuitously, plants eat carbon dioxide and exhale oxygen; animals do the reverse. It's great synergy.

Some foods capture the Sun's important quantum energy better than others. Oils (fats) are important in the oxygen transportation process, as Warburg deduced. Some fats (not all) retain the Sun's energy in the form of special double bond electrons called "pi electrons". These are pretty oxygen-friendly electrons and make good super "food" for living organisms.

Butyric acid wasn't good at this, unfortunately for Warburg. There were no double bonds with pi electrons. But there are two plant oils that do it very well: linoleic acid and linolenic acid. Although these substances are technically acids, they are essentially fats, hence the term fatty acids. Because the pi electron bonds are on the 3rd carbon position on the chain, we know these as omega-3 oils (omega is ancient Greek for the one at the end, as in alpha and omega).

So now some of what you already know will start to draw together.

In fact it was Johanna Budwig, of the Budwig diet fame (see section 3.2), who joined all the dots for us. A first-class scientist, she was well aware of Otto Warburg's discovery and his problem finding the answer. She looked for the richest plant source of pi electrons and found...

> Flaxseed oil (aka. Linseed oil). The key ingredients are linoleic acid and linolenic acid.

Strictly speaking, Budwig wasn't the first. 1922 Nobel Laureate Otto Meyerhof conducted fascinating experiments in which linseed oil increased recovery times of frog muscle depleted of oxygen by 1,000 times!

Szent-Gyorgy earned the Nobel prize in 1937 by showing that linoleic acid, in combination with sulphur-rich proteins, stimulated the vital oxygenation processes of the body.

But Johanna Budwig takes the main credit. She published her book "Komische Krafte gegen den Krebs" in 1951 (unusual arts against cancer, currently published as *Komische Kräfte gegen Krebs*, Elektronen-Biology , Freiburg im Brisgau, Hyperion-Verlag, 1966). Yet despite support from other scientific greats, like Fritz Popp and Albert Szent-Gyorgi, her work has been suppressed and ignored by mainstream ascientists.

In fact there is more to this story. Budwig meticulously collected blood samples of thousands of patients and analyzed them. Uniformly, she found that sick people were deficient in linoleic acid, whereas healthy people had acceptable levels.

But she also found that sick people lacked phosphatides. These substances are essential for normal cell division; cancer, of course, is corrupted cell division.

She also noticed a greenish tinge to the blood of very sick people, where it should be bright red. The greenish tinge was caused by lack of adequate oxygen. Without adequate linoleic acid, the body cannot produce an effective oxygen carrying system. Budwig theorized that supplying the essential fatty acids in combination with sulphurated proteins could restore health.

So, she reasoned, supplying the missing linoleic acid, together with sulfur proteins, should restore health. When she tested the theory, sure enough, within weeks the healthy phosphatides and lipoproteins began to appear in the blood. And, not surprisingly perhaps, the tumors of terminally ill cancer patients began to diminish.

## Bad Fats Kill

Now, I hope, you see why Budwig's program of flaxseed oil and quark (a kind of cottage cheese) has been so successful. It is, in effect, pulling down the Sun's energy to heal your reluctant cancer cells! The presence of protein and sulfur compounds is required and that is quickly supplied by the quark.

Also this tells you why high fat diets are deadly and cause cancer (orthodox medicine too is quite clear on this point). Today "fats" mean almost entirely synthetic altered substances what cannot be metabolized properly and clog up metabolic pathways. Worse than that, they squeeze out any presence of good fats.

Not that there is much good fat out there. As we eat a diet so removed from that of a hunter-gatherer, we have too little natural food in our diet. Nowhere is this more important than concerning so-called "essential fatty acids". They are very unstable and just do not survive storage, transportation and cooking.

We have to eat them. Plants are not the only source: grass-fed beef is actually the richest natural source of omega-3s.

## Fresh Food Is The Answer

You can grind your own flaxseeds (get a coffee grinder). Unground seeds are worthless and pass straight through the alimentary canal.

You can also buy quality supplements but you need to be warned: *real quality flax-seed oil is rare and expensive*. The usual junk that is peddled, even in health food stores, is rendered useless before it even leaves the bottling plant.

Take only unrefined, cold-pressed virgin flaxseed oil, otherwise you won't get well. It must be kept in darkened glass bottles and stored in a chiller in the store. When you get it home put it straight in the refrigerator. Vitamin E may sometimes be added, as an antioxidant to keep it fresh.

Of course there are good marine sources of omega-3s but beware of mercury contamination and other issues with modern ocean products.


## How to take your sulfur!

Johanna Budwig's idea was for people to take quark (or cottage cheese), ladled with flaxseed oil.

I don't like dairy products and many people cannot tolerate them. As an alternative, use eggs. I take a frequent breakfast of omelet with fresh berries; I just pour lashings of flaxseed oil over the lot. Usually I add a half teaspoon of maple syrup too! Delicious!

You can serve steel-cut oats porridge with the fruit and flaxseed oil. Tastes great. It's not a cancer treatment. You'll just need to get your sulfur from something else (like N-acetyl cysteine, s-Adenosyl methionine (SAMe).

Finally, you don't actually have to swallow the oil at all. Just rub it on your skin! I find the inside of the thighs, where the skin is thinnest, works best. You can have someone give you a loving massage and rub in the oil. But remember it will stain clothing and sheets. You've been warned!


# 3.4 Mind Your PQQs!

PQQ is something everyone should know about and supplement. In a phrase: it creates new mitchondria for you. Mitochondria are the little energy units inside a cell. The more you have, the better they work, the more your energy is boosted, the healthier you are and able to conquer disease, including, of course, cancer.

PQQ is an extremely powerful antioxidant capable of catalyzing continuous cycling (the ability to perform repeated oxidation and reduction reactions) to a much greater degree compared to other antioxidants. For example, PQQ is able to carry out 20,000 catalytic conversions compared to only 4 for vitamin C.

Although PQQ is not currently viewed as a vitamin, its involvement in cell signaling pathways, particularly those important to mitochondriogenesis in experimental animal models, may eventually provide a rationale for defining PQQ as vital to life (much more believable than vitamin B17—which does not exist in real life).

[Rucker R, Chowanadisai W, Nakano M. Potential physiological importance of pyrroloquinoline quinone. *Altern Med* Rev. 2009 Sep;14(3):268-77]

Without going into detail, this capability of extracting more energy cycles during aerobic respiration is totally in line with the Warburg hypothesis.

But it seems that PQQ (pyrroloquinoline quinone) has extra benefits for cancer, at least according to a new Chinese study, published in the Journal Of Cancer. Turns out it encourages cancer cells to self-destruct in the vital process called "apoptosis." One of the things that makes cancer cancer is that these cells stop responding to signals to behave normally.

So anything that makes them toe the line and self-destruct when they should is a good thing.

But that's not the only benefit of PQQ. It also restricts tumors by cutting off or reducing their blood supply. It turns off genes that promote the spread of cancer.

And that's not all! It combats cancer-causing inflammation (see section 1.6).

In a study published in the Journal of Cancer, Chinese researchers were stunned that PQQ worked so well at destroying cancer cells without toxicity. They even suggested its use as a widespread anti-cancer therapy.

[Zhihui, M., et al. "Pyrroloquinoline quinone induces cancer cell apoptosis via mitochondrial-dependent pathway and down-regulating cellular Bcl-2 protein Expression." *Journal of Cancer*. 2014; 5(7): 609–624]

Our bodies can't produce PQQ. We have to get it from food or supplements.

The richest natural source is Japanese natto, a pretty malodorous foodstuff, made of fermented soy beans. Eggs, parsley, green peppers, kiwi fruits and papaya are also good sources.

You can also take a PQQ supplement. I recommend 10 mg a day.

# Section 4
## Enzyme-Based Therapies

In the entire history of man, no one has ever been brainwashed and realized, or believed, that he had been brainwashed. Those who have been brainwashed will usually passionately defend their manipulators.

**Dick Sutphen**

# 4.0 Dr. Beard

In 1902 a Scottish doctor, John Beard, published an interesting paper. He drew attention to the fact that when the placenta implants into the uterus, the way it burrows in and invades the mother's tissue is exactly like a cancer does.

Why didn't the placenta just keep going and take over everything – like a cancer does? Nobody knew at the time but then John Beard noticed that the placenta stops invading at exactly the moment when the infant's pancreas starts to secrete digestive enzymes. If that doesn't happen, the deadly cancer of pregnancy - chorion-carcinoma - ensues which is capable of killing the mother and baby very quickly (today there is an excellent cure rate for chorion-carcinoma).

The cells of the placenta which invade are called the trophoblasts. Whenever you see the word "tropho" or "trophic" in science, it means feeding. A -blast is a cell which gets something going; so these cells set out to establish the food supply line for the baby fetus.

Beard began to ask himself whether cancer cells, which look exactly like trophoblast cells—young, vigorous, unspecialized—could also be turned off by enzymes from the pancreas. In fact he went even further and speculated that cancer came from hidden trophoblasts cells in the body, left over from days in the womb, which got activated again, by stress and toxins. Perhaps normally these get picked off by enzymes but sometimes they do not and cancer is the result. So Beard called this **the trophoblastic theory of cancer.**

I think he hit the target right on bullseye and it's worth making sure you understand the implications of this theory and the treatments which result. Because it does work. Within a few years there were hundreds of clinics which sprang up offering pancreatic enzyme treatments for cancer patients. In the early 20th century, there were 40 centers in London alone. Their results were remarkable.

Of course it was attacked as nonsense by the medical establishment. They attack everything, as history shows, from good diet, to surgeons washing their hands and keeping everything clean, to anesthetics. But it wasn't that which saw Beard's work disappear. Not long afterwards Madam Curie came along and convinced people that X-ray was the way to go because it was so "safe" and "effective" and the pancreatic enzyme cancer cure was quickly abandoned. Marie Curie became famous and John Beard was promptly forgotten (that's called "scientific progress"!)

# 4.1 Dr. Kelley

But the story didn't die totally. William Donald Kelley, a dentist from Grapevine, Texas, cured himself of pancreatic cancer in the sixties, largely using Beard's theories, and went on to develop a nutritionally-based, do-it-yourself home cure for cancer which is probably over ninety per cent effective in patients who have not been overly destroyed by chemotherapy and orthodox treatments.

Dr. Beard believed the enzymes had to be injected, to prevent destruction by hydrochloric acid in the stomach. However, recent evidence demonstrates that orally ingested pancreatic proteolytic enzymes are acid stable and pass intact into the small intestine, where they are absorbed. Dr Kelley had his own enzymes compounded and they certainly worked.

The late Dr Nicholas Gonzalez, one of the doctors you should check into if you are interested in this line of treatment, took the time to evaluate Kelley's work, while still a medical student. Eventually, what began as a student project developed into a two-year formal research effort which he pursued during formal immunology training.

Gonzalez reviewed nearly 10,000 of Dr. Kelley's patient records and interviewed over 500 patients with appropriately diagnosed advanced stages of cancer. This included 50 of his patients initially diagnosed with a variety of poor prognosis cancers, all of whom had enjoyed long term survival and/or apparent regression of disease while following their nutritional regimen.

Gonzalez also studied 23 cases that came into Kelley's office.

Of these, 10 of them met him once, and never did the program. They were dissuaded by family members or doctors who thought that Kelley was a quack. The average survival for that group (which became a good control group of untreated patients) was about 60 days.

The second group of 7 patients who did the therapy partially and incompletely (again, they were being dissuaded by well-intentioned but misguided family members or doctors), their average survival time was 233 days. Almost a four-fold increase!

The third group consisted of 5 patients who were appropriately diagnosed, with biopsies, who did the program fully, all with advanced pancreatic cancer, and *their average survival was eight and a half years*. It was just unheard of in medicine.

One of those remarkable patients first went to see Kelley in 1982. She had undergone surgery which had revealed a tumor in her pancreas and a tumor in her liver. The surgeons biopsied her liver and removed her gall bladder but the pancreatic tumor was so extensive, they didn't even attempt to excise it.

She was then sent to the Mayo Clinic where they reviewed the slides and confirmed that it was stage four pancreatic cancer and gave her six months, maybe a year to live.

Says Gonzalez, she was really lucky to be discouraged from chemotherapy; it probably saved her life! A fine joke... but probably true.

To the Mayo Clinic's great credit, if they know that chemo doesn't work, they're not going to push it onto somebody. In this woman's case, they said —don't waste your time and money on chemo; it will just make you sick.

She learned about Kelley through a health food store, in her local town in Wisconsin, underwent the treatment and she was still alive in 2011. I personally know of no patient with stage 4 pancreatic cancer, confirmed at the Mayo Clinic with liver metastasis, who could be alive 29 years later.

Despite the careful documentation of these amazing successes, no one in academic medicine could accept that a nutritional therapy might produce positive results with advanced cancer patients.

In 1986, probably as a result of endless harrassment, Dr. Kelley gave up research and patient care, and I myself have not spoken to him or any of his associates since 1987. He passed away in January 2005.

# 4.2 Dr. Gonzalez

But Gonzalez pressed on. He carried out a pilot study in 10 patients suffering inoperable cancer of the pancreas, with survival as the endpoint. Pancreatic cancer cases were chosen because the prognosis for the disease is so poor, the disease so rapidly fatal, that an effect could be seen in a small number of patients within a short period of time.

Gonzalez was told by Robert Good, then president of Sloan-Kettering, that if 3 of the 10 patients lived a year, that would be considered a positive result. What actually happened was that over 80% of the patients, some with only weeks to live, made it to one year!

9 (81%) lived one year, 5 lived two years (45%), 4 lived three years (36%) and 2 lived longer than four years.

# 4.3 The Right Enzyme Products

Let me now give you some understanding, which makes it almost imperative that you take at least some quality enzymes.

There are many enzymes in biology, indeed a dazzling array for every function of the cell. Enzymes make important chemical reactions occur at body temperature, which otherwise might need heat. But here we mean digestive enzymes or their equivalent, usually from animal pancreas sources. Bromelain (from pineapple) and papain (from papaya) are also able to digest proteins and other complex biological molecules, safely and effectively. Why is this important?

Most tumors and cancer cells are covered by a sticky resistant mucous/protein coating, which makes them safe from immune cells and even protects them to a degree, from chemotherapy. We can use a mixture of enzymes to dissolve away this protective coat, leaving the cancer cell naked and vulnerable. It can then be poisoned and quickly gobbled up by the body's defences. So it will help chemo because the deadly chemical will be more likely to reach the core of the cancer cells and choke it to death.

There are many enzymes replacement products on the market. Look for preoteolytic enzyme (trypsin) or pancreas-type names (Pancreatin, or such), or even pancreas extract.

Enzyme mixtures of this sort also cool inflammation and so they also have a use against heart disease and blood clotting disorders, arthritis, asthma, and inflammatory bowel disorders. Alternative doctors will take an enyme formula after sports exertion, to curb the aches and pains (which are also largely inflammatory in nature).

Stalling inflammation is part of any good anti-cancer program, so there is that benefit as well from taking enzymes.

But the important role here is that of stripping off the protective coating from cancer cells, allowing the immune cells to get at 'em.

A number of proprietary brands exist, of which I can recommend German brand Wobenzym, available widely. A typical dose regime would be 12- 20 capsules a day. As a proprietary product, it tends to be expensive but it's good. Wobenzyme contains bromelain, papain, as well as trypsin, chymotrypsin and pancreas extract. [http://www.wobenzym.com/en/]

Of course you may explore your own substitutes but be very careful not to get hogwashed by the misleading and frankly dishonest claims of many Internet suppliers, whose "enzymes" wouldn't dissolve a wet biscuit, never mind attack cancer cells.

**The best test I know for quality digestive enzymes is to put one tablet (or some of the contents of a capsule) on your tongue. If it hurts, that's good! It means the enzymes are starting to digest you!**

# 4.4 The Fiasco of The Gonzalez/ Columbia Enzyme Study

In 1993, the National Cancer Institute (NCI), as part of a legitimate effort to reach out to alternative practitioners, invited Nicholas Gonzalez to present 25 cases from his own practice.

Although there was obvious hostility form some at NCI, the then-associate-director of the NCI, Michael Friedman, was very open-minded.

Again Gonzalez was challenged with a bunch of "unsurvivable" cancer of the pancreas cases. A pilot study was proposed (no controls) and Gonzalez was told that, if he could get even three patients to live one year, it would be considered an official miracle.

Incidentally, all these patients were approved by a team of really good cancer researchers, so there would be no doubt that they did really have pancreatic cancer (another way orthodox medicine has of effacing effective cures: claim the patient never really had the disease!) There's no question these patients had pancreatic cancer. They were properly diagnosed and their slides were properly reviewed

In this small NCI pilot study, with initially 11 subjects, 5 patients lived two years, 4 lived three years, and 2 lived five years. One patient quit the program and died of a heart attack. Another quit because she was just tired of living and went off the program; it's hard work and, since she was elderly, she didn't want to keep doing the work. But even these 2 lived five years.

So out of 11 starters, 5 five lived two years or more.

The pilot study was published in June 1999 in the medical literature, and showed the best results for the treatment of pancreatic cancer in the history of medicine.

You can compare that with a study at about the same time, of the newly approved drug gemcitabine. Of 126 patients with pancreatic cancer —more than 10 times as many patients—not a single patient lived longer than 19 months and yet that was considered a "successful" drug.

## Gonzalez Vs. The Cancer Industry

Based on the results of the pilot study, the NCI decided to fund a large scale clinical trial, gemcitabine vs. the Gonzalez/Kelley protocol. They allocated $1.4 million to do the study — it was going to be run at Columbia University.

According to the agreed protocol (Nestle put up the money for the study) patients were to receive either gemcitabine therapy or Gonzalez's regimen of "proteolytic (digestive) enzymes, nutritional supplements, detoxification (coffee enemas ), organic diet (70% raw or minimally cooked); skin brushing and cleansing; salt and soda baths, liver flush, clean sweep, etc."

It turned out to be a huge scientific scam. The alternative approach was thoroughly sabotaged.

The fighting started early and amid violent acrimony and counter-accusations, the much-awaited trial finally collapsed and was forgotten. See Ralph Moss's very insightful Newsletter of June 21, 2008, "A Great Opportunity Lost" at:

http://www.cancerdecisions.com/content/view/122/2/lang,english/

Then, to everyone's complete surprise, the falsified trial results were abruptly published on August 17th, 2009: "Pancreatic Proteolytic Enzyme Therapy Compared With Gemcitabine-Based Chemotherapy for the Treatment of Pancreatic Cancer."

[J Clinical Oncology, vol 28, no 2, Apr 20, 2010]

The published study reported that 32 patients chose Dr. Gonzalez's Enzyme regimen and were managed by him; 23 patients chose conventional chemotherapy and most of them were managed at Columbia University-19 of those 23 received Gemcitabine (Gemzar), Capecitabine (Xeloda) and Docetaxel (Taxotere).

The claimed outcome was as follows: "Those who chose gemcitabine-based chemotherapy survived more than three times as long (14.0 months) vs 4.3 months median survival for those on the enzyme protocol. The chemo patients also had a better quality of life than those who chose proteolytic enzyme treatment."

## Gonzalez version:

What Gonzalez says happened is different altogether and shows the sad state of appalling corruption in the cancer "industry", dictated by Big Pharma control...

All started well, with Richard Klausner, the then-director of NCI. But unfortunately, about a year after the study was approved, Klausner left NCI. From then on the tone changed; unveiled hostility to alternative medicine and a Big Pharma agenda emerged. All the original staffers left or were removed and hard-line anti-nutritionists took the stage.

The paranoia and hostility became so bad, says Gonzalez, that one of their staff couldn't even talk to him, fearing that she'd be fired if she took his phone calls!

Despite this unpleasant negative environment, Gonzalez decided not to quit but to stick it out. With hindsight, that may have been a big mistake. The study was sabotaged and yet made it to the literature. It emerged eventually that the principal investigator at Columbia had an interest in a competing chemo regimen. This outrageous conflict of interest was never declared.

**How the Gonzalez protocol was sabotaged**
Patients were put into the study who did not meet the stated requirements for the protocols. It was understood that patients must be able to follow the program, otherwise the results were invalid. Those admitted to the trial had to be able to feed themselves. The enzyme protocol is, essentially, a nutritional program.

Moreover it is carried out at home. It's a vigorous protocol; patients have to be able to prepare food and administer regular coffee enemas. They have to take 200 pills a day. Patients have to be able to eat. If they can't eat, they can't do therapy. This is not like chemo, where you show up to your doctor's office, stick your arm out for the IV and watch TV while they give you chemo.

At first, requirements were met but, says Gonzalez, there was a sudden change at around 2000 to 2001, when the Columbia group had total control of the entry of patients in the study. Absurdly, Gonzalez and his team found themselves excluded from that process of selection.

So the chief investigator, the dishonest clinican with a financial interest in destroying this trial, Dr. John Chabot of Columbia Presbyterian Medical Center, started sending over patients who could hardly eat. Some patients were so sick they would never have been accepted into Gonzalez' private practice.

But the Columbia team and the NCI started insisting that the moment a patient was accepted into the trial, they were to be considered treated, even if they never received the therapy! In fact, several died before receiving any enzyme therapy but they were considered to have treated by the protocol. In Gonzalez view, only a half dozen of the 39 patients assigned actually did the protocol.

In 2005, the NIH did a review of the study and actually, to their credit, came out in writing with an official statement saying that so many patients had been entered for treatment that couldn't honestly do the program properly, that the data would have no meaning. And there things should have ended. And Gonzalez thought they had.

But that didn't stop the hatchet job. The study was deliberately manipulated to make chemo look better and then, without warning, it was published in the Journal of Clinical Oncology in 2009. This is the journal that would most like to have seen natural therapies discredited.

Gonzalez filed a complaint in 2006, with the Office of the Human Research Protection (OHRP), which is an oversight group responsible for making sure that federally-funded clinical trials should be run properly, and a two-year long investigation ensued, which found that that 42 out of 62 patients had been admitted inappropriately. This has never made its way into the media.

Among other irregularities the OHRP found that for 40 of 62 subjects it appeared that informed consent was not documented with a signed written consent form prior to the initiation of research activities involving human subjects."

This was a really criminal trial, masquerading as science.

You can read the correspondence, regarding the violation of protocols, on the OHRP website, which is part of the Department of Health and Human Services of the NIH. Go here: http://www.hhs.gov/ohrp/detrm_letrs/YR08/feb08e.pdf

I have covered this at length, to show you the depths of depravity of commercial greed and fake science that is current today in the United States and the world-wide pharmaceutical industries. It's all in pursuit of profits and none of these hoods seem to care a jot how many patients die unnecessarily in the process.

Despite the total discrediting of this fiasco of a scientific study, the shameless Journal of Clinical Oncology has never retracted the article. It never will. If it tried to "go honest", Big Pharma funding would be withdrawn, the Journal closed down (or taken over) and the honest editors left without a job.

$1.4 million was wasted, all the money went to Columbia. It's all gone. The data, as far as Gonzalez is concerned, is utterly worthless. Yet the NIH and NCI are using it to show that enzyme therapy—and by wider inference ALL holistic alternatives—don't work.

# Section 5

## Promising New Therapies

The medical and scientific establishments have (largely through the fact that they have sold out to the enormously wealthy and powerful international pharmaceutical industry) obtained more or less complete control over politicians and the media.....advertisements for my book *Food for Thought* are still banned by Britain's Advertising Standards Authority because the book contains advice on what sort of diet to eat in order to reduce the chance of developing cancer.... Because we refused to accept the ban the ASA (which, quite bizarrely, will not accept scientific research papers or even government publications in evidence) has warned newspapers not to accept any of our advertisements.

The ASA claims to exist to protect the public but I find it difficult to see how banning a book that contains a summary of proven clinical advice on how to avoid cancer can possibly protect the public.

It seems to me that, wittingly or unwittingly, the ASA is simply protecting the cancer establishment. I find it difficult to avoid the observation that the cancer industry would undoubtedly find it much harder to raise money if the incidence of cancer were cut.

**Dr Vernon Coleman**

# 5.1 Vaccination Against Cancer

## It's coming, so wise up

It's a constantly recurring theme from medically-untrained alternative "health researchers" (who just read and steal other people's notes in Google): that vaccines don't work. Of course they work. It's only the homeopathic principle, after all—a little of the substance trains the body to respond in a healthy way.

I'm always glad of the smallpox vaccine; and rabies, as I have said many times. My first mother-in-law was a nice lady who, as a child, had a brush with death via smallpox. That's how real the disease was in our modern world.

Influenza vaccine is more or less a waste of time because the virus mutates so fast, by the time the vaccine is manufactured, it is out of date.

And some, of course, are very dangerous, like Gardasil, which should never have come to market.

But proper vaccines continue to save lives. They are, after all, an intelligent interaction with one of our main defence mechanisms, the immune system.

So why not engage the vaccination tool against cancer? It could mean the end, once and for all, of ghastly chemo, radiation therapy and mutilating surgery.

Why am I optimistic? Because we will be using Nature's own mechanisms to strike down the cancer. That's got to make sense.

## How could this work?

Most people, I think, understand the receptor principle. Receptors are small fragments of molecules sticking out from a cell, which lock in with specific messenger chemicals. No receptors and the messenger can't do its job.

So what if we could wreck the necessary receptors on the surface of a cancer cell, those which fuel growth and proliferation? It would cripple cell function. And choosing only receptors in this way means a much smaller target to hit than trying to wreck a whole cell. In theory it should work better.

Well, it's coming. Animal studies have demonstrated it's entirely feasible to knock out valuable receptors on the surface of cancer cells by cultivating T-cells that react to them as a specific antigen. In other words, they produce antibodies against those receptors *highly selectively*.

With persistence Mary Disis of the University of Washington and her research team developed several targeted cancer therapies and after more than a decade of laboratory and animal testing, they have developed the first ever human anti-breast-cancer vaccine.

Over 60 women who received the experimental vaccine against metastatic breast cancer and most are doing very well.

In 2010, the U.S. Food and Drug Administration approved the prostate cancer vaccine, called Provenge.

In 2011, researchers at the University of Pennsylvania unveiled what they call a cancer "breakthrough 20 years in the making": a vaccine against chronic lymphocytic leukemia (CLL) that has brought about remissions of up to a year and counting—and which its inventors believe can be tweaked to attack lung cancer, ovarian cancer, myeloma, and melanoma.

Scores of other vaccines are in the pipeline.

So if you are battling cancer and someday soon get offered the chance to try vaccination, take it. Eventually the technique will be formidable—because we are relying on Nature's own mechanism—our own body wisdom—to solve the problem of the intruder.

That's how we beat cancer naturally and why large numbers of people never develop it; it's nipped in the bud by our wily immune systems.

The future of these "natural" anti-cancer therapies is so bright that makes it worth working very hard, applying as much as you can of the advice in this book, and make sure you survive till the vaccine becomes a clinical reality.

Vaccines might even tame pancreatic cancer. A clinical trial at the Cancer Institute of New Jersey showed great promise.

The first patient treated started injections in March 2010. By December, scans detected no tumors anywhere; three of five other patients with inoperable pancreatic cancer are also stable. 13- 19 months later the patients were doing remarkably well. None have liver or other metastases, which is surprising because pancreatic cancer likes to spread everywhere.

Brain cancer is as deadly as pancreatic cancer, but at least one experimental vaccine is showing promise against glioblastoma multiforme, the most common and aggressive form. That's the one that killed Ted Kennedy.

A glioblastoma contains bits of the antigen called epidermal growth factor receptor variant III, which studs brain cancer cells. In a clinical trial, 18 patients whose tumors had been surgically removed received the vaccine; median survival was 26 months, scientists at Duke University reported in 2010, compared with the usual 14. That's almost double.

And in July, Larry Kwak of M.D. Anderson and colleagues reported that in patients given an experimental vaccine against follicular lymphoma, a form of non-Hodgkin's lymphoma, their cancer also remained in remission almost twice as long as expected, and counting, as did unvaccinated patients. Biovest International plans to seek FDA approval for the vaccine, BiovaxID, in 2012.

# 5.2 The End Of Chemo Resistance?

Vaccines have the potential to revolutionize cancer treatment because their effects do not stop with existing tumors. Cancer is notorious for its craftiness, changing the biological pathways by which cells proliferate so much that chemotherapies and even targeted molecular therapies soon stop working. Chemo resistance it's called.

Vaccines could match the cancer cells move for move. In women who received Mary Disis's vaccine, after T cells destroy breast cancer cells they gobble them up and spit them out. That floods the body with more of the antigens, stimulating the immune system to target this second wave of tumor antigens. This spreading immunity creates locked-and-loaded T cells that can destroy tumor cells years after years vaccination—the same kind of lifelong immunity that, say, a smallpox vaccine confers.

Remember, T cells never forget. Once the immune system has targeted a threat, be it cancer or smallpox, it keeps a reserve team ready to attack should that threat return. In principle, that should confer immunity against breast cancer and possibly other cancers as well—forever.

Note: don't mix this approach up with vaccinations against viruses relevant to cancer, such as the deplorable Gardasil vaccine against papilloma virus, which is neither safe nor effective.

[SOURCE: http://www.thedailybeast.com/newsweek/2011/12/11/could-this-be-the-end-of-cancer.html accessed 10/24/2012 12.00 pm PDT]

# 5.3 Avemar. It's Good!

Studies have shown that Avemar is a potent natural compound is effective against a wide variety of cancers including, breast, colorectal and skin cancers. You can safely use it while receiving chemotherapy. So if you want to combine conventional treatments and alternatives, this one is especially good to know.

It may also be preventative. Too early to make claims.

Avemar is often said to be the brain child of Hungarian doctor and Nobel Prize winner Dr. Szent Györgyi (the guy who discovered vitamin C) but was actually originated by Dr. Mate Hidvegi. Hidvegi holds the patent.

[http://www.matehidvegi.com/]

More than 100 papers published in prestigious journals have reviewed clinical and experimental results with this extract, and it's now a medically approved substance for cancer treatment in Europe.

In Hungary, where the product was developed, the mortality rate of cancer stopped rising and began declining after its introduction and in the wake of its increasingly wide-spread use. In Hungary's neighboring countries, where they have not learned of Avemar, the cancer death rate has continued to rise.

Researchers and oncologists from points all around the globe, including UCLA (University of California at Los Angeles), the Universities of Sheffield and Barcelona, Israeli clinics, the University of Tel Aviv, the Blokhin Oncological Center in Moscow and the University of Genoa —some 20 countries in all—joined in the research.

Avemar comes from a patented process that ferments wheat germ with baker's yeast (but it's NOT a brad!). The result is a supplement that performs three vital functions in the body:

1. Helps the body regulate metabolism and more efficiently create energy from the nutrients we eat

2. Boosts the body's immune system and helps create stronger T-cells and macrophages (the cells that eat invaders)

3. Helps the body target "bad" cells and eliminate them by shutting off the "cloaking mechanism" that tells the body not to kill cancer cells

Let me explain this last: Your body has a miraculous frontline defense of natural killer (NK) cells. These are the cells that jump on invading bacteria and viruses as well as mutated cells like cancer. An NK cell has receptors that tell it to either kill or move on, once it attaches to a potential invader.

The NK cell is like a cop that stops someone suspicious, demands to see an ID, and asks a few questions. If it decides the target cell is "innocent," it moves on. If not, it will zap the rogue cell!

This means any kind of invading or mutated cell is only able to grow and thrive if it convinces the body's NK "police" that it's a normal cell. Unfortunately, that's exactly what cancer cells do.

Cancer "lies" to the NK cells, telling the NK's receptors, "It's okay, I'm a good guy." It does this with a surface molecule called MHC-1 that acts like a "fake ID". Once the NK cell sees this disguise molecule, it accepts the intruder and moves on.

This is where Avemar comes into play. Avemar suppresses the cancer cell's ability to display the MHC-1 molecule, so it can no longer fool the NK cells. The result? Cancer cells get destroyed swiftly and removed.

Also, according to a 2002 study, American and Spanish researchers showed Avemar has a direct influence on the metabolism of tumor cells which prevents the cancer cells from reproducing themselves and from carrying out the all-important DNA synthesis. As a result, the tumor does not develop further and the cancer cells, owing to Avemar's effect in other areas, die off, either on their own or under the influence of the body's cancer-killing mechanisms. [*J Biol Chem* 277: 46408–46414]

## Worldwide Acceptance For Avemar

The Hungarian medical authorities registered Avemar as medical nutriment for cancer patients on 1 July 2002 with the following approved label: 'Indications: Avemar is recommended for use by patients suffering from cancer as a supplement to clinical oncological treatments (surgery, radiotherapy, chemotherapy, immuno-therapy, etc.'

After Avemar's registration in 2002, it was not long before the Czech medical authorities also registered it as a medical nutriment for cancer patients. Soon after this, the Bulgarian authorities also registered and approved Avemar as a medical nutriment for cancer patients. In Australia, the product falls into the category of therapeutic products for use in immune-modulation therapy, while, in Austria, it is already paid for entirely by the National Health service.

In Europe (including in Hungary), Avemar is currently the only non-prescription product with an officially approved label available on the market specifically for cancer patients.

The FDA classifies Avemar as GRAS (Generally Recognized as Safe), which means is can be used in foods, beverages and dietary supplements. Avemar is not that different from bread (so wheat and gluten allergics beware!)

The great thing is you can take Avemar alongside conventional therapy (surgery, chemotherapy and radiation therapy). It's not a "one or the other" choice.

This universal acceptance is simple to explain: Avemar works!

A report given by Prof. Ferenc Jakab, the department director and chief physician at the Uzsoki Street Hospital in Budapest, was even featured on CNN news. Prof. Jakab discussed a test performed at the hospital, again emphasised that significant differences can be observed in patients undergoing treatment which includes Avemar when compared with those who do not receive Avemar.

The conclusions of the test were that, when combined with surgery, radio- or chemotherapy, Avemar was able to reduce significantly the formation of metastases and lengthen survival time in colorectal cancer patients.

Prof. Miklós Kásler, director general of the National Oncological Institute, said, "It is not a dietary supplement, but it is a very important new treatment, registered for cancer treatment."

**You can find Avemar in the U.S. under the brand name Avé. It's recommended as a dietary supplement in a once-a-day, instant drink mix.**

# 5.4 GcMAF

Now here's a tangled story. It runs from fake science to alleged assassination!

GcMAF recently hit the news when a slew of holistic doctors died in quick succession, several murdered violently. It was claimed (I think erroneously) that all were in some way connected with this promising new cancer cure. That must be proof it works; because it threatens the cancer industry's revenues ($174 billion dollars in the US alone)!

Well, there are those that look for conspiracies in everything out of the ordinary. I personally don't believe the 8 deaths were statistically significant (about average for that period). The murderers were found and apprehended in 2 cases and the suicides seemed genuine enough.

But it does add spice to the story of GcMAF!

It stands for globulin component macrophage activating factor. In 2008-2009, four human studies appeared claiming fantastic results for a groundbreaking new cancer treatment. The studies were conducted Dr. Nabuto Yamamoto, who at the time was a Professor of Biochemistry at Temple University Medical School in Philadelphia. He was assisted by a team of other researchers.

Dr. Yamamoto looked at a number of diseases, including AIDS. More importantly, his team treated 16 metastatic breast cancer patients with a single injection of 100 nanograms of GcMAF per week for 22 weeks. The treatment resulted in tumor eradication. Patients were well after four years follow-up. This was published in the International Journal of Cancer [Int J Cancer. 2008 Jan 15;122(2):461-7]

In another study, 16 metastatic prostate patients were tumor-free after 24 weeks and remained so at seven years follow-up. [Transl Oncol. 2008 Jul;1(2):65-72] And in another, all 8 metastatic colorectal patients were cancer-free after 48 weeks and remained so at seven years follow-up as confirmed by CT scans. [Cancer Immunol Immunother. 2008 Jul;57(7):1007-16]

This is astonishing, if proven. That means Professor Yamamoto achieved a 100% remission rate in metastatic cancer patients.

But trouble is just around the corner. The $174 billion Cancer Industry does not want cures. It will attack, cripple, deride and undermine any research which could suggest such amazing recoveries. Why, every oncologist who didn't use it would be out of business overnight! And those who did use it would cure patients quickly and earn buttons on the dollar!

The assassination part of this story is really the attack on Yamamoto and his discoveries. Is it justified?

Well, just for once, I am willing to share the views of The AntiCancer Fund which are as follows:

The IJC article reports the use of GcMAF in 16 breast cancer patients. All patients had previously mastectomy or lumpectomy and all but one received radiotherapy or chemotherapy, prior to the initiation of the treatment with GcMAF.

The authors do not give any information on the staging of these patients. However, they determined that these patients had metastatic disease, based on an elevated level of serum Nagalase. Elevated Nagalase level is not a criterion to define metastatic disease in the TNM classification of cancer, 7th edition. There is therefore no proof that the patients had residual disease after the standard treatment they received.

According to the information presented in Table 1, no patient received both radiotherapy and chemotherapy, which is rather unusual in the management of breast cancer patients. Especially, two patients who had lumpectomy did not receive radiotherapy which is recommended after lumpectomy.

The Anticaner Fund tried to contact Yamamoto's co-authors. They found out that Hirofumi Suyama, a co-author affiliated to the Nagasaki Immunotherapy Research

Group in Japan, passed away in 2009. Pr. Hirofumi Suyama was a professor of Forensic Medicine at the Nagasaki University who retired in 1987 and did not publish papers from 1991 until 2007, when he suddenly co-authored several papers together with Nobuto Yamamoto.

The co-authors affiliated to the Socrates Institute for Therapeutic Immunology in Philadelphia, an organization of which Yamamoto appears to be director, are untraceable.

The Nagasaki and the Hyogo Immunotherapy Research Groups that gave IRB approvals for these trials do not exist anywhere, except in the papers from Nobuto Yamamoto. Moreover, *three people listed in the approval documents denied being part of those groups or having ever participated in Yamamoto's work.*

The purported sponsors of this trial denied having supported clinical research on GcMAF. They supported Yamamoto's preclinical work, in the 90s. The US Public Health Service from 1992-1994 and the Elsa E. Pardee Foundation only in 1998.

The Anticancer Fund also found that Yamamoto forged the name of Pr. Charles E. Benson from the University of Pennsylvania, when he presented further results of GcMAF to treat some types of cancer and HIV to FOCIS meetings.

The most worrisome problem, claimed the Anticancer Fund, is that this article, and others published in other peer-reviewed journals, is used by some GcMAF manufacturers to support their claims and sell it "illegally" to patients.

Americans love to throw around this word "illegally", which they liberally use to mean something that isn't sanctioned officially. But that's NOT the same as illegal.

Same with the word "unapproved". Approved by who? When there's no science, they say "unproven" but when there are lots of papers published in reputable journals, they switch to "unapproved", to make it sound criminal.

### So What's The Story Here?

GcMAF is something that every one of the 7 billion humans produce in their bodies. It is NOT a special substance.

The foundations of GcMAF as a possible cancer therapeutic agent began in 1979 when Dr. Yamamoto started basic research in molecular biology and immunology. The first publication in a peer-reviewed journal on GcMAF appeared in 1994, in the *Journal Of Immunology*. Dr. Yamamoto and colleagues at Temple University demonstrated that GcMAF activated macrophages. These are vital immune cells that kill pathogens and cancer cells and switch on other aspects of the immune system. [*J Immunol*. 1994 May 15;152(10):5100-7]

A year later he showed that a defect in the production of GcMAF inside the body contributes to a poorer immune response in AIDS patients. In 1996 he demonstrated that this was also the case in cancer patients.

### How Does It Work?

Professor Yamamoto discovered that cancer cells and some viruses, but not normal cells, secrete an enzyme called Nagalase. This enzyme is able to block the production of a protein that activates macrophages to attack the cancer cells. He named this Gc-protein-derived Macrophage Activating Factor — GcMAF for short. In other words, nagalase and GcMAF are antagonists. Whichever wins could be good or bad for cancer cells.

Cancer's ability to block macrophages by secreting nagalase can be bypassed by injecting GcMAF, so the theory goes. The treatment restores normal immunity and the body is then able to attack tumor cells.

Professor Yamamoto demonstrated that when macrophages are activated by Gc-MAF their activity increases by 30-fold. There is also a 15-fold rise in superoxide ions. These also attack pathogens and cancer cells.

The probable answer to the seemingly amazing results he got were that it is no use trying it on the majority of patients; only carefully selected categories of patients:

> GcMAF is least likely to work in patients who have a large tumor burden and in those whose tumors are well differentiated (i.e. look similar to normal cells). It works best in those with a low tumor load and in poorly differentiated (highly abnormal) cells.

> GcMAF can be stopped from working by opiates, patients lacking sufficient red blood cells, or those with low white blood cell counts.

Dr. Yamamoto's subjects had undergone conventional therapies to reduce the tumor burden to a very low level. They were also at an early stage of metastasis and had no conditions that could block the protein. They were all selected as *non-anemic*, which is crucial.

## Other Actions of GcMAF

Until 2002 it was believed GcMAF activated only macrophages. Then Professor Yamamoto, together with researchers from Japan, discovered that GcMAF blocks angiogenesis. Angiogenesis is the process whereby cancer tumors form their own network of extra blood vessels, needed for rapid growth.

This finding was confirmed the following year by the highly distinguished doctor Judah Folkman and others at Children's Hospital in Boston.

That's good in itself. But there's more:

In 2010, researchers from the University of Kentucky showed for the first time that GcMAF directly inhibits the migration, proliferation and metastatic potential of human prostate cancer cells. This happened independently of macrophage activation.

And in 2012 a team under Marco Ruggiero, a professor of molecular biology at the University of Florence, Italy, confirmed this effect in breast cancer cells. The Florence team showed something else remarkable, too: GcMAF was able to cause cancer cells to revert to normal cells. [Anticancer Res. 2012 Jan;32(1):45-52]

## The Big Aha!

Professor Ruggiero and his wife Dr. Pacini realized that the enzymes that act on Gc protein to turn it into GcMAF also occur during the fermentation of milk.

They therefore set about creating an "anti-cancer super-yogurt" called MAF314. This contains over 30 microorganisms and strains of bacteria designed to create a potent immune-enhancing food product that, they say, can also restore a healthy human microbiome.

Professor Ruggiero one day experienced a sudden insight. He realized that GcMAF needs to combine with oleic acid to function. He said, "This neglected association between oleic acid and GcMAF was the missing link that more than a thousand researchers including Dr. Yamamoto and myself had been seeking for the past 20 years."

Prof. Ruggiero and Dr. Pacini then went on to combine GcMAF with oleic acid to create GOleic.

Unlike GcMAF, which has to be injected, or MAF314, which can be either eaten or administered into the colon, GOleic, in addition to these methods of administration, can be taken as sublingual drops, a spray, suppositories or even as an ointment.

Ruggiero claims to have demonstrated that GOleic is far more potent than GcMAF and has effects at a molecular level that cannot be reproduced with the protein alone.

## The Swiss Protocol

Unfortunately, Ruggiero also got involved in the AIDS controversy, opposing the orthodox view. I have had a saying for over 30 years: if you say you can cure cancer, they will bankrupt you; if you say you can cure AIDS, they will murder you. Maybe AIDS is less defensible these days (but still a multi-million dollar scam). Sure enough, this was Ruggiero's downfall; he was attacked and had to leave Italy.

He and his wife went to Switzerland, where they they met an entrepreneur, David Noakes. Noakes manufactured GcMAF and GOleic and made them commercially available. The therapy was offered in Swiss and German clinics. International conferences on GcMAF took place. Research facilities and funding for Professor Ruggiero were provided.

Ruggiero developed a more comprehensive approach to treating cancer, which is called The Swiss Protocol. Great claims are made for it. You must investigate it for yourself. I have never used it but it makes sense, in view of all you have been reading.

1. A high protein, low carbohydrate diet (can be as low as 2% depending on the type of tumor). As readers of this newsletter know, I strongly advocate a low-carbohydrate diet for all, and especially for cancer patients.

2. High absorption and rapidly utilized amino acids in the form of Master Amino Acid Pattern (MAAP) proteins

3. MAF314 taken either by mouth or into the colon depending on the type of cancer

4. GOleic. The practitioner may inject this substance at the site of the tumor or administer it in other ways.

5. Vitamin D. Up to 20,000 IU a day may be recommended. Note that this is far more than even alternative doctors recommend, and is in line with what I've suggested previously in my newsletters. Blood tests are the only way to determine how much vitamin D a patient needs, and the amount is nearly always far more than the four or five thousand daily IUs that even "aggressive" alternative doctors recommend.

6. Water. Two liters a day may be suggested.

7. Low dose acetylsalicylic acid (aspirin) may be prescribed.

Interestingly, only the day I revized this section (Sep 2015), *MedScape Daily News* informed me of the US Preventive Services Task Force (USPSTF) recommended that adults 50 to 69 years of age should take daily low-dose aspirin for at least 10 years to reduce their risk for colorectal cancer, as well as lower cardiovascular risk. Predictably, the USPSTF statement has drawn criticism from a number of experts as potentially confusing and lacking in clear evidence. [http://www.uspreventiveservicestaskforce.org/Page/Document/draft-recommendation-statement/aspirin-to-prevent-cardiovascular-disease-and-cancer]

## The Ongoing Story

Examples of the Ruggiero team's work in patients using the new protocol were presented at the 9th International Conference of Anticancer Research in Greece in October, 2014.

During the last 25 years a large number of scientists in eight countries have published research on GcMAF, and thanks to David Noakes it has now been supplied to 350 doctors in 30 nations. Professor Ruggiero estimates that over legally-licensed 200 doctors worldwide are following his protocols.

Notwithstanding, early in 2015, in a quite English village, ten investigators burst into Immuno Biotech's lab unannounced, and terrified two female scientists before removing 10,000 vials of GcMAF, a chemical that occurs naturally in milk and blood, remember. Immuno Biotech is apparently owned or controlled by Mr. Noakes. This sort of thing we are used to seeing in the USA but in the UK this can be taken as firm evidence that the Cancer Mafia has links high up in the UK government.

The Medicine and Healthcare Products Regulatory Agency (MHRA) - the UK equivalent of the FDA - claimed the product "may pose a significant risk to people's health."

This is absurd. GcMAF is in everyone's bodies and has definitely proven health benefits. It's like shutting down the blood bank, saying blood is dangerous for humans.

The backlash continues. Other scientists have attacked both the Yamamoto and Ruggiero research and claim to have identified irregularities in the way some of the studies were conducted, reviewed and published. At least one Yamamoto study, published in the *International Journal of Cancer*, has been retracted by the publication's editor.

Bearing in mind my caution above, about the elusiveness of some of the figures mentioned in Yamamoto's published studies, I think it's right to say this treatment is not a fully accredited miracle. Being attacked by authorities is not "proof" that is really works, as some naïve supporters of holistic therapies seem to think.

About the only definite comment I could make is to say you must bear in mind the restrictions on its usefulness for cancer cases at large. If Yamamoto and Ruggiero proved anything, it's that *GcMAF will only work on a small tightly defined subset of cancer cases: those who have had their cancer cell burden reduced by chemo and/or radiation just before administration of GcMAF*. It doesn't work for the majority cases.

If you want to try it, I can assure that the official position that it's potentially harmful is utter nonsense. However you will have great difficulty obtaining it in the near future.

**Lee Euler of CancerDefeated.com has informed me of the following:**

At the time of writing, the IAT Clinic in the Bahamas includes GcMAF as part of its cancer protocols, as does the Rosenberg Integrative Cancer Treatment and Research Institute in Florida. Other clinics in Nevada, Arizona, and California also prescribe it, as well as health centers in Japan.

The original European clinics appear to have closed, but there are now two in the Netherlands; their exact location is not disclosed.

As Lee says, "Let's hope this exciting treatment turns out to be everything its adherents claim, and that the regulators don't succeed in quashing it as they have so many therapies in the past."

Let's also pray that someday we will all be able to get at all unadulterated scientific truth, without it being sterile, false, politically-correct pap, put out by those who want to manipulate the facts to protect their vested interest.

# Section 6

## Herbs Against Cancer

The only accepted legal medical diagnosis of cancer is by biopsy. This is not 100% accurate, for there are false positives as well as false negative biopsies. We, that is you and I, are not permitted to make a diagnosis of cancer. Nor are we permitted by law to use any system of diagnosis except biopsy for cancer diagnosis. The Medical Establishment tightly controls the diagnosis of cancer.

**Dr Donald Kelley DDS**

Next, let's come onto herbs and related matters. Herbal cures have been around for centuries and you can bet a good few are effective against cancer. Some have even been specially formulated to treat cancer.

Most famous of all is probably Essiac. But first let me introduce a startling study from China. A lot of good medical science is coming out of Asia these days. They certainly don't have the prejudices against traditional therapies that are prevalent in the West.

Recently a keynote Chinese clinical trial was undertaken to study the anti-cancer benefits of two herbs formulas, "Y" and "C". These mixtures were:

**"Y" Formula: schidigera yucca, licorice root, fennel seed, clove buds, anise seed, cinnamon bark, etc.**

**"C" Formula: burdock root, rhubarb root, slippery elm bark, sheep sorrel.**

This article has summarized 583 cases of taking "C" Formula and "Y" Formula (288 cases of cancer, 84 cases of asthma, 176 cases of rhinallergosis, 35 cases of lupus erythematosus). Of the 288 cases of cancer patients, 145 cases were "highly effective", accounting for 50.37%; 100 cases were "effective", accounting for 34.70%.

The most effective results were observed in the patients with intestinal cancer, malignant lymphoma, nasopharyngeal carcinoma, leukaemia. In everyday figures 85% great success, 15% moderately effective, 15% not much use. This is better than chemo anyway but don't forget the added bonus: these herbs were shown to be harmless in test doses administered to mice which were 555 higher than the clinical herbal dose! No hair loss; no vomiting!

Of the 84 cases of asthma, 11 were healed, 30 were notably effective, 36 were effective, and the total effective rate was 92.47%. Of the 176 cases of rhinallergosis, the total effective rate was 94.89%. For the 35 cases of lupus erythematosus, the total effective rate was 92.86%.

Generally speaking, the combined use of "C" Formula and "Y" Formula on the same patient was very effective on strengthening /adjusting immune function. Otherwise, the independent use of either of the drugs was not as effective. For more than seventy years, the two drugs have been indeed effective in cancer prevention and treatment.

Herb tea, in fact, can be medicine with good taste and enjoyable. However, since the essential ingredients of "C" Formula and "Y" Formula are pure herbs, "C" Formula and "Y" Formula should be classified as effective herba; medicine.

Remedy "C" above is essentially the Essiac formula...

# 6.1 Essiac

Probably the most famous herbal cancer remedy is Essiac, named after Canadian nurse Rene M. Caisse (her surname in reverse). She claimed it was an ancient Ojibway Indian formula. Wherever it came from, its claim to success is riding high.

There are many stories of its efficacy though, until the above trial in China, no actual scientific studies. It may help, it's harmless and at worst would be a waste of money, so you may care to try it. There are hundreds of sources on the Internet and you will have to satisfy yourself of their potency and authenticity. In recent years, this formula has gained notoriety.

There are interesting, substantiated accounts of its recent use in the treatment of cancer. Dr. Gary Glum has investigated and written extensively about the Essiac Formula in his book, "Calling of An Angel."

In the early 1920's, Caisse began giving the preparation to any one who requested it as a treatment for cancer. It is reported that even the worst cases were cured or lived longer than expected and were free of pain. As one would expect, the government became involved. She was attacked and faced jail. But more than 55,000 signatures were collected on her behalf, thus allowing her to continue her work.

As in so many instances of a similar nature, the cases were limited to certified and well-documented terminally ill patients declared incurable by the establishment. In other words, they only allowed her to work on orthodox failures that were virtually certain to die. She was not allowed to charge for her services. Contrary to expectations, many hopeless patients lived more than thirty-five years after Essiac treatment.

When Caisee finally died in 1978, the Canadian Ministry of Health and Welfare destroyed all of her documents. Isn't it amazing that there are so many well-documented cases of the destruction of records of this nature that have occurred in nations where free speech is supposedly protected?

"Book burning" is obviously not just an historical event that happened in Nazi Germany! One has to wonder why democratic countries feel compelled to suppress knowledge of any kind?

Dr. Charles Brusch, personal physician to President John F. Kennedy, treated thousands of patients with cancer, including this remedy. Dr. Brusch stated that Essiac was an excellent cure for cancer and was placed under a "gag-order" by the Federal Government. Dr. Brusch treated and cured his own cancer with Essiac and his records are still preserved.

The most important herb in the formula is Sheep's Sorrel and it is non-toxic. Nevertheless, this herb is "banned" in Canada and in the United States. That's pretty silly because it is a common weed and is easily found by anyone who can recognize it! It is not the only herb that has been banned when news of its use in cancer got out. See Hoxey's Herbs in the next section.

## The ESSIAC FORMULA

Sheep's Sorrel (*Rumex Acetosella*) - 16 ounces in powdered form

Burdock Root (*Arctium Lappa*) - 6 1/2 cups in cut form

Rubarb Root (*Rheum Palmatum*) - 1 ounce in powdered form

Slippery Elm Bark (*Ulmus Fulva*) -.4 ounces in powdered form

# 6.2 Hoxsey Herbs

For over three decades, Harry Hoxsey (1901-1974), a self-taught healer, cured many cancer patients using an herbal remedy reportedly handed down by his great-grandfather. By the 1950s, the Hoxsey Cancer Clinic in Dallas was the world's largest private cancer center, with branches in seventeen states. Born in Illinois, the charismatic practitioner of herbal folk medicine faced unrelenting opposition and harassment from a hostile medical establishment.

Nevertheless, two federal courts upheld the "therapeutic value" of Hoxsey's internal tonic. Even his arch-enemies, the American Medical Association and the Food and Drug Administration, admitted that his treatment could cure some forms of cancer. A Dallas judge ruled in federal court that Hoxsey's therapy was "comparable to surgery, radium, and x-ray" in its effectiveness, without the destructive side effects of those treatments.

But in the 1950s, at the tail end of the McCarthy era, Hoxsey's clinics were shut down. The AMA, NCI, and FDA organized a "conspiracy" to "suppress" a fair, unbiased assessment of Hoxsey's methods, according to a 1953 federal report to Congress.

Attacks even included an unprecedented "Public Warning Against Hoxsey Cancer Treatment" which the Commissioner of the FDA ordered mounted in 46,000 US post offices and substations in 1956 (Young, 1967, 387; Larrick, 1956).

Hoxsey's Dallas clinic closed its doors in 1960, and three years later, at Hoxsey's request, Mildred Nelson, R.N., his long-time chief nurse, moved the operation to Tijuana, Mexico.

# 6.3 The Truth About Herbs

In the years since that time science has discovered anti-cancer substances in virtually all Hoxsey's herbs. For instance, bloodroot contains an alkaloid, sanguinarine, that has powerful anti-tumor properties.

Medical historian Patricia Spain Ward reported "provocative findings of antitumor properties" in many of the individual Hoxsey herbs when she investigated the Hoxsey regimen in 1988 for the United States Congress's Office of Technology Assessment. Ward noted that "orthodox scientific research has by now identified antitumor activity" in most of Hoxsey's plants.

[Patricia Spain Ward, "History of Hoxsey Treatment," contract report submitted to U.S. Congress, Office of Technology Assessment, May 1988, p. 8.]

Another example, two Hungarian scientists in 1966 reported "considerable antitumor activity" in a purified fraction of burdock (also in Essiac). Japanese researchers at Nagoya University in 1984 found in burdock a new type of desmutagen, a substance that is uniquely capable of reducing mutation in either the absence or the presence of metabolic activation. This new property is so important, the Japanese scientists named it the B- factor, for "burdock factor."

[Kazuyoshi Morita, Tsuneo Kada, and Mitsuo Namiki, "A Desmutagenic Factor Isolated From Burdock (Arctium Lappa Linne)," Mutation Research, vol. 129, 1984, pp. 25-31, cited in Ward, op. cit., p. 7]

The basic ingredients of Hoxsey's internal tonic are potassium iodide and such substances as licorice, red clover, burdock root, stillingia root, barberis root, pokeroot, cascara, prickly ash bark, and buckthorn bark.

Again the formula is no secret and there are plenty of people willing to sell it to you on the Internet.

# 6.4 One Gramm of Lemon Grass!

If there was a natural plant (food) substance that had powerful properties which caused cancer cells to undergo apoptosis (programmed suicide), you would think it pretty remarkable.

You would also expect the medical profession to jump on this "miracle cure" and start promoting it. Well, it hasn't happened—yet.

So what is this wonder treatment I'm referring to?

It's lemon grass; or more exactly, citral extract, which comes from lemon grass. And to be precise about this discovery, what I am saying is that Israeli researchers at Ben Gurion University (BGU) have found that one gram of lemon grass contains enough citral to prompt cancer cells to commit suicide in the test tube. It does this without harming normal cells.

The findings were published in the scientific journal Planta Medica, which highlights research on alternative and herbal remedies. Shortly afterwards, the discovery was featured in the popular Israeli press. Of course you never heard it on CNN and other US stations.

Citral is the key component that gives the lemony aroma and taste in several herbal plants such as lemon grass (*Cymbopogon citratus*), melissa (*Melissa officinalis*) and verbena (*Verbena officinalis*)

The Israeli investigators checked the influence of the citral on cancerous cells by adding them to both cancerous cells and normal cells that were grown in a petri dish. The quantity added in the concentrate was equivalent to the amount contained in a cup of regular tea using one gram of lemon herbs in hot water. While the citral killed the cancerous cells, the normal cells remained unharmed.

As they learned of the BGU findings in the press, many physicians in Israel began to believe that while the research certainly needed to be explored further, in the meantime it would be advisable for their patients, who were looking for any possible tool to fight their condition, to try to harness the cancer-destroying properties of citral.

The best way to consume the citral is to put the loose lemon grass in hot water, and drink several glasses each day.

**However don't go crazy and assume it's a done deal.** Science is rarely that easy!

One study I found suggested citral might *cause* cancer (lymphoma) in female mice fed citral in their food.

Citral was nominated by the National Cancer Institute for study as an antigen because of its widespread use in foods, beverages, cosmetics, and other consumer products and its structure as a representative beta-substituted vinyl aldehyde. Citral is used primarily as lemon flavoring in foods, beverages, and candies. It is also used as a lemon fragrance in detergents, perfumes, and other toiletries.

Male and female rats exposed to significant doses of citral exhibited listlessness, hunched posture, absent or slow paw reflex, and dull eyes. But there was no increased incidence of any cancers.

However, the incidences of malignant lymphoma in female mice exposed to citral at 2,000 ppm was significantly greater than that in the control group. Tissues most commonly affected by malignant lymphoma were the spleen, mesenteric lymph node, thymus, and, to a lesser extent, the ovary.

The researchers described this incidence of lymphoma in mice as "equivocal" evidence of cancer-causing properties. If the testing was done properly, it should not, in my view, be dismissed as equivocal. It would be grounds for further research.

For you (reader), it depends if you want to go with the rats or the mice!

[Natl Toxicol Program Tech Rep Ser. 2003 Jan;(505):1-268]0.

# 6.5 Ginseng (Eleutherococcus etc.)

It helps to know there are several plants by the name "Ginseng". The one grown on the islands of the Indian Ocean is *Hydrocotylee asiatica*; *Panax quiquefolius* or American ginseng has been shown effective against liver cancer. Classic Siberian ginseng is *Eleutherococcus sentiocus* boost white cells and so logically helps against cancer.

Ginseng is an adaptogen—a substance that regulates various body functions depending on individual needs. Eastern medical practitioners have used this Chinese herb to treat a variety of ills and renew energy.

Now a growing body of scientific research has focused on a specific chemical in ginseng—aglycolin sapogenin or AGS—and it's apparent anti-cancer properties.

For example, AGS completely destroyed melanoma cancer cells within 24 hours of contact, with nearly zero toxicity and no side effects. AGS could turn out to be one of the safest cancer treatments available. Study after study has reported virtually no side effects.

Other names: the AGS group of sapogenins is also sometimes called R-family sapogenins, so if you see this term, it means the product is same thing as AGS.

The good thing about taking AGS on its own is that you avoid the sugary ginsenosides. As you know (section 16), sugar is the last thing you want around cancer cells. This is one rare case when an extract may be better than taking the whole herb.

There is good science to show that AGS enhances apoptosis. AGS can also work with other anti-cancer agents to prevent drug resistance in cancer cells.

But there's more! AGS is even able to change cancer cells back into normal cells. [Odashima, S., et al. "Induction of phenotypic reverse transformation by plant glycosides in cultured cancer cells," *Gan To Kagaku Ryoho*, 1989 Apr;16(4 Pt 2-2):1483-9. Retrieved from http://www.ncbi.nlm.nih.gov/pubmed/2658830]

It may also be helpful because of the diversity of cancer cells, even within a specific tumor. This is often why chemo doesn't work well: it's the wrong agent for that particular phenotype, as these different cells are called.

AGS solves that by attacking a wide variety of cancerous cells, making them chemo-sensitive; in other words MORE sensitive to chemo. That makes AGS an important player in the increasing problem of chemo-resistance.

Oh, and AGS can also protect you from developing harmful cancer cells in the first place...

## Products:

According to one estimate, it takes about 100 pounds of ginseng to make just one gram of AGS! So AGS supplements are not cheap. Also, remember my warning: beware of the science from people who are trying to sell you something!

That said, here are two sources to start you off:

> Pegasus Pharmaceuticals Group, Inc. of Canada. They produce AGS in both liquid and soft gel formulas. Called Careseng, the product contains a combination of ginseng-derived AGS.

> Another AGS product, called Force C, is available at www.HealthSecretsUSA.com without a prescription.

# 6.6 The Maackia Tree Stalls Some Cancers

An international team of scientists led by Gary Goldberg, PhD, of the University of Medicine and Dentistry of New Jersey-School of Osteopathic Medicine (UMD-NJ-SOM), has found that a protein from the seeds of a plant used for centuries in traditional medicines may be able to halt the spread of melanoma, a lethal form of skin cancer.

On average, melanoma kills one person nearly every hour in the USA, and many more in other countries. The American Cancer Society, with its usual breathtaking lies, claims the overall 5-year survival rate for melanoma is 91%. For localized melanoma, the 5-year survival rate is 97%. BUT THAT'S NOT AN "OVERALL" FIGURE AT ALL! It applies to the tiny percentage that are picked up in time. Once it spreads (stage IV), it's nearer 15%.

Now there may be a solution; a very simple solution at that.

In fact, this new remedy kills or blocks the growth of many other cancers too. But melanoma is particularly dismal because it kills very fast and, apart from maybe Abnoba's homeopathics (section 8.1f) there is no specific treatment; only the general anti-cancer measures I give here.

The remedy in question comes from the seeds of a legume tree, *Maackia amurensis*, a native to parts of Asia.

References to Maackia being used medicinally can be found in ancient Chinese documents that date back more than 400 years. Dr. Goldberg and his colleagues believe that MASL, a specific component found in the plant's seeds, interacts with a particular receptor (PDPN) that is carried by many types of cancer cells.

This is great news, because the PDPN allows tumor cells to break out of their microenvironment, invade new areas and metastasize (metastasis is what causes the vast majority of cancer deaths).

In other words, MASL from the Maackia seeds blocks cancers from doing what cancers do that is most dangerous: spreading to other parts of the body.

But according to Dr Goldberg, that's not all. MASL not only significantly reduces cell migration and metastasis, it also inhibits cancer cell growth.

MASL works at non-toxic doses and levels requires to inhibit tumor growth had no noticeable side effects at doses necessary to inhibit cancer cell growth and migration. Moreover, it can be taken orally. This is good news indeed.

[The findings appeared in the July 23, 2012, edition of PLoS ONE]

Although these studies focused on melanoma, MASL may also be useful to treat and prevent a variety of other cancers that express PDPN. Dr. Goldberg's group has collaborated with the Developmental Therapeutics Program at the National Cancer Institute of the NIH to find that MASL can effectively suppress the growth of lung, breast, prostate, colon, and brain cancer cells that are often resistant to current therapies.

[Gary S. Goldberg *et al.*, Plant Lectin Can Target Receptors Containing Sialic Acid, Exemplified by Podoplanin, to Inhibit Transformed Cell Growth and Migration. PLoS ONE, 2012; 7 (7): e41845 DOI: 10.1371/journal.pone.0041845

# 6.7 Turmeric

Add spice to your years!

The death of Steve Jobs in 2011 added yet another name to the list of celebrities who have died from pancreatic cancer, a group which includes star names, such as Patrick Swayze, Michael Landon, Luciano Pavarotti, and Jack Benny. Pancreatic cancer is the fourth leading cause of cancer-related deaths in the United States and has the highest mortality rate of all cancers, killing 95 percent of its victims, according to the American Cancer Society.

So imagine if a humble Indian spice could help these dismal statistics. Consider Turmeric!

Dr. Robert Wascher, MD, a surgical oncologist from California often prescribes turmeric for his cancer patients. This natural food spice contains a powerful anticancer substance, *curcumin*.

A Phase II clinical trial at MD Anderson Center involved 25 patients with pancreatic cancer who were given 8 grams of turmeric a day for two months. Tumor growth stopped in two patients, one for eight months and another for two-and-a-half years. Another patient's tumor temporarily regressed by 73 percent. Since the only two drugs approved by the FDA are effective in no more than 10 percent of patients, turmeric's effectiveness was similar with no side effects.

In another study, turmeric reduced tumor growth in mice with pancreatic cancer by 43 percent. When combined with fish oil, tumor growth was reduced by 70 percent.

Since turmeric is poorly absorbed by the body, experts advise mixing it with olive oil or a combination of olive oil and black pepper to increase absorption.

Wascher, is author of book "A Cancer Prevention Guide for the Human Race."

[SOURCE: http://www.newsmaxhealth.com/headline_health/ avoid_pancreatic_cancer/2011/10/13/411622.html]

# 6.8 Got Cancer? Take An Aspirin You'll Feel Better!

*Aspirin (salycylic acid), as you may know, was originally a product from willow bark (Salyx alba); that's why I decide to put this fascinating development here among herbal remedies!*

Remarkable as it may seem, humble aspirin has a strong effect against cancer cells. This is in part due to the fact that cancer is part of the picture caused by our "inflammatory fire" (see section 1.6); partly because it has a specific cytotoxic effect—see below.

A study published 2011 showed taking aspirin (salicylic acid) significantly reduced the risk of colorectal cancer. 434 subjects taking just a placebo had an incidence of 30 cancers; 427 subjects taking aspirin daily for at least 2 years had an incidence of only 18 cancers.

That's a remarkable 40% reduction. No fancy expensive drugs can do that, or even come close!

The trouble is, as you know, that aspirin has its problems: it causes intestinal bleeding and ulceration.

But now a "new aspirin" gets round that problem.

Here goes the science: the gut lining protects itself from inflammation ("Fire in the Belly") by secreting nitric oxide (NO) and hydrogen sulfide (SH, stinking rotten eggs gas!) So now Khosrow Kashfi at The City College of New York has developed "NOSH aspirin", a variant that releases its own nitric oxide and hydrogen sulfide, on the spot, where it's needed, so protecting the gut to some degree from the ravages of aspirin.

Great—but does it still knock out cancer? Yup!

Kashfi's team tested their NOSH aspirin against 11 human cell lines, including colon, breast, lung, prostate and the deadly pancreas cancer.

It was not just "as good as" aspirin alone: it was 100,000 more potent! With colon cancer, for example, it caused cancer cells to stop dividing, to wither and die.

Nobody knows yet why NOSH aspirin should have such potent anti-cancer properties. But the good news is that it suggests a far lower—and therefore non-toxic dose of aspirin—would suffice, thus preserving the gut living.

It's very non-toxic in any case. In mice transplanted with human colon cancer, they were fed daily doses sufficient to reduce the tumor size by 85%, yet there was no sign of gut damage.

We could be looking at a human cancer trial within a few years. This is exciting. Who would have thought it; humble aspirin?

[SOURCE: http://pubs.acs.org/doi/abs/10.1021/ml3000020m]


# 6.9 Boswellia carterii (Frankincense)

Famous as one of Christ's first gifts, frankincense may surprise you with possible anti-cancer benefits.

It originates from Africa, India, and the Middle East, and has been important both socially and economically as an ingredient in incense and perfumes for thousands of years.

Frankincense (*Boswellia carterii*) was considered to be a very precious commodity than gold in the time of Christ. In the Middle East, it has been used for religious purposes for centuries and is known as the holy anointing oil. Frankincense also receives a mention in the *Ebers Papyrus*, an ancient Egyptian record of the use of plants for medicinal and aromatic purposes.

Frankincense oil is prepared from aromatic hardened gum resins obtained by tapping Boswellia trees. It contains boswellic acids (various), which have been shown to cause apoptosis of cancer cells, particularly brain tumors and cells affected by leukemia or colon cancer. [http://en.wikipedia.org/wiki/Boswellic_acid - cite_note-1 [Liu, Jian-Jun; Nilsson, A., Oredsson, S., Badmaev, V., Zhao, W., Duan, R. (December 2002). "Boswellic acids trigger apoptosis via a pathway dependent on caspase-8 activation but independent on Fas/Fas ligand interaction in colon cancer HT-29 cells" (abstract page). Carcinogenesis (Oxford University Press) 23 (12):

2087–2093

The goal of another study published in March 2009 was to evaluate frankincense oil for its anti-tumor activity and signaling pathways in bladder cancer cells.

Researchers again found that Frankincense attacked cancer cells vigorously but appeared not to harm normal cells.

The researchers tested Frankincense against mutant human bladder cells (J32) and compared its effects to normal but immortalized bladder cells. What's more it appeared to have a direct genomic effect.

Comprehensive gene expression analysis confirmed that frankincense oil activates genes that are responsible for cell cycle arrest, cell growth suppression, and apoptosis in J82 cells.

However, frankincense oil-induced cell death in J82 cells did not result in DNA fragmentation, a hallmark of apoptosis. So not a total success.

You can read about this study here at the BioMedCentral site:

http://www.biomedcentral.com/1472-6882/9/6/abstract

Since Frankincense is so delightful and it can calm and de-stress the mind, I'm tempted to recommend it specifically as a soothing agent for all cancer cases. It can do no harm.

Lowering stress will do immense good and allow the oppressed immune system to catch it's breath.

# 6.10 And Watch Out For Myrrh!

Myrrh is a yellow gum, which has for centuries been used as a herbal painkiller and for treating stomach complaints and diarrhea (Lord knows why the Wise Kings thought baby Christ needed a bunch!) The bitter-tasting, fragrant resin has also been used for thousands of years as an ointment, perfume, incense and embalming fluid, it can even ward off bad breath.

Now, American scientists are reported to have discovered a new anticancer compound in the resin of the plant *Commiphora myrrha*, which could make it a powerful weapon against prostate and breast cancers.

Chi-Tang Ho of the Department of Food Science, Rutgers University is working with chemists there and colleagues at the University of Medicine and Dentistry of New Jersey and Osaka City University, Japan. The researchers have discovered a property of an extract from myrrh that is a potent anticancer compound.

The researchers have shown that this compound from myrrh kills breast tumor cells in the laboratory, even those that resist current anticancer drugs. Obviously, it will need animal and human trials before it amounts to a therapy. But I thought I'd slip in that interesting Biblical note!

# 6.11 Zyflamend

Zyflamend, developed by a company called New Chapter, is a formulation containing ten different herbs. It is marketed as a dietary supplement for healthy inflammation response and normal cardiovascular and joint function. According to the Sloan-Kettering website, preliminary studies suggest that the ingredients in Zyflamend have anti-inflammatory, antiangiogenic, and antiproliferative properties, so logically it should benefit cancer cases.

Zyflamend is shown to inhibit the proliferation of oral squamous carcinoma, pancreatic cancer and melanoma cells *in vitro* (in glass, meaning in a test tube).

In an animal model, it inhibited the growth of both hormone-sensitive and hormone-insensitive prostate cancer, and reduced levels of prostate specific antigen (PSA).

Zyflamend may potentiate the cytotoxic effects of certain chemotherapeutic agents, including gemcitabine, taxol, doxorubicin and bicalutamide.

You can follow up all 8 citations on the Sloan-Kettering website, noting it does say human data are lacking. [http://www.mskcc.org/cancer-care/herb/zyflamend accessed 10/24/2012 3.10 pm PDT]

According to the National Cancer Institute (USA) website (cancer.gov):

Zyflamend is a dietary supplement that contains extracts of rosemary (Rosmarinus officinalis L.), turmeric (Curcuma longa L.), ginger (Zingiber officinale Roscoe), holy basil (Ocimum sanctum L.), green tea (Camellia sinensis [L.] Kuntze), hu zhang (Polygonum cuspidatum Siebold & Zucc., a source of resveratrol), Chinese goldthread (Coptis chinensis Franch.), barberry (Berberis vulgaris L.), oregano (Origanum vulgare L.), and Baikal skullcap (Scutellaria baicalensis Georgi). The individual components of Zyflamend have anti-inflammatory and possible anticarcinogenic properties.

The individual components of Zyflamend have anti-inflammatory and possible anticarcinogenic properties.

In other preclinical studies, Zyflamend has demonstrated single-agent anticancer activity, and the capacity to be combined with hormonal and chemotherapy agents for improved cancer suppression.

Zyflamend was well tolerated in the previously described 2009 clinical study. Mild heartburn was reported in 9 of 23 subjects, but it resolved when the study supplements were taken with food.

New Chapter, the originators of Zyflamend, has been bought up by Proctor and Gamble, with ties to Monsanto, and the politically-correct loonies have suddenly decided this herb maybe isn't so good, after all. **YOU DON'T CARE**. You want to survive cancer and this stuff has some good pedigree.

I drink Tulsi tea, one of the chief ingredients of Zyflamend, every day. It has almost a holy inscence odor, with just a hint of India. It's manufactured by Organic India and makes a very pleasant change from peppermint, green tea and chamomile.

Read some research apers here: http://www.cancer.gov/cancertopics/pdq/cam/prostatesupplements/healthprofessional/page7

# 6.12 Grapefruit Juice May Aid Anti-Cancer Meds

Some early studies suggest that sirolimus may have tumor-fighting effects. Derivatives of the drug are used in kidney cancer and breast cancer.

But sirolimus has poor bioavailability, meaning it isn't absorbed well and not much gets into the blood (14% or so).

When grapefruit juice is taken concomitantly, absorption was much higher. Do as well as increasing the benefits of this drug, it could allow lower doses and hence cost saving.

Sirolimus costs around $1,000 a month. If it could be combined with drinking grapefruit juice, the cost would drop to about $300 a month.

With cancer drugs costing anywhere from $3,000 to $10,000 per month, here is a mechanism that might allow us to significantly reduce the cost.

But there are wider implications. This is a proof of principle that grapefruit juice could be used in this way.

The report was published Aug. 7 in the journal Clinical Cancer Research. It compared the benefits of adjunct therapy, using grapefruit juice and ketoconazole. The ketoconazole did slightly better, allowing the sirolimus to be reduced to 16 mg a week. With grapefruit juice, 25 mg a week was needed.

That's far less than the toxic standard dose of 90 mg. Serious side effects, such as nausea and diarrhea started above 45 mg weekly, so this is good news for some sufferers.

No-one (including me), is saying that grapefruit juice might make a cancer treatment on its own. But it would certainly be something to take in addition to whatever therapy you may have opted for, whether chemo or holistic alternatives.

[Aug. 7, 2012, Clinical Cancer Research]

# 6.13 Skullcap: Scutellaria baicalensis

One of the most highly regarded herbs in traditional Chinese medicine, and an ingredient of Zyflamend incidentally (page 6.11), is skullcap (*Scutellaria baicalensis*)

It has been extensively researched and shown to have definite anti-cancer properties. You may want to add it to your diet program and supplement regime.

Chinese skullcap is a member of the mint family and grows in China and Russia. Its root is a rich source of over 35 flavonoids, giving it a yellow color - hence its traditional name of golden root or *huang qin*, the Chinese term for yellow gold (known as *ogon* in Japanese).

One of the major flavonoids contained in the root of the plant is baicalein, which is being studied for its anti-cancer, anti-inflammatory, antiviral, antibacterial and anti-allergy effects. Among other effects, skullcap is able to halt the replication of various human cancer cell lines, via the inhibition of the 12 lipoxygenase enzyme system, and this is attracting a great deal of attention from the scientific community.

Skullcap appears to be able to block cell proliferation, induce apoptosis (voluntary cell death) and prevent experimental metastasis. It aids in DNA repair. It is also a powerful antioxidant.

Very interestingly, baicalein inhibits the enzyme 5 alpha-reductase. This is the enzyme which converts testosterone to dihydrotestosterone (DHT), the "male estrogen". DHT is strongly associated with the development of prostate enlargement (benign prostatic hyperplasia) and prostate cancer and so not a good thing.

Great then, that skullcap puts a stop to it. As such, it is potentially useful for the prevention and/or treatment of androgen-dependent (testosterone-driven) disorders, including prostate enlargement and prostate cancer.

# 6.14 Astralagus the Herb That Beats Cancer

Astragalus is a useful immune-boosting herb found in most parts of the world (many species). Chinese version is *Huangqi*; in the Western US, where I live, it's milk vetch or locoweed.

Sloan-Kettering website has interesting well-referenced information:

http://www.mskcc.org/mskcc/html/69128.cfm

Two studies showed it helped block the reduction in immune function that takes place after chemo.

Derived from the root of the plant. This product is primarily used for its immune stimulating properties. In vitro, animal, and anecdotal human data show reduction of immune suppression following chemotherapy.[1] [references at the end of this section] Astragalus-based herbal formulas may enhance the effect of platinum-based chemotherapy (drugs such as cisplatin).[2]

One Chinese analysis (poor standard) showed Astragalus increases the effectiveness of platinum-based chemotherapy for advanced non-small-cell-lung cancer. Thirty-four randomized studies involving 2,815 patients were analyzed. Results suggest that when used in conjunction with platinum-based chemotherapy, Astragalus compounds improved survival, tumor response, performance status, and reduced chemotherapy toxicity when compared with chemotherapy alone.

However, the low quality of the studies analysed is a drawback and the results are therefore, not conclusive. Well-designed studies are warranted.[3]

Astragalus can also delay chemical-induced liver cancer in rats.[4]

Four clinical trials were reviewed to assess the effectiveness of Astragalus compounds on the quality of life, side effects of chemotherapy, and on adverse effects in colorectal cancer patients. A decoction of Astragalus compounds was used in combination with chemotherapy in three studies, whereas the fourth study compared Astragalus compounds with two other Chinese herbal formulas.

Patients who were given Astragalus compounds experienced a reduction in nausea and vomiting along with a decrease in the typical loss of white cells after chemo. Patients receiving chemotherapy alone were controls.

Sloan-Kettering keeps complaining that Chinese studies are of poor quality (true); but what about the very poor quality indeed of most orthodox papers that are trying to hustle in new expensive drug therapies? Those are so bad they are misleading (by intention).

Astragalus appears to work by stimulating several factors of the immune system. The polysaccharides *in vitro* potentiate the immune-mediated antitumor activity of interleukin-2, improve the responses of lymphocytes from normal subjects and cancer patients, and enhance the natural killer cell activity of normal subjects and potentiate activity of monocytes.[6,7]

To date, no significant adverse events have been reported. Patients on immuno-suppressants (e.g., tacrolimus or cyclosporin) should not take this supplement; it wouldn't make sense.

Herbal astragalus preparations should be administered only by oral route.

## References:

1. Qun L, Luo Q, Zhang ZY, et al. Effects of astragalus on IL-2/IL-2R system in patients with maintained hemodialysis. Clin Nephrol. 1999 Nov;52(5):333-4.

2. Tang W, et al. Chinese Drugs of Plant Origin. Berlin: Springer-Verlag; 1992.

3. McCulloch M, et al. Astragalus-based Chinese herbs and platinum-based chemo-therapy for advanced non-small-cell lung cancer: Meta-analysis of randomized trials. J clin Oncol 2006;24(3):419-430.

4. Cui R, He J, Wang B, et al. Suppressive effect of Astragalus membranaceus Bunge on chemical hepatocarcinogenesis in rats. Cancer Chemother Pharma-col. 2003 Jan;51(1):75-80.

5. Taixiang W, et al. Chinese medical herbs for chemotherapy side effects in colorectal cancer patients (Review). The Cochrane Database Syst Rev 2005; (1):CD004540.

6. Shi R, He L, Hu Y, et al. The regulatory action of radix astragali on M-cholinergic receptor of the brain of senile rats. 1 Tradit Chin Med 2001;21:232-5.

7. Cho WC, Leung KN. In vitro and in vivo anti-tumor effects of Astragalus mem-branaceus.Cancer Lett. Jul 8 2007;252(1).43-54.

# 6.15 Graviola

An exciting anti-cancer herbal preparation comes from the seeds, leaves, bark and stem of the South American plant *Annona muricata*, generally known as Graviola. In fact there are many other plants in this genus, various of which yield extremely potent cytotoxic substances. These are especially effective against prostate and pancreatic cancers and work well even against lung cancer.

Much of the research on Graviola focuses on a novel set of phytochemicals called *annonaceous acetogenins* (annonaceous just means from Graviola plants). The potent antitumor properties of these annonaceous acetogenins have been reported and patented.

Purdue University has conducted a great deal of research on annonaceaous ace-togenins, much of which has been funded by The National Cancer Institute and/or the National Institute of Health (just test-tube; none of it clinical trials, please note).

In 1997, Purdue University published information with promising news that several of the Annonaceous acetogenins: "not only are effective in killing tumors that have proven resistant to anti-cancer agents, but also seem to have a special affinity for such resistant cells."

You will hear claims that one exciting study at Purdue showed that an acetogenin in Graviola was selectively cytotoxic to colon adenocarcinoma cells in which it showed "10,000 times the potency of Adriamycin (doxorubicin, a chemotherapy drug)". Once again, the level-headed Ralph Moss comes in with the the real facts:

What Dr. X.X. Liu and colleagues actually stated in 1999 was that: "Annoglacins A and B were selectively 1,000 and 10,000 times, respectively, more potent than Adriamycin against the human breast carcinoma (MCF-7) and pancreatic carcinoma (PACA-2) cell lines in our panel of six human solid tumor cell lines."

**But these were annoglacins, from a different tree altogether!** *Annona glabra*, a Polynesian tree called the pond or alligator apple, NOT Graviola.

There is no question, however, of the power of derivatives of the annona species. Another study showed that six acetogenins (four previously known and two newly discovered) exhibited significant activity in cytotoxic tests against two human hepatoma cell lines.

[tJ Nat Prod. 2002 Apr;65(4):470-5].

Another review in the *Skaggs Scientific Report* 1997-1998 states, "Annonaceous acetogenins…. have remarkable cytotoxic, antitumor, antimalarial, immunosuppressive, pesticidal, and antifeedant activities."

The great thing is that Graviola is pretty non-toxic. The dose required to kill cancer cells is way below that which will injure healthy human cells.

Although the often-quoted finding "10,000 more powerful than chemo" is an over-generous mis-quotation of one narrow finding, there is no reason to doubt that Graviola will benefit more than just colon cancers.

Given it's low toxicity, good science backing it and reasonable market price, I recommend anyone working against their cancer might try it.

But please remember what you get in capsules bought from sleaze-medicine sites on the Internet may bear little relation to the strength of substances used in these trials. That's the problem.

# 6.16 Cranberry Fights Cancer For You

Cranberries deserve a further look. A study by Canadian researchers reporting that cranberry juice inhibited breast tumor growth appeared in 2000 [Guthrie N. Effect of cranberry juice and products on human breast cancer cell growth. *San Diego: Experimental Biology*; 2000] and was followed by a more detailed study showing that an extract of cranberry presscake inhibited proliferation of certain breast cancer cells. [Ferguson P, Kurowska E, Freeman DJ, Chambers AF, Koropatnick DJ. A flavonoid fraction from cranberry extract inhibits proliferation of human tumor cell lines. *J Nutr.* 2004;134:1529–35]

A study published in the *Journal of the Science of Food and Agriculture* showed that cranberry extract (*Vaccinium macrocarpon*) prevented cancer cells from breaking off and spreading to healthy cells. [http://onlinelibrary.wiley.com/doi/10.1002/jsfa.2347/abstract] In addition, it inhibited the growth of human lung, colon, and leukemia cancer cells.

A more recent study from Canada confirmed cranberry's cancer-fighting properties. It causes apoptosis (programmed cell death). Prostate cancer cells self-destructed when exposed to the berry extract. [*Nutr Cancer.* 2011;63(1):109-20. doi: 10.1080/01635581.2010.516876]

Probably best known for treating urinary tract infections, cranberries are a powerhouse of antioxidants. Two flavanols found in cranberries are quercetin and ursolic acid. Both have shown to prevent inflammation and inhibit tumors. [http://nutrition.highwire.org/content/137/1/186S.full]

Cranberries also contain anthocyanins and proanthocyanidins (PACs). It's these compounds that give the berries their scarlet color. They are also potent factors in cancer inhibition. Especially PACs.

Cranberry PACs have a special structure that blocks enzyme activity and pathways leading to cancer. [*J Cell Biochem.* 2010 Oct 15;111(3):742-54. doi: 10.1002/jcb.22761]. As the authors stated in their published paper: " This study further demonstrates that cranberry PACs are a strong candidate for further research as novel anti-cancer agents."

They also interrupt cell signaling that could be harmful to the body.

You definitely don't get apoptosis with chemo; it's just a poison. This is better.

I found another study from the Department of Chemistry and Biochemistry, University of Massachusetts, North Dartmouth, MA which said: "Results from *in vitro* studies using a variety of tumor models show that polyphenolic extracts from *Vaccinium macrocarpon* inhibit the growth and proliferation of breast, colon, prostate, lung, and other tumors, as do flavonols, proanthocyanidin oligomers, and triterpenoids isolated from the fruit. The unique combination of phytochemicals found in cranberry fruit may produce synergistic health benefits. (*in vitro* (in glass, literally) means in a test tube)

"Possible chemopreventive mechanisms of action by cranberry phytochemicals include induction of apoptosis in tumor cells, reduced enzyme activity, decreased expression of matrix metalloproteinases associated with prostate tumor metastasis, and antiinflammatory activities, including inhibition of cyclooxygenases" [cyclooxygenases are the inflammatory substances that NSAIDs block].

This article concluded: "These findings suggest a potential role for cranberry as a dietary chemopreventive and provide direction for future research." [I lightly edited some of the technical words for you]

[http://nutrition.highwire.org/content/137/1/186S.full]

## How To Utilize Cranberries

You can enjoy them fresh, dried, and frozen. Maybe you prefer the juice but it's rather sour; you won't want to be sweetening it with sugar if you are fighting cancer.

When selecting fresh cranberries choose those that are plump and firm to the touch. And don't forget—the deeper the color, the higher the concentration of healing antioxidants.

Cranberries lose some of their nutritional value when cooked. So whenever possible, eat them fresh.

Worst choice is to buy them in pill, liquid, or powder form but they are available that way.

# 6.17 Kanglaite

If you haven't heard already, you will soon come across an anti-cancer therapy called Kanglaite. It's manufactured in China and is pushed by incredible hype and fanfares as a "proven" and "miracle" cure. But we've been there before, haven't we? When commercial interests get on the bandwagon, the inconvenient matter of truth and integrity suddenly get lost in all the brouhaha.

So what are the facts?

Kanglaite was developed by a pharmacist, Li Dapeng. It is made from a plant called Job's tears, a relative of maize. We might think of it as "Chinese pearl barley". The botanical name, for those interested, is Coix lachryma-jobi. Its Chinese name, yi-yi-jen, or yi-mi (in southeast China) is the same as that used for barley, or yang-yi-mi, 'yang' meaning 'foreign', or 'across the ocean'.

Yi-mi is used in soups and gruel and is a common ingredient in many Chinese traditional herbal medicines for treating a variety of ailments including cancer. It has also been widely used as a diuretic, analgesic and antispasmodic agent.

No one knows exactly how Kanglaite works, but the drug has been enthusiastically promoted by Chinese sources.

Standard treatment course for KLT is 200 ml (2 bottles) per day via intravenous drip x 42 days (84 bottles). There is a break for 4-5 days after 21 days. And clinical experiences in China and Russia suggest 2 treatment courses for those with late stage advanced and metastatic tumors for better therapeutic effect and evident prolongation of life.

Both Chinese and overseas clinical experiences have shown that KLT has proven effect in the treatment of cancers mainly at sites of lung, breast, liver, nasopharynx, esophagus, stomach, pancreas, kidney, colon-rectum, ovary and prostate. This agent is also applied in the treatment of malignant lymphoma and acute leukemia. KLT has brought great benefits to over 500,000 cancer patients in more than 2,000 big or medium hospitals in China since 1997.

# Scientific trials of Kanglaite

So what is Kanglaite, exactly? It is a "neutral lipid" of the endosperm of Job's tears, extracted with an organic solvent, such as acetone, and then combined with glycerol and lecithin from soy or egg to make an emulsion in water that can be injected intravenously into patients.

I am always wary of Chinese medicine studies, especially on substances they sell for foreign exchange. Most of it is awful science and a lot of it bordering on ham.

But I can report on an intersting animals study: it was tested against grafted pancreatic cancers in mice and Kanglaite dramatically inhibited the growth of pancreatic cancer xenografts and induced apoptosis simultaneously.

[BMC *Complementary and Alternative Medicine* 2014, 14:228]

There are numerous references to a study supposedly carried out at John Hopkins University, USA, showing tumor-inhibitive rate of KLT on transplanted breast carcinoma induced by cell strain MDA-MB-231 of over 50%. However, I can find no external references to this paper, other than in Kanglaite's own propaganda.

Another study experimental study of counteractive effect of kanglaite injection on cancer cachexia was supposedly successful. But it has never been published and appears only on the website kanglaite.com [http://www.kanglaite.com/images/Basic/12.pdf]

In 2003, FDA approved a US phase I trial. Kanglaite was given to 16 people who had different types of cancer including lung, prostate and oesophageal cancers. The results showed that people did not have many side effects but the effect on their cancer varied. Some people showed no response, and their cancers continued to grow. But in others the cancer stopped growing for a few months.

You can search for data at PubMed (http://www.ncbi.nlm.nih.gov/pubmed) and you will probably come to a similar conclusion to me: articles about kanglaite trials are frustratingly vague, all in Chinese and not totally convinving as to standards.

So, if you buy into the story, I recommend you just get hold of Job's tears seeds, plant some at home and eat it! I'm all for nutritional sources that fight cancer. But if it's that good, why not just incorporate it in everyone's diet. It's cheap and readily available almost everywhere. It ranks—along with wheat and barley in Europe; beans, corn, squash and pepper in the Americas.

# Section 7

## Fungi and Mushrooms

Throughout his career Dr John R. Christopher spent his life in and out of court and in and out of jail. He was handcuffed and taken away after one of his lectures for giving herbs to ease the suffering of a woman with terminal cancer. Usually the jury acquitted him against the instructions. Finally in 1969 he was not so lucky and was given a suspended sentence, because prescribing (suggesting herbs) without a license was a felony.

**Dr Richard Shulze, N.D.**

# 7.1 Reishi

Let's start with the Reishi mushroom (*Ganoderma lucidum*). To the ancient Chinese this mushroom was called *Lingzhi* meaning "spirit plant". According to legend, Taoist priests in the first century were supposed to have included the mushroom in magic potions that granted those who consumed them longevity eternal youth and immortality. In Chinese art the Reishi mushroom is a symbol of good health and long life; symbols of it abound everywhere.

Clinical studies have confirmed Reishi has properties as an anti-inflammatory, antioxidant, BP and blood sugar moderator and cholesterol reduce. Reishi contains over 100 bioactive immunomodulatory substances, along with the beta glucan. One of Reishi's additional properties is that it protects the patient from the side effects of radiation, especially protecting from lowering of white blood cells which can be disastrous.

More importantly, studies have shown that Reishi significantly increases three immune signalers known to help the immune system destroy cancer cells. The macrophages and monocytes and T-lymphocyte all increased their production of TNF alpha, interleukin-1-beta and interleukin-6—but not above normal levels which would be toxic to healthy cells.

Reishi inhibits angiogenesis (the development and growth of blood vessels feeding the cancer) in prostate cancer. It's also effective against bladder cancer, lung, breast and the dreaded hepatoma (liver cancer).

When I say "effective" beware I do not mean it has as good an effect in killing cells as chemo does. But there is a strong measurable effect, due to the increased immune activity it stimulates and, of course, without the obvious toxicity of chemo.

# 7.2 Maitake

Next let's look at Maitake (*Grifola frondosa*). Maitake means "dancing mushroom". In Europe it is known as "Hen Of The Woods " and is sometimes called the King Of Mushrooms because of its size.

Maitake is a delicious culinary mushroom but also valued for its medicinal properties. Once again it has benefits in blood sugar control, cholesterol levels and hypertension. Maitake has been shown to be especially effective in prostate cancer. Scientists tested cancer cells *in vitro* (in a test-tube) against a purified beta glucan extract from Maitake called Grifon-D. After only 24 hours all the prostate cancer cells were dead. What's really interesting is that the scientists then went on to test the mixture of Grifon-D and vitamin C. When vitamin C was present *only 1/8 of the dose of vitamin C was necessary to kill the cancer cells*.

It seems likely then that Maitake combined with chemotherapy could be highly effective and that's exactly what is found. Even when there was little effect on the tumor, the unpleasant side-effects such as loss of appetite vomiting nausea hair loss and pain were much reduced. Maitake is most effective against breast, lung and liver cancers, though less effective against bone and stomach cancers or leukemia.

# 7.3 Turkey tail

Next comes the Turkey Tail mushroom (*Trametes* or *Coriolis versicolor*). Turkey tail is the only known medicinal mushroom with habitats throughout forests worldwide and in North America is the most common wood-recycling mushroom. Its presence in ancient forests here in the USA (now down to just 4% of the primordial forest) makes these remaining woodland habitats a critical scientific, medical and sociological treasure, as well as an awesome botanical heritage.

Turkey Tail mushroom has been the focus of over 400 clinical studies which have demonstrated meaningful antitumor chemo protective and immunomodulating effects. Turkey Tail mushroom contains a unique polysaccharide called polysaccharide-K (PSK) that increases gamma interferon production, improves T-cell proliferation and enhances immune function. Interestingly it has very little effect on normal healthy cells.

You might recognize PSK as the chemo drug "Krestin".

Recent studies indicate that PSK is powerful at destroying tumors by setting up an antigen-antibody specific response. It is usually prescribed to cancer patients who have had a tumor removed surgically and are undergoing subsequent chemotherapy or radiotherapy. It's particularly useful for colon, lung, stomach and esophageal cancer and has virtually no side-effects.

In a 10-year study of 185 lung cancer patients 39% of patients who took PSK survived compared to only 16% in the non-PSK group; that's almost treble the survival rate. Of stage III cancer patients, 22% survived with PSK but only 5% of patients who did not take PSK. That's more than quadruple the survival rate.

In another 10 years study 81% of patients who took PSK survived while only 64.5% of patients with chemotherapy alone survived.

There was a certain amount of euphoria early on about PSK. This needs to be moderated and the current wisdom in the conventional arena is that PSK can very significantly increase survival rates when used in conjunction with chemo or radiotherapy but not necessarily on its own.

I'm speaking about the attitude of my colleagues in Japan, of course. Here in the USA mushrooms are just laughed at or declared a dangerous fraud by the medical profession.

# 7.4 Shiitake

The most famous of all!  It produces a growth inhibiting beta glucan called Lentinan (from shiitake's scientific name *Lentinula edodes*).  Scientific trials of Lentinan organized by the Japanese government's Health and Welfare Ministry (like the FDA) have shown that Lentinan is effective in treating many kinds of cancer. However it does not have any direct anticancer activity.  In other words when Lentinan is put in a test-tube with cancer cells they are not harmed.  But when injected into the body, Lentinan triggers the production of T-cells and natural killer cells which are murderous to cancer.  Thus Lentinan is often prescribed to patients who have undergone chemotherapy and radiotherapy as a means of revitalising the patient's immune system.

Regrettably Lentinan has not been approved by the FDA and so is not available in the USA.  This is ridiculous; Lentinan is very safe and has no significant side-effects at clinical doses.  So you would have to eat a lot of shiitake, but hey, this mushroom is delicious!

# 7.5 Phellinus linteus

*Phellinus linteus* has been a little known mushroom outside the Korean peninsula until recently, so it has no common name. However it's health properties have been long known. Traditionally the mushroom is boiled in water and drunk as a tea but it is also sometimes soaked in wine or whisky before drinking. *Phellinus* is used as an active ingredient in skin creams because of its beneficial effects.

Scientists in South Korea tested *Phellinus* to see if it could work alongside Adriamycin, a common chemotherapy drug (doxorubicin). They especially studied the problem of metastasis—that's the way in which cancer spreads beyond its original site to other parts of the body.

They tested *Phellinus* on mice and found the animals which took only the mushroom had the highest survival rate. With Adriamycin alone, tumor growth was inhibited but it did little to stop metastasis.  The combination of the two was effective in inhibiting tumor growth but did not inhibit the spread.

The scientist's conclusion was that *Phellinus* might be of use in conjunction with chemotherapy drugs such as Adriamycin. I find this baffling, since it did little to prevent the spread of metastasis and the study showed quite clearly that *Phellinus* alone had the best results. But perhaps it's too much to expect that a conventional doctor would recommend a mushroom over orthodox chemotherapy.

*Phellinus*, like most mushrooms, doesn't work by directly killing cancer cells, but by enhancing the immune response. Examples like this tell you, over and over, that the immune system is what kills cancer and it is your most precious resource. Unfortunately it risks harm from chemo poisons and radiation, which is why I counsel you to protect your immune system with every nutrient you can muster, if you choose to go that route.

Incidentally, the website of the Democratic People's Republic of Korea (North Korea) is said to present a table summarizing the clinical results observed in 50 patients with diverse malignancies such as long liver stomach: larynx breast and survival cancers as well as lymphoma. I couldn't find it (very user unfriendly site). In any case, you would expect me to warn young that the Korean government may be trying to enhance the potential export product with fake science. But if it was totally reliable information it would not surprise me, since it aligns with what we already know from credible scientific sources.

Let me now just name a few more species. You can research more of these yourself. Or wait for version 2.0 of Cancer Confidential!

# Other mushrooms with recognized anti-tumor capability are:

Lion's Mane (*Hericium erinaceus*), *Cordyceps sinensis*, Royal Sun Agaric (*Agaricus blazei*), *Agaricus bisporus* (portobello strain) is good for skin cancers, and Chaga (*Inonotus obliquus*).

It just remains to enter a few words of caution:

Firstly, on no account go out and start harvesting mushrooms yourself and trying to make home-brew extracts. You'll likely kill yourself. The Fungi are an enormously large range of organisms and the difference between safe ones and those which kill can be very subtle. It takes an expert to safely identify edible mushrooms.

Of course if you live in France or anywhere civilized which really *knows* food, you can go into any pharmacy and they will identify any mushrooms you gather. But really, you are safer not collecting your own, unless you are a botanist or better still a mycologist (fungologist).

There is an additional problem, which may not be obvious to you, which is getting a predictable dose. It's something which bugs even commercial fungi extracts which you may find for sale on the Net. Let me warn you that the vast majority of products offered are totally worthless, no matter even if the vendor is sincere and well-meaning. It is very difficult to get a regular, effective dose and keep it consistent. Most mushroom "extracts" tested contain little or nothing of worth to you in your fight against cancer.

See, part of the difficulty is that fungi are protected by a membrane coat of chitin. That's same stuff insect cases and your fingernails are made of. Just grinding up mushrooms isn't going to get at the best of the content. It needs a heat extraction process to get at the good stuff, by breaking down the chitin. This, of course, is counter-intuitive to most alternative healers and practitioners, who know that heat normally destroys nutrients.

Let me assure that in this case it's a waste of money, if not extracted properly, and 99% or manufacturers don't even know this, never mind practice it!

My friend Eric Cerecedes in Oregon is the man I most trust for advice and products from fungi. His business is called Mycoformulas:

http://www.mycoformulas.com

Tell him I sent you over!

# 7.6 AHCC and BB12

AHCC stands for Activated Hexose Correlated Compound. BB-12® is a probiotic strain from Denmark that has remarkable immune-enhancing properties.

Let me tell you how powerful this is:

A lady with pancreatic cancer (the worst), a 3 inch tumor, was told it's over; she would die. But she tried this combined remedy and within weeks, the tumor was down to half the size. WITHIN 6 MONTHS IT WAS GONE.

Another woman with inoperable breast cancer took AHCC + BB-12® and her tumor too just vanished. The oncologists at The Memorial Sloan-Kettering Cancer Center were flabbergasted as they called her in to tell her the cancer was totally gone.

## So What Is It?

There are two key ingredients in this revolutionary discovery; each has effects that seem to focus on both the innate and adaptive immune system, including antigen presentation, cytokine production, and immunoglobulin secretion. Each has already been proven to work. But it's when you put them together, you get one of those explosive synergistic things... each one multiplies the other, over and over. It's like 1 + 1 = 2 transformed into 1 + 1 = 88 or 137, or whatever!

In this case, one of the ingredients is a probiotic (haven't I been telling you for years about the power of shutting down the fire in your belly?) Probiotics are BIG; and this one is even bigger than lcr35, the famous probiotic from Aurillac in France (*Lactobacillus rhamnosus* 35). The other coupled agent is a fungus derivative.

BB-12® is a probiotic strain registered to Chr. Hansen Company in Graasten, Denmark and is identified as *Bifidobacterium animalis subsp. lactis*. The strain is classed as GRAS (Generally Recognized As Safe) by the FDA and approved by the Danish Medicines Agency as a natural health product.

The fungus is a mushroom derivative, already known to science: AHCC. Active Hexose Correlated Compound (AHCC) is an alpha-glucan rich nutritional supplement produced from the shiitake mushroom (Lentinula edodes). Lentinan is an intravenous anti-tumor polysaccharide drug, also derived from this mushroom. Lentinan has been approved as an adjuvant for stomach cancer in Japan since 1985.

[Spierings, EL; Fujii, H; Sun, B; Walshe, T (2007). "A Phase I study of the safety of the nutritional supplement, active hexose correlated compound, AHCC, in healthy volunteers". J Nutr Sci Vitaminol 53 (6): 536–539]

AHCC is one of the world's most researched specialty immune supplement and is supported by 20 human clinical studies, by over 30 papers published in PubMed-indexed journals and by more than 100 pre-clinical and in vitro studies.

AHCC was originally designed to lower high-blood pressure. However, researchers at Tokyo University found that AHCC increased natural killer (NK) cell activity in cancer patients, and also enhanced the effects of killer T-cells, and cytokines (interferon, IL-12, TNF-alpha).

When AHCC and BB12 are paired together, that's when this amazing combination emerges. Nobody has seen the like of it before.

## Anti-Cancer Effect

There have been reports of tumor reduction and even cures of cancer using mushrooms and their derivatives, called *beta-glucans*. It has been observed that these traditional remedies may work by up-regulation of the immune system.

[Wasser S, Weis A, Therapeutic effects of substances occurring in higher Basidiomycetes mushrooms: a modern perspective, Crit Rev Immunol 19: 65-96, 1999]

A study published in the Journal of Hepatology compared the outcomes of 113 post-operative liver cancer patients taking AHCC with 156 patients in the control group. The results showed the rate of recurrence of malignant tumors was significantly lower (34% versus 66%). That's down by half!

Patient survival was significantly higher in the AHCC group (80% vs. 52%). That's up by 153%!

It's almost impossible for the naysayers to argue, because actual survival figures were recorded and the patients had all been carefully observed internally at the time of surgery with photographs of tumors and lesions.[ Matsui Y, Uhara J, Satoi S, Kaibori M, Yamada H, Kitade H, Imamura A, Takai S, Kawaguchi Y, Kwon A, Kamiyama Y, Improved prognosis of postoperative hepatocellular carcinoma patients when treated with functional foods: a prospective cohort study, J Hepatology 37(1): 78-86, 2002]

Of course the don't-want-it-to-work faction still try to trash the findings.

In Japan, AHCC is the 2nd most popular complementary and alternative medicine used by cancer patients. Agaricus blazei is the most popular (but it's very liver toxic and I wouldn't take it).

AHCC is widely used in Japan and China. It is used to protect the immune system of cancer patients undergoing chemotherapy and radiation in over 700 clinics and hospitals in Japan alone. Even the Memorial Sloan-Kettering Cancer Center website admits, "In cisplatin-treated mice, AHCC increased its anti-tumor effects while reducing side effects." But as usual complains that "large human studies are lacking".

AHCC is available to the general public in Japan, Asia, the USA and the EU without a prescription and many people use it for general health maintenance and treatment of acute infections. AHCC is marketed as a "functional food", to stay under the radar.

Incidentally, beware MLM companies selling "beta-glucans" which are derived from yeast, NOT mushrooms, and are piggy-backing mushroom science, without any evidence the same properties apply to their cheap-to-make products.

## This Is So Good It Can Master Liver Cancer

Most patients with liver cancer are not operable by the time they are diagnosed. All that orthodox doctors can do is what is called "palliative" treatment, meaning try to keep the patient as comfortable as possible, while they die. It's grim.

Recently, in clinical trials, AHCC was found to improve the prognosis of hepatocellular carcinoma patients following surgical treatment.

Let me report on a 2006 study which investigated whether AHCC could prolong survival and improve the prognosis of patients with advanced liver cancer. Survival time, quality of life, clinical and immunological parameters related to liver function, cellular immunity, and patient status were determined.

Of the 44 patients, 34 received AHCC and received 10 placebo (control) orally, respectively. Patients in the AHCC treated-group had a significantly prolonged survival when compared to the control group. Also, quality of life in terms of mental stability, general physical health status, and ability to have normal activities were significantly improved after 3 months of AHCC treatment.

1.      Unlike the control patients, AHCC treated-patients with longer survival time had the tendency of better outcomes since liver function tests did not show rapid deterioration. This study suggests that AHCC intake could prolong the survival and improve the prognosis of patients with advanced liver cancer and delay the gradual decline of their physiological status. [Asian Pac J Allergy Immunol. 2006 Mar;24(1):33-45]

## The Probiotic

BB-12® (Bifidobacterium lactis 12) is a remarkable strain of probiotic. Bif makes sense, rather than lactobacillus, because about 90% of our natural flora is Bif.

Certain cancers (eg. Colon cancer) can be favored by the introduction of BB12. [Am J Clin Nutr February 2007 vol. 85 no. 2 488-496]

In one study, consumption of BB12 for 3 weeks resulted in doubling of the number of circulating phagocytes showing phagocytic activity [Schiffrin et al., 1997].

## Where Do I Get It?

The combination is called Enhanced AHCC. To get past regulations and appear as a functional food, they call it mushrooms plus yoghurt. Having read this far, you know better than that!

Each sachet of Nn Enhanced AHCC® contains 600mg high potency AHCC® from shiitake mushroom (equivalent to 1,000 mg regular strength AHCC®).

It comes in convenient travel packets, 20 per pack. Each sachet contains 2 gr.

You can get it from www.organiccareproducts.org, an online division of eCosway (launched in 2002), an MLM company with headquarters in Malaysia and outlets throughout Asia, Australia, UK and US. Cosway, the parent company, was founded in 1979 and is a member of the Berjaya Group.

AHCC alone can be ordered from Amino Up in Sapporo, Japan. It's twice the strength of that sold in the USA and elsewhere. Insist you want theirs. It's your life!

[http://www.aminoup.co.jp/e/products/AHCC/]

# Section 8

## Homeopathy: The Safe Approach

While writing the story of Gerson, I couldn't help feeling it was too shocking to believe. The friends with whom I discussed it became almost angry in their denial that anything of the sort could happen in this day and age.

It developed that we were all naïve...there had been dozens of lone scientists...who had been stamped out of existence and driven to spending their last days in solitude and bitterness.

**S.J. Haught**
(Dr. Max Gerson, Censured for Curing Cancer)

# 8.1 Homeopathic mistletoe (Iscador etc.)

A special case of herbal medicine is homeopathy and homotoxicology.

Homotoxicology is a more modern form of homeopathy and is widely used in Germany and elsewhere. Homeopathy was once a major medical discipline in the USA, until the Flexner report of 1910 which closed down 80% of medical schools and recommended that all homeopathic medical schools be closed down because they were not based on real science—he said.

This overlooks that most so-called "science" in medical schools is really propaganda and marketing of drugs, not science. It also overlooks many studies showing that homeopathy is as effective or even more effective than drugs.

The fact is that homeopathy has been around for centuries—a lot longer than drug-based medicine. Moreover homeopathy was getting good results at a time when conventional physicians were still blood letting and using leeches.

Homeopathy is a system that has been described as using like to treat like. It uses diluted therapeutic preparations of substances like *Carcinominum*, which is made from actual cancer cells, to treat cancer.

## 8.1a Mistletoe as Iscador

Did you know that Iscador (homeopathic preparation of mistletoe) is the most commonly prescribed oncological drug in Germany? Actually, according to an entry in Wikipedia entry, some 60% of all oncological treatments in central Europe include some form of mistletoe! That's now been deleted, as the hacks of anti-holism have got their claws into the editing.

Any inconvenient truths are suppressed by the US medical mafia and their media allies.

They cling here to the feeble obsession that the US way is the "only way" and by inference, therefore the correct way. Of course this has more to do with protecting profits than any subsumed moral or scientific right. But it's curious, isn't it, that all humble and inexpensive treatments are "bad", "unproven" or even "dangerous"!

Iscador was originally introduced by German philosopher, educationalist and healer Rudolph Steiner (1861- 1925). Steiner went on to found a whole healing system called anthroposophic medicine—literally "human-loving".

Iscador is actually a lactobacillus-fermented extract of the European mistletoe plant, *Viscum album* and is available here in the USA, by prescription, as the drug Iscar. None of what is written here applies to the American mistletoe, *Phoradendron serotinum* (we just don't know).

# 8.1b History of Mistletoe

Do you know why we kiss under the mistletoe at Christmas? Millennia ago, in the days of the Druids in Europe, Yuletide was a highly celebrated event (it survives as our Christmas, which has nothing to do with Jesus' supposed birthday). The drink and partying went on for days. So did the wild promiscuous sex!

Mistletoe was the chosen contraceptive. A decoction of this sacred plant taken by women gave them a few days in which they could make whoopee, without the inconvenience of becoming pregnant.

Fast forward 3,000 years or more and today we settle for a coy little kiss under a sprig of mistletoe. My, how times have changed!

# 8.1c Anti-cancer properties

The tumor-fighting possibilities of mistletoe have been known for centuries.

As I reported, the use of mistletoe is still widespread in Europe, where it does not need to prove itself. Many cancer patients use natural supplements in conjunction with cytotoxic chemotherapy, but little is known about their potential interaction.

One survey showed that over 60% of all German cancer patients used mistletoe in some form — frequently in conjunction with standard cancer treatments such as radiation, chemotherapy, or surgery.

> [Bussing A: Mistletoe: A story with an open end
> Anticancer Drugs 8:S1-S2, 1997 (suppl 1)]

Formulations are sometimes labeled based on the tree from which the mistletoe was harvested; M for Malus (apple); P for Pinus (pine); Q for Quercus (oak); and U for Ulmus (elm) with different effects attributed to each. Each varietal is considered right for different cancers.

A number of studies published along with two other related papers, in the *European Journal of Integrative Medicine*, showed much the same thing (not quite such good survival):

Renatus Ziegler, a research scientist at Institute Hiscia in Arlesheim, Switzerland and co-author Ronald Grossarth-Maticek studied cervical and ovarian cancer patients to see how they might benefit in the long run if fermented mistletoe extracts, such as Iscador, were added to their treatment regimes.

Over the course of a few decades, cancer patients who received mistletoe preparations lived an average of half a year longer and experienced reduced drug reactions, could better withstand chemotherapy, and had prolonged remission periods.

So the best take-home for this recent study is that it definitely prolongs survival but also improves the quality of life.

On this note, I found a 2005 paper studying the immune system of ear, nose and throat carcinoma patients treated with radiation and chemotherapy that was interesting in the context. It found that adverse effects of radiotherapy and chemotherapy on the microcirculation and the immune system were significantly decreased and reconstitution processes were accelerated by complementary administration of a standardized mistletoe extract (Iscador).

[Anticancer Res. 2005 Jan-Feb;25(1B):601-10].

# 8.1d Potential side effects of Iscador

Side effects at recommended doses are very mild and benign. They include flu-like symptoms, gingivitis, fever, local erythema, and eosinophilia.

Anaphylactic reactions have been reported but they happen with virtual any substance. None of this seem to me to be worth worrying about.

Sometimes there is a skin sensitivity reaction, especially with sun-exposure. Severe reactions are said to have occurred with the use of methotrexate, but that's pretty evil stuff on its own!

This is all that is known and therefore makes Viscum a proven much safer drug than anything in the conventional armoury against cancer. Oncologists take note!

# 8.1e Dosing

Let me make it clear right off that Viscum in all its forms, including Iscador, and especially referring to decoctions of the plant berries, is not a matter for self-administration. This stuff is potentially toxic.

Get yourself a knowledgeable herbalist, homeopath or, better still, an alternative MD who knows all the wider issues of cancer markers etc.

The usual route of administration is by injection of the Viscum just under the skin. Each day of therapy a more concentrated version is administered. After the first few daily doses, a red swelling often appears at the injection site. There may be a transient fever, which most CAM doctors would theorize plays a positive role in the beneficial action of Iscador. Once the maximum-strength dose is reached, the injections are continued regularly, the length of time judged by the treating physician.

Generally speaking, I prefer HEEL's preparation *Viscum compositum*. It is usually recommended to take it with *Echinacea compositum* (from HEEL), alternating every couple of days.

I found this often provoked a fever response, reminiscent of Coley's toxins fever therapy. So it may have a  multiple mode of action.

## 8.1f Abnoba Viscum

Latterly (well, 1990s), Dr. Patrick Kingsley, who I regard as a mentor in this domain, taught me the use of Abnoba's Viscum range.

Abnoba suggest different host trees for different cancers:

So, for example, the apple tree (Malus) is said to be good for breast cancer; oak (Quercus) is used for the gastrointestinal tract and the male sex organs; ash (Frexini) has a high concentration of viscotoxins and lectins in Viscum album, Fraxini can be recommended for the treatment of metastatic tumor diseases.

Dr. Kingsley reported to me a remarkable case of recovery. A man with multiple melanoma had presented as a bowel blockage, caused by a melanoma the size of a baseball in his gut. After resection the patient started on Abnoba Viscum, injected into one of the skin lesions; it began to shrink steadily after each shot. It quickly disappeared and Dr. Kinsley had to choose another site for injection. There were scores of these skin lesions but the interesting thing that happened was that, although the shots were only to one site each time, soon all of them started to recede at once. Eventually, they all disappeared.

To conclude, I found one reasonably well done conventional trial for Abnoba Quercus in the Journal of Oncology, vol 21, no 3, 2004, which said it didn't work. This was on a bunch of cases resistant to all other therapy, so not quite a fair trial! Still, we must acknowledge they tested it (and they chose the correct varietal).

Perhaps the advisory from Abnoba is critical: the selection of the host tree by your doctor, however, also depends very substantially on the treatment plan and above all on the individual disease. In individual cases it may occur that in the treatment of breast cancer that mistletoe from the pine tree (Pini) or Viscum album Abietis (fir tree) is used instead of the frequently employed "Mali" species (apple tree). This is done in order to make the body react in a different way to the different compositions of the ingredients.

# 8.2 Homeopathy Beats Brain Tumors!

It's quite a historic day when a study showing homeopathy works as well as a major (very expensive) drug gets published in a prestigious peer-reviewed journal (*International Journal of Oncology*).

Please believe me, there are some decent doctors and honest scientists out there. Yes, even here in the USA! The spirit of science lives on and good people everywhere want to know the truth about human lives and human health.

It's just the Big Pharma monopoly and their vicious allies in the media that are perverting the real meaning of science.

The study was arranged by Moshe Frenkel MD of the MD Anderson Cancer Center, Houston, Texas. He travelled to India to meet two remarkable doctors: Prasanta Banerji and his son Pratip at their clinic in Kolkata (formerly Calcutta)

In India, homeopathy is BIG. The pharmaceutical industry does not have its stranglehold of lies over medicine there, unlike here in the USA. Doctors are free to tell the truth; they won't lose their jobs. What's more the whole ethos of medicine is looking for simple, safe, effective cures, NOT PROFITS over patient health.

Speaking of his visit to the Banerji Clinic, Dr. Frenkel said, "I saw things there that I couldn't explain. "Tumors shrank with nothing else other than homeopathic remedies...X-rays showing there is a lesion on the lung and a year after taking the remedy it has shrunk or disappeared."

Also impressed was Barbara Sarter, Ph.D., Associate Professor in Advanced Practice Nursing at the University of San Diego, who also travelled to India.

"For the most aggressive and lethal of brain tumors they are able to cure one out of three patients, compared to the five percent cure rate with conventional treatments of surgery, chemotherapy and radiation," she said.

According to the Banerjis' own data, between 1990 and 2005 they treated 21,888 patients for malignant tumors. Although these patients did not undergo any conventional treatment, there was complete regression in 19% and tumors were static or improved in 21%.

Believing he was onto something big, Dr. Frenkel decided to return to the USA and mount a proper study

So: what did this landmark paper show? Four homeopathic remedies, Carcinosin 30C; Conium maculatum 3C; Phytolacca decandra 200C and Thuja occidentalis 30C, had a pronounced cytotoxic effect against two breast cancer cell lines. All four remedies were capable of inducing apoptosis, the "cell suicide" effect that causes cancer cells to self- destruct.

*Phytolacca* is better known as pokeweed root, which grows as a towering weed in the US and elsewhere. *Conium maculatum* is poison hemlock, while *Thuja occidentalis* comes from the Eastern Arborvitae tree. *Carcinosin* is the only non-botanical in the group. It is made from a highly diluted extract of breast cancer tissue.

The trial was conducted by scientists from the Integrative Medicine Program, the Department of Molecular Pathology, and the Department of Melanoma Medical Oncology of MDA, with the cooperation of the Banerjis. The findings appeared in the February 2010 issue of the International Journal of Oncology.

What was especially interesting to me was that the cell-killing effects of Carcinosin and Phytolacca appeared similar to the activity of paclitaxel (Taxol), the most commonly used chemotherapeutic drug for breast cancer, when it was tested in the same two adenocarcinoma cell lines investigated in this study.

The use of poisonous plants to treat cancer is commonplace in orthodox medicine. The periwinkle plant (Vinca) has given us vincristine and vinblastine, two very powerful chemo drugs. The aforementioned drug paclitaxel (Taxol) is derived from the bark of the Pacific Yew tree.

But these compounds are used at full strength and are very toxic to the patient, as well as the tumor. The great benefit of homeopathy is that it is so dilute (which is why orthodox doctors and scientists say "It can't work"), that it is pretty harmless.

"The remedies exerted preferential cytotoxic effects...causing cell cycle delay/arrest and apoptosis [cancer cell death]," the scientists reported. They even found that two of the remedies were similar in their effects to the activity of Taxol, a chemotherapy drug commonly prescribed for breast cancer.

So, next time you hear somebody claim there is no proof that homeopathy works, just remember this study, published in a major peer-reviewed journal!

[Int J Oncol. 2010 Feb;36(2):395-403. Cytotoxic effects of ultra-diluted remedies on breast cancer cells. Frenkel MI, Mishra BM, Sen S, Yang P, Pawlus A, Vence L, Leblanc A, Cohen L, Banerji P, Banerji P.]

Meantime, the British medical establishment has just pronounced there is "no proof" that homeopathy works and has removed financial support for it as a therapy. Taxol costs $20,000 US for 6 rounds of therapy. The homeopathic remedies, $20 for all four! Do you think this makes sense? It makes perfect sense if the British Establishment is controlled by Big Pharma money and takes bribes!

# The NCI Approves

The doctors Banerji began testing homeopathy for cancer patients in 1992. In late 90s they gave a six hour presentation on 16 cases of brain tumor regression before oncologists from leading American cancer centers at an international conference. I wasn't there.

But the National Institutes of Health (NIH) asked them to submit records of successful cases for their "Best Case" program. This allows practitioners outside conventional medicine to present data for appraisal.

After detailed evaluation by the National Cancer Institute (NCI), four cases were accepted for publication in the journal Oncology Reports in 2008. Two of these patients presented with cancers of the esophagus and two with lung cancer. All four became symptom free and enjoyed highly positive outcomes. None of the four patients received any conventional treatment.

The NCI found the results were "sufficient to warrant further research". So don't say that all of orthodoxy is on a mission to destroy viable alternatives.

There's more: in a study also published in the International Journal Of Oncology, homeopathy was proven highly effective against glioma. An incredible 6 out of 7 patients made a total recovery!

Glioblastoma multiforme is a highly aggressive brain tumor whose prognosis is very poor. Due to early invasion of brain tissue, its complete surgical removal is nearly impossible, and even after aggressive combined treatment (association of surgery and chemo- and radio-therapy) five-year survival is only about 10%.

All the more remarkable then that homeopathy worked at all. But such staggering success is a triumph for natural healing methods. Of course the orthodox criticism is that the number of patients in the group was small. Nevertheless, the authors were bound to admit, the outcome of homeopathic treatment was highly encouraging and novel. [*International Journal Of Oncology* 23: 975-982, 2003]

Naturally, this outstanding result has been totally ignored by the medial fascists, who still scream and roar that homeopathy is "totally implausible" and a fraud.

[Scientific paper, University of Texas: http://www.virtualtrials.com/pdf/ruta6.pdf]

# 8.3 Mulla Mulla (Ptilotus)

We've been hearing good things about *mulla mulla*, a flower essence remedy. You can get it from Ian White of Australian Bush Flower Essences and Healing Waters in the USA. He's a Naturopath and fifth generation Australian herbalist.

Flower Remedies are not new. The Australian Aboriginals have always used flowers to heal the emotions, as did the Ancient Egyptians. There has also been a very long tradition of use of Flower Essences in India, Asia and South America and they were also very popular in Europe in the Middle Ages.

Hildegard von Bingen (12th century) and Paracelsus (15th century) both wrote about how they collected dew from flowering plants to treat health imbalances.

This healing method was rediscovered by Dr. Edward Bach sixty years ago through the use of English flowering plants.

Today, according to White, our society and its needs are totally different to that of sixty years ago. There has been a great need for remedies that would help people deal with the issues of the 21st century - sexuality, communication skills, cancer, pollution and spirituality to name but a few.

Mulla Mulla is used for burning and heat. That would include sunburn, fire burns and radiotherapy burns. It can also be used, incidentally, for hot flashes, fevers or any kind of burning body sensation.

The obvious use for cancer patients is as a protective against radiation burns from the therapy. It can be very harsh and burn the gullet and internal organs, as well as the obvious surface burns. Mulla mulla reduces this unpleasant side effect and can quickly heal any lesions that may occur.

If you accept the radiotherapy route, order some immediately:

**From the formulator:**
Ian White
Bush Biotherapies Pty Ltd, trading as Australian Bush Flower Essences
45 Booralie Road, Terrey Hills NSW 2084,
Australia
Phone: 61 2 9450 1388


**And for those in the USA:**
Healing Waters

1933 Meadowview Drive NW
Albuquerque, New Mexico 87104  USA
505-934-3861
HealingWaters@EssencesOnline.com

Take 7 drops in the morning of treatment and repeat the dose again, just before you go in for the radiotherapy.

PS. Do not forget the radiation healing effect of n-butanol, discovered by the greatest cancer genius, Emanuel Revici (see chapter 10.1). It has been shown especially effective in cases of clumsy overdoses and burns (not rare!).

# 8.4 Homotoxicology

Homotoxicology requires less specialist and intuitive skills than its older homeopathy counterpart.

Despite a clumsy name, homotoxicology is a wonderful natural healing science. It is a therapeutic branch which enables deep cleansing of the body tissues, removing old toxins, disease processes and degenerative debris, leaving the fluids clean, fresh and able to function as intended.

Based on homeopathy, but not quite the same thing, homotoxicology is the brain child of German doctor Hans-Heinrich Reckeweg (1905-1985). Drawing on a vast knowledge of herbal lore and medicines, he compounded a store of remedies which trod a line between folk medicine and basic plant pharmacology. In the course of time it has proved itself so well that tens of thousands of German doctors use it in daily practice, although less well known in the rest of the world. It has been also called the German system of homeopathy, though this is slightly comical, since the original system of homeopathy was also invented by a German, Samuel Hahnemann.

Whereas so much molecular medicine is aimed at the cell, as if it were the sole seat of disease, Dr. Alfred Pischinger, then professor of Histology and Embryology in Vienna, saw with great insight that the extracellular fluids were the key to health. These fluids, which Pischinger called the "matrix", or ground, because it supports everything else, brings nutrition, oxygen, hormone messengers and other vital substances to the tissues and removes excretion products, toxins and the residue of old diseases.

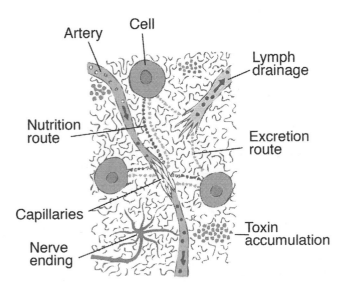

Cells may be important but not a separate entity, because they cannot exist without being nurtured in this matrix.

Reckeweg adopted Pischinger's matrix idea and devized ways to use natural substances to support, clean and revitalize the extracellular matrix. Most of the classic homeopathic remedies are still there, though used slightly differently.

The key difference from "classical" homeopathy is the use of mixtures, which classical homeopaths frown upon. But Reckeweg ignored the dogma and carried out decades of practical research, demonstrating conclusively that the mixed formulations worked and worked well. He made compounds which would support the liver and kidneys, which would work for flu, diabetes, women's problems, stimulate metabolism, tone up the immune system, retard tumors, repair inflammation, act as pain-killers and so on. In other words these are function-based medicines. The mixtures give rise to yet another name you may encounter "complex homeopathy". Not all remedies are mixtures of substances however; some are single remedies in a mixtures of potencies (called a "chord", after the musical term for several notes sounding at once).

Homotoxicology has a lot to offer in the battle against cancer. I have explained how progressive deterioration of the body's own cleansing system leads to gradual compromise of the defence mechanisms. Eventually, as the process nears an end and the "biological age" of the body tissues (the biological vitality of the tissues, as opposed to the calendar age), neoplasms or cancer changes are seen as almost inevitable on this model. It makes sense, then, that reversing this process will gain valuable points in the fight against a tumor. The more you help the body recapture its lost biological age, the better it can compete with the invasive cells. It's like turning back the clock!

A basic attack would be to use a detox formula and liver support (there are several), Lymphomyosot, or similar mesenchyme cleanser, and a general anti-viral (more and more cancers are being found to have a viral basis), specific detoxes for acquired vaccine abuse of the immune system (a complex job, requiring skilled medical advice), then tissue stimulants, such as glyoxal and Psorino-heel, and finally, as the situation warrants it, some Viscum preparation. I use HEEL's own Viscum compositum, and alternate it with an Echinacea complex (again, this is a compounded formula, with 25 other ingredients than the Echinacea).

# 8.4a Viscum Comp. and Other Ingredients

Viscum comp. contains two other active ingredients which are important. The first is adenosine tri-phosphate (ATP), which is there to bring cell metabolism back into line. Cancer cells misbehave and if they can be persuaded to act more like normal cells, then we are getting somewhere. ATP stimulates hormonal and cell membrane activity right inside the cell itself.

Mercury iodide is also included, which has strongly anti-viral properties. Quite simply, almost all switched-on doctors today believe that many (maybe even all) cancers are mediated by viruses, such as the papilloma virus. Remember viruses are bits of DNA bad news creating mischief, like alien genes, as I've seen them called. It's a small step for them to get locked into cellular DNA and when that goes wrong...why that's all cancer is, really: unruly DNA leading to loss of cell integrity and runaway multiplication.

One further detail, mercury is administered as the iodide because that stimulates the thyroid gland (homeopathically) and speeds up the metabolic process. But it goes deeper than this; there is some unknown cross-over between thyroid disorder and cancers. Thyroid malfunction comes up time and time again with malignancy. I can't explain it, but somebody will, some day soon. Certainly thyroid function bears importantly on the performance of the immune system, so it makes plenty of sense.

You see there are many powerful herbal modalities which may help you safely overcome cancer, using Nature's own natural and gentle recovery methods. It brings real healing, not brutal slash and burn and poison, like surgery, radiation or chemo!

I repeat what I said several times already: there is absolutely no reason why you can't run these alternative modalities side by side with orthodox treatments if you feel too scared to abandon them. HEEL does a wonderful detox remedy of three components. You can find them at www.heelusa.com or www.biopathica.co.uk

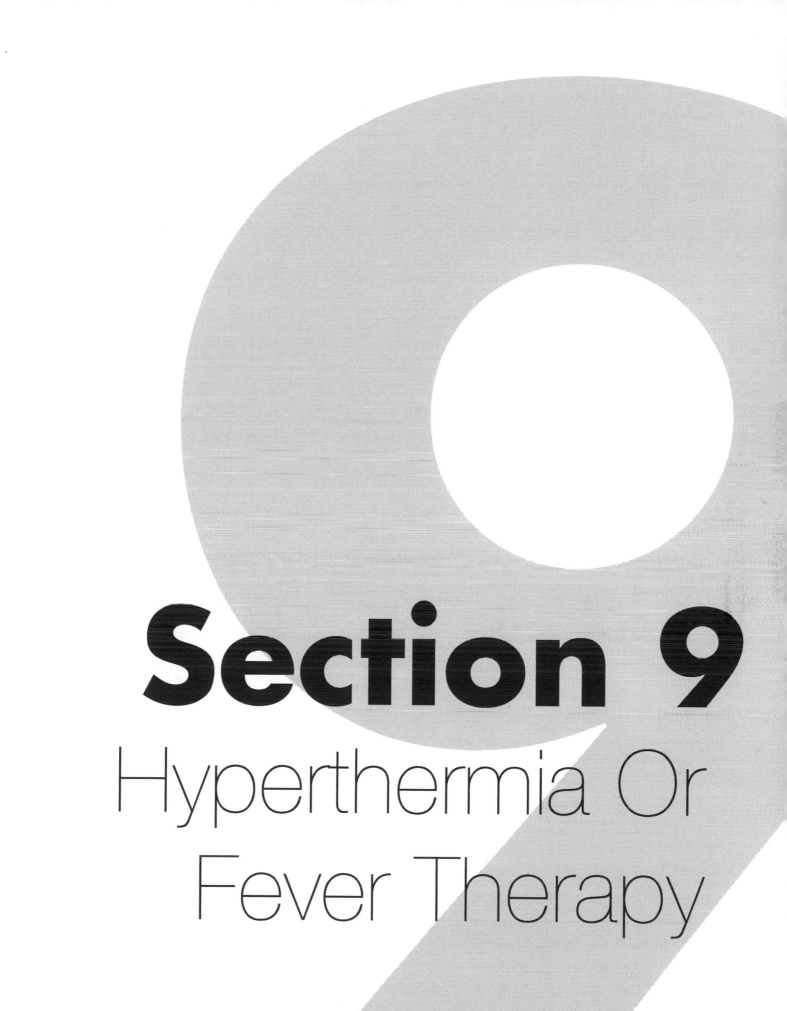

# Section 9
## Hyperthermia Or Fever Therapy

On two occasions Gerson became violently ill...
Lab tests showed...arsenic in his urine. Some
of Gerson's best case histories mysteriously
disappeared from his files...Gerson was invited
on a talk show by host Long John Nebel...Nebel
was fired the very next day and the radio
network was threatened by the AMA.

**Norman Fritz**

# 9.1 Coley's Toxins Treatment

Hyperthermia as a treatment specifically for cancer was first proposed by nineteenth century US physician Dr. William B. Coley, MD. He used very toxic bacteria waste products from *Streptococcus pyogenes* to generate the high temperature. The results were very encouraging and the treatment still, rightly, bears the name of Coley's Toxins Fever Therapy.

In 1888, Coley (1862-1936), a Harvard Medical School graduate, and eminent New York City surgeon and Sloan-Kettering researcher, stumbled across one of the most intriguing findings ever made in cancer research: high body temperature seems to help the knockout process.

Frustrated after losing his first patient at Memorial Hospital, a 19 year old female bone cancer patient, despite an early detection followed by prompt amputation of her arm and a good prognosis, Coley began methodically searching the patient records at New York Hospital. He went back 15 years and examined records of all bone cancer patients. Most cases ended in failure and death. However he discovered one patient who had been given up for lost by his doctors and yet had walked out of the hospital apparently cured.

This patient had suffered two attacks of erysipelas, a severe skin infection caused by bacteria *Streptococcus pyogenes*. Coley reasoned that this might have been what led to the cure.

He decided to try and induce delibaterate fever with *Strep. Pyogenes*. His first attempts ended in failure. Later, working with a more virulent mix, he was able to develope a severe case of erysipelas with high fever. Within a few days the patient's tumors completely disappeared.

In 1893 Coley published his first paper on the new method.

[Coley, William B. "A Preliminary Note on the Treatment of Inoperable Sarcoma by the Toxic Product of Erysipelas."Post-graduate 8:278-86, 1893]

Using live bacteria was very dangerous (this was in the age before antibiotics, remember) and Coley later tried to and succeeded in improving his method. Instead of using live bacteria, he mixed the toxins of the strep with those of another germ, *Bacillus prodigiosus*, which today is called *Serratia marcesens*. This seemed to work similarly to the live culture.

Pharmaceutical company Parke-Davis produced the toxins commercially for many years, but they heated the formula, which reduced its effectiveness. Despite that, even this weakened form of toxins, *Parke-Davis formula IX, showed 37 percent cure rate for inoperable patients.*

A randomized trial of patients with nodular lymphoma (now known as follicular lymphoma) was discussed at a 1983 conference. Of the patients who received Coley toxins and chemotherapy, 85% had a complete response, in which all signs of cancer disappeared. This was compared with a 44% complete response rate in the patients who did not receive Coley toxins. Nodular lymphoma is among the cancer types that respond well to modern immunotherapy with monoclonal antibodies, however, so the relevance of this study to modern oncology practice is uncertain.

The FDA finally denounced Coley's therapy and Parke-Davis ceased production. It survives now mainly as an adjunct of Issel's therapy (see section 10.2).

It isn't a pleasant therapy to undergo, by any means, and the patient feels just as you would expect: feverish, chills, shaking, muscle aches and even nausea. But it passes, and is considerably less unpleasant than chemotherapy!

# 9.2 Viscum Fever Therapy

A slight variation on fever therapy I like and have used a lot combines a mild fever therapy with the properties of viscum related above (section 8.1). I use *Viscum compositum* from HEEL-GMbH in Germany.

The BIG advantage, to my mind, over Coley's toxin therapy is that even if you don't get the unpleasant fever, you are still doing an immense amount of good against the cancer (see section 9.1), whereas bacterial toxins have little else to offer beyond raising the temperature.

Because of the essentially low-dose composition of the homeopathic medication, we can give it in a sustained way, pushing the defences until they get mobilized. This is seen by the onset of the patient's own curative fever, which is a sure sign that the body is fighting back (another important medical principle which drug-handy doctors seem to overlook).

This fever is so valuable that I do not give even biological or herbal remedies to counter it but try to pour the fuel on somewhat and get it higher! The exact details vary from patient to patient and need not concern us here. But by alternating with another very powerful immune stimulant *Echinacea comp. forte* (a fortified homeopathic preparation, not the common herbal drops you may buy at the health shop or pharmacy), we can generally stoke up the fire quite well. It's one of those odd moments for a doctor when the patient feeling rough is what we want.

# 9.3  Hyperthermic Technology

Finally, the idea of hyperthermia as a treatment has been taken into the technological domain. Treatment centers are using different types of energy to apply heat, including microwave, radiofrequency, and ultrasound in order to deliberately create high tissue temperatures. Radiofrequency ablation (RFA) is a type of interstitial hyperthermia that uses radio waves to heat and kill cancer cells. This is reminiscent of Rife technology (section 11.9).

A number of cancer centers also offer treatment based on perfusing the tumor itself with heated liquids, avoiding the need to heat up the whole body. That's a relief!

Hyperthermia (also called thermal therapy or thermotherapy) is a treatment in which body tissue is exposed to high temperatures (up to 113°F). Research has shown that high temperatures can damage and kill cancer cells, usually with minimal injury to normal tissues (US cancer-gov site: http://www.cancer.gov/cancer-topics/factsheet/Therapy/hyperthermia accessed 9/24/2015, 1.51 pm PDT).

It is almost always used with other forms of cancer therapy, such as radiation therapy and chemotherapy. Hyperthermia may make some cancer cells more sensitive to radiation or harm other cancer cells that radiation cannot damage. When hyperthermia and radiation therapy are combined, they are often given within an hour of each other. Hyperthermia can also enhance the effects of certain anticancer drugs.

Most clinical trials have studied hyperthermia in combination with radiation therapy and/or chemotherapy. Many of these studies, but not all, have shown a significant reduction in tumor size when hyperthermia is combined with other treatments.

As the NCI website says, "A number of challenges must be overcome before hyperthermia can be considered a standard treatment for cancer. Many clinical trials are being conducted to evaluate the effectiveness of hyperthermia. Some trials continue to research hyperthermia in combination with other therapies for the treatment of different cancers. Other studies focus on improving hyperthermia techniques."

However, at least they are not hostile to the idea.

## What are the different methods of hyperthermia?

Several methods of hyperthermia are currently under study, including local, regional, and whole-body hyperthermia.

In local hyperthermia, heat is applied to a small area, such as a tumor, using various techniques that deliver energy to heat the tumor. Very high temperatures can be used, since most of the body is not affected.

Depending on the tumor location, there are several approaches to local hyperthermia:

In regional hyperthermia, various approaches may be used to heat large areas of tissue, such as a body cavity, organ, or limb.

Deep tissue approaches may be used to treat cancers within the body, such as cervical or bladder cancer. External applicators are positioned around the body cavity or organ to be treated, and microwave or radiofrequency energy is focused on the area to raise its temperature.

Regional perfusion techniques can be used to treat cancers in the arms and legs, such as melanoma, or cancer in some organs, such as the liver or lung. In this procedure, some of the patient's blood is removed, heated, and then pumped (perfused) back into the limb or organ. Anticancer drugs are commonly given during this treatment.

Continuous hyperthermic peritoneal perfusion (CHPP) is a special regional technique used to treat cancers within the peritoneal cavity (the space within the abdomen that contains the intestines, stomach, and liver), including primary peritoneal mesothelioma and stomach cancer. During surgery, heated anticancer drugs flow from a warming device through the peritoneal cavity. The peritoneal cavity temperature reaches 106–108°F.

Whole-body hyperthermia is used to treat metastatic cancer that has spread throughout the body. This can be accomplished by several techniques that raise the body temperature to 107–108°F, including the use of thermal chambers (similar to large incubators) or hot water blankets.

There are few side effects, the obvious one being burns and blisters.

# 9.4 Scientific proof

Here are some selected references I culled from the US official cancer.gov site:

1. van der Zee J. Heating the patient: A promising approach? Annals of Oncology 2002; 13:1173–1184.

2. Hildebrandt B, Wust P, Ahlers O, et al. The cellular and molecular basis of hyperthermia. Critical Reviews in Oncology/Hematology 2002; 43:33–56.

3. Wust P, Hildebrandt B, Sreenivasa G, et al. Hyperthermia in combined treatment of cancer. The Lancet Oncology 2002; 3:487–497.

4. Alexander HR. Isolation perfusion. In: DeVita VT Jr., Hellman S, Rosenberg SA, editors. Cancer: Principles and Practice of Oncology. Vol. 1 and 2. 6th ed. Philadelphia: Lippincott Williams and Wilkins, 2001.

5. Falk MH, Issels RD. Hyperthermia in oncology. International Journal of Hyperthermia 2001; 17(1):1–18.

6. Dewhirst MW, Gibbs FA Jr, Roemer RB, Samulski TV. Hyperthermia. In: Gunderson LL, Tepper JE, editors. Clinical Radiation Oncology. 1st ed. New York, NY: Churchill Livingstone, 2000.

7. Kapp DS, Hahn GM, Carlson RW. Principles of Hyperthermia. In: Bast RC Jr., Kufe DW, Pollock RE, et al., editors. Cancer Medicine e.5. 5th ed. Hamilton, Ontario: B.C. Decker Inc., 2000.

The most recent study I could find is from Rolf Issels, MD, PhD, professor of medical oncology at the Klinikum Grosshadern Medical Center at the University of Munich (not to be confused with Josef M. Issels, in the next section). He presented the results of regional hyperthermia (RHT) at a press conference in Berlin (September 23, 2009). This was part of Europe's largest cancer congress. The final results were surprisingly robust.

Prof. Issels reported on 341 patients with high-risk sarcomas who received a standard chemotherapy regimen consisting of three drugs: etoposide, ifosfamide and Adriamycin. Half of the patients were then randomized to receive hyperthermia before and after their chemotherapy. The median follow-up time was 34 months.

Adding RHT to chemotherapy reduced the risk for recurrence or death by an astonishing 42 percent. Patients who were assigned to the combination treatment survived an estimated 120 months before progressing compared to 75 months for those who were assigned to chemotherapy alone.

There were other signs of the benefit of adding heat to conventional treatment. After two years, 76 percent of patients assigned to the combination therapy were alive without local progression compared with 61 percent of those assigned to chemotherapy alone. Tumor shrinkage occurred in just 12.7 percent of patients assigned to chemotherapy alone vs. 28.8 percent assigned to combination therapy. In addition, tumor growth occurred in 6.8 percent of those assigned to combination therapy vs. 20 percent of those assigned to chemotherapy alone.

Prof. Issels described this as "the first - and the only completed - randomized study on neo-adjuvant chemotherapy in high-risk soft tissue sarcoma showing that the addition of regional hyperthermia significantly improves the overall response rate, time to progression, local progression free survival, and disease free survival."

# Section 10

## The Good, The Controversial and The Not-So-Bad

Gaston Naessens's trip to hell was a direct consequence of his having dared to wander into scientific incognita...In 1985 he was indicted on several counts, the most serious of which carried a potential sentence of life imprisonment.

**Christopher Bird**

# 10.1 Emanuel Revici: The Doctor Who Cured Cancer

Emanuel Revici's contribution to the cancer story is unsurpassed by any other doctor and, yes, I include Otto Warburg, who received a Nobel prize for his work; Revici never did, not because he wasn't worth one--he was worth several--but he lived and worked in the USA, where he was fought almost to a standstill by powers that did not want a cancer cure.

Revici has now passed on. But his legacy hasn't. The amazing work and cures he succeeded with are still around. You can share and benefit from learning about them.

Most who knew Revici considered him to be a towering genius. Even Albert Einstein was reported to have referred to him as the "greatest mind he'd ever come across in his lifetime." And you can be sure Einstein met some serious smarts!

Gerhard N. Schrauzer, Ph.D. (Professor of Chemistry, University of California, San Diego), an authority on selenium, credited Revici with "having discovered pharmacologically active selenium compounds of very low toxicity." Schrauzer went on to acclaim Revici as "an innovative medical genius, outstanding chemist and a highly creative thinker."

Another notable scientist counted 113 new scientific discoveries by Revici, at least 7 or 8 that could have won him a Nobel Prize, had he better connections and more mainstream support. Instead, Revici chose to battle alone against the Cancer Establishment, which brought nothing but bitterness and hostility, instead of the acclaim he so justly deserves.

As a Jew, he left Germany to avoid Hitler's reign of terror. For a time he served with the French Resistance. He was twice offered the French Legion Of Honor, a prestigious medal of recognition, almost equivalent to the British knighthood. He declined on both occasions.

Eventually, Revici settled in Mexico City in 1941, where he established and directed a FREE clinic for cancer patients. Throughout the 60-year long "there is no cure for cancer" scam of America perpetuated via the FDA, the CDC (Centers for Disease Control and Prevention), and the AMA (American Medical Association), several renowned doctors and scientists have recognized Revici for the genius he was. Professor Joseph Maisin, Director of the Institute of Cancer, and former Director of the International Union Against Cancer, found Revici's medications "effective in numerous terminal cases refractive to other treatment."

During World War II, Revici successfully treated the cancer of the wife of the Soviet Ambassador to Mexico. He was offered the Stalin Decoration and $50,000. He turned them both down. That's the measure of the man.

## Short Bio

Dr. Emanuel Revici (1897- 1998), the Scientific Director of the *Institute of Applied Biology*, N.Y., from 1946 to 1990, was no "quack." Many of Revici's findings predate ideas that are now widely accepted. Revici received his doctorate in medicine and surgery from the University of Bucharest (Romania) in 1920. He concentrated on biochemical research, specializing in the relationship between lipids and normal and abnormal cellular metabolism. Many of his studies took place at academic and hospital laboratories. Five papers deposited in the National Academy of Sciences summarize his observations about the influence of lipids in pathological pain and cancer.

He died in 1998 at the grand old age of 101. I have sledom regretted not meeting a colleague so much as never making it to the USA while he was alive.

## Revici Found That Alkalized Blood Will KILL 50% Of Patients

The dangerous and underperforming Internet fools, who like to tout their pet theories without a shred of scientific support, have repeatedly claimed that Revici proved that alkalizing blood is a sure-fire cure for cancer.

IN FACT HE DID NO SUCH THING. Read the rest of this paragraph carefully, or you may end up putting yourself or someone you love at risk, due to circulating ignorance on this topic. What he did show was that HALF the patients will benefit from this approach. But the other HALF needed to acidify to beat the cancer. If you mix up the two halves and alkalize or acidify the wrong bunch, you will greatly accelerate their cancer.

Revici came by this important effect by noticing that some of his patients reported pain in the morning while others suffered at night. Some patients relieved pain by eating, but for others, pain was intensified by eating. Revici surmised that this could be associated with physiologic cycling, so he studied a variety of aspects of blood and urine.

He found healthy patients had daily rhythmic fluctuations with urinary pH and their levels of free potassium in the blood, where the cancer patients did not have these normal fluctuations and exhibited patterns of either acidic or alkaline imbalances.

He developed a test which consists of measuring urine pH from two specific time periods: 4.00 am to 4.00 pm (daytime) and 4.00 pm to 4.00 am (nighttime). Normally, Revici found, urine is acidic (6.0 or below) in the 4.00 am to 4.00 pm 12 hours; but then at 4.00 pm the pH of urine moves to over 6.2 (more alkaline).

This in itself was an interesting discovery; science had always believed the pH variation was random (so nobody bothered to check, till Revici came along)!

The obvious step was to compare this healthy pattern with what happens with cancer patients. He also had the patients record their pain symptoms.

What he found was fascinating: patients who lost the acidic part of their cycle in the daytime, experienced more pain in the mornings and early afternoons. Revici called this the "acid pain pattern". The other group, who lost the alkaline part of their cycle (nighttime), experienced much more severe pain in the late afternoon and evening hours. He called this the "alkaline pain reaction".

What is worth noting is that each group of patients experienced their worst pain at the time when the abnormal urinary pH set in. There was a quantitative element to this too: the worse the pain, the larger the pH abnormality.

Revici went on to experiment and found that administering alkali (bicarbonate) to patients with the acid pattern was helpful and similarly administering acid (dilute phosphoric acid) to alkali patients helped. The pain was dramatically reduced... but only temporarily. Still, it was a start.

[W. Kelley Eidem, *The Doctor Who Cures Cancer*, Huge Health Secrets Publishing, 1997, pp. 35-37]

# Why Cancer Surgery Can Be Dangerous

There are implications to this far beyond just tumor growth. For example, Revici found that certain things consistently produced the alkaline pain reaction: trauma to the tissues, broken bones, burns or surgery. He thought that this was the probable reason why the cancer of some people flares rapidly after surgery. If these people were in the alkaline pain pattern group, surgery could almost condemn them to death. He published a suitable warning as long ago as 1961 but he was ignored.

Today, if a patient experiences a fast recurrence at the site of a surgery, or a new cancer arising somewhere else, surgeons and oncologists respond with a shrug and the attitude that it was just "bad luck". The idea that the surgery itself was to blame is unthinkable to a conventional doctor.

Revici's advice was that surgery could have a limited place: for patients with localized tumors, with no metastases and whose pattern is acid. Outside of that group, it's far more risky than ignorant surgeons can admit.

And might not this effect also apply to tissue trauma caused by chemo and radiation. Why not?

Having read this, you would be crazy to subject yourself to any kind of intervention, without insisting on Revici's acid-alkali urine test protocol.

## Lipids For Relief

Recognizing that interventions based on amino acids, ions, or proteins would not change pH long enough for meaningful relief, Revici then developed a method of altering pH with lipids. Lipids provide important functions in the body, including storing energy, insulating the body, and serving as a cushion to protect organs (as with phospholipids). Revici was the first pioneer to understand just how valuable essential fatty acids are for immune health, as well as cell-wall integrity and top condition of the nerve trunks.

He redefined these important substances, describing the importance of the polar (charged) and non-polar regions of these molecules which is a key component of currently accepted definitions. In contrast to the prevailing wisdom concerning bioactive molecules, he observed that many of these molecules contained adjacent carbon atoms that carried identical charges, and this played a crucial role in his design of medicines.

Decades before Bengt Samuelsson reported on leukotrienes, earning a Nobel Prize, Revici essentially described them, indicating their crucial role in inflammation. [Samuelsson B, Leukotrienes. Science. 1987;237:1171-1176]. Revici was so far ahead of his time (1950), he was mocked and hounded but, of course, modern science backs up everything he was saying—because he was right! [Revici E, The influence of irradiation upon unsaturated fatty acids. Paper read by Robert Ravich, MD, before the Sixth International Congress of Radiology, London, 7/26/50]

It's a sad injustice.

## Two Kinds Of Cancer

These are already more than enough discoveries for a lifetime. One can see the point, that he could have been awarded several Nobel prizes, if he had been given the right support he deserved.

But there's more. He basically identified two types of cancer: the *catabolic* and *anabolic* types. Don't be scared of these two words: anabolic means building up the tissues (like the anabolic steroids that athletes use when cheating); catabolic means breaking down tissues. Our bodies function best as a balance of the two. We need to break down old, unwanted tissues and replace them with built up new substance.

Catabolic agents cause an alkaline shift. Anabolic agents cause an acid shift. These pH observations are not causative but secondary. It is pointless taking alkaline solutions (or acid solutions, if you have the alkaline pain pattern). You need to remedy the cause, not the result. Duh!

However the administration of catabolic agents in laboratory animals appeared to markedly reduce the spontaneous appearance of cancers. Conversely, the administration of anabolic agents seemed to bring on cancers. Sodium chloride is anabolic; magnesium and bivalent sulfur or catabolic.

But it was not totally simple.

Either form of cancer is essentially a break with nature's harmonious balance. Each type needs a different approach. Revici developed non-toxic preparations from both catabolic and anabolic substances, in various proportions and strengths. Agents included selenium, copper, sulfur, zinc, calcium, nickel, beryllium (recognized as a carcinogenic substance), and poisons, such as lead and mercury.

The point is that Revici used very small traces of these substances, with a general toxicity level of less than 1/1,000th of the normal.

His ingenuity went further than that. For example selenium is a recognized anti-cancer mineral. But it becomes very toxic at doses above 200 mcg. Yet Revici found a way to get 1 gram (1,000 mcg) into patients, without harmful effects, by combining selenium with lipids, creating a product suitable for injection. Lipids are not soluble in blood, which is aqueous; toxicity problem solved! (actually the selenium-lipid compound of Revici's has been used at does of 1 million mcg. quite safely).

## Metabolic Tuning

It is important to understand that Revici's answer to cancer is not the "killer compound" approach, in the way that Laetrile purports to be, or Ukrain or 714-X.

Instead, the idea is to eliminate the dysfunction that allowed the cancer to develop in the first place. His approach has been validated numerous times by peers. In 1984 Edouardo Pacelli MD, a physician practicing in Naples, Italy, presented his findings on the use of Revici Therapy with 372 cancer patients, representing six different types of cancers. None of the patients studied were considered curable at the start of the treatment. Of these patients, 186 had lung cancer. Revici Therapy produced a cessation of the coughing up of blood for 75% of the lung cancer patients, pain reduction or elimination for 80%, and regaining of proper body weight after three months for 75%. Average survival time increase from 80 days 272 days; however 45% survived well beyond the expected years.

Of 53 stage IV breast cancer patients, 80% received either pain reduction or elimination with a doubling of survival time. For 57 patients with intestinal cancers, life expectancy jumped from an average of 60 days to 245 days, with 21 patients outlasting the study.

Uterine cancer accounted for 27 patients. Their life expectancy had been estimated at 90 days, but under Revici Therapy, this extended to 270 days, with some outlasting the study. In addition, 71% experienced significant pain reduction and a doubling in their quality-of-life from 35 to 70 (out of 100). Results of an equivalent nature were obtained for patients with liver and stomach cancers.

Seymour Brenner, MD, a board certified radiation oncologist practising in New York City, examined the medical records of 10 patients treated by Dr. Revici. In presenting these case at the March 1990 meeting of the advisory panel for the *US Office of Technology Assessment*, Dr Brenner publicly stated that he believed these 10 patients to be examples of successful treatment with Revici Therapy, citing evidence of tumor regression, survival greater than expected, and enhanced quality-of-life.

[Office of Technology Assessment. Emanuel Revici And Biologically Guided Chemotherapy (Washington, DC: US Government Printing Office, 1990)

In 1996 Dr Brenner declared: "Dr Revici has cured many people who were otherwise considered incurable. It is my professional opinion that his medicines have worked for many of the patients whose records I have examined."

Its interesting to note that Dr Brenner at one time allowed Revici to treat him for elevated prostate specific antigen (PSA). His PSA at the time was 6.2 (less than four is considered safe). After taking Revici's medication for one year, his PSA had dropped to 1.6 and stayed low thereafter, even after discontinuing therapy.

The largest study of Dr Revici's work was fairly early on and was conducted by Robert Ravitch MD, who worked with Revici at his *Institute Of Applied Biology*. Dr Ravitch's study focused on 1,047 cancer patients who were treated at the Institute between 1946 and 1955. Most were either "far advanced" or "terminal" cases and had already been treated by conventional means, but without success. Accordingly, the majority of this study population were expected to die.

When they were treated with Revici Therapy, 206 responded well to the treatment and of these, 100 had both favorable objective and subjective responses.

[Ravitch, RA. Revici method of cancer control: evaluation of 1,047 patients with advanced malignancies treated from 1946 to 1955. New York Institute of Applied Biology, unpublished manuscript, cited in the definitive the *Alternative Medicine Definitive Guide To Cancer*, Diamond, Cowden and Goldberg, Future Medicine publishing, Tiburon, CAA, 1997)

## Further Reading:

There really is too much to write about this remarkable man. To learn more, you are advized to get and read The Doctor Who Cures Cancer, by Kelley Eidem, Huge Health Secrets Publishing, 1997]. You can get a copy here:

It is also worth reading Revici's entry in Burton Goldberg's massive compilation: The Alternative Medicine Definitive Guide To Cancer, Diamond, Cowden and Goldberg, Future Medicine publishing, Tiburon, CAA, 1997.

Revici's own book is, to own the truth, very difficult to read. You won't stand a chance with an errata sheet. The Crazy Pharmacist (a pseudonym) has produced one, which you can download here: http://thatcrazypharmacist.com/?author=1

To find out more about current manufacture of Revici's formulations, contact Lynn August. She worked directly with Revici and has the secret of his methods. She can be reached at:

Health Equations
P.O. Box 323
Newfane, VT 05345
Ph: (802) 365-9213
Fax: (802) 365-9218

Toll free: (800) 328-2818

e-mail: service@healthequations.com

## Conclusion of the Story

NCI and AMA collaborated to ruin Revici. In 1962 they laid a trap. They convinced Revici to collaborate with two separate oncologist groups associated with two medical institutions in New York City. Their protocol divided the investigators into two groups - one group observed patients who were resistant to mainstream therapy and were treated by Revici himself, but the other group observed patients that who administered Revici's treatment at a different hospital. Of course, the unsupervized group did not conduct the protocols correctly.

Each group was supposed to publish their conclusions separately. But instead the sneaky oncologists combined both reports into one, concluding that "no benefit resulted" from Revici's treatment of any of the 33 patients studied. The lousy group wiped out the obvious benefits from the group Revici personally supervized. Another triumph for grubby medical "ethics".

The findings were published in JAMA (Journal of the American Medical Association) in November of 1965. The National Cancer Institute (NCI) and the AMA simply conspired to bury the cure for cancer.

This deprecatory conclusion devastated Revici's practice and his rebuttal, outlining the mischief, was of course rejected by JAMA. Revici later proved that several patients in the study had tumor remissions that the study group allegedly failed to recognize. In his published rebuttal, documents did show that the two clinical assessment groups violated the protocol by merging into one group and signing their names to one report.

Ironically, New York's Office of Professional Medical Conduct (OPMC) later revoked Revici's license to practice in 1993 for "not adhering to conventional oncology practice". What? Was he supposed to criminally manipulate findings too, like his attackers? One concludes that in the cancer arena, lying, criminality and cover ups are not grounds for professional discipline; only honest success will get you into trouble!

# 10.2 Issels Immunotherapy

Cancer is seen, in many ways, as a disease of the immune system. With a fully functioning immune system, cancer would never get started. The most intelligent breakthroughs in conventional medicine are also leaning in this direction.

Things will change fast (I hope) and you may not be limited to the treatments in this report for very long (except in the USA, where you may be waiting indefinitely). Meantime, though, if you want to check out Dr Josef M. Issels immunotherapy treatment, it has a good history. From 1981 until his retirement in 1987, Dr. Issels served as an expert member of the German Federal Government Commission in the Fight Against Cancer.

Issels therapy is well-respected for success with patients who had exhausted all standard treatments. The range has included advanced cancers of the bladder, bones, brain, breast, cervix, colon, liver, lung, ovaries, prostate, stomach, testicles, thyroid, sarcomas, lymphomas, and leukemias.

Treatment also significantly reduced the rate of recurrence from 50 percent, according to world statistics, to 13 percent thereby increasing the cure rate from 50 to 87 percent.

The Issels treatment has also been able to reverse or improve chronic degenerative diseases such as arthritis, Grave's disease, systemic lupus, Sjoegren's syndrome, etc. No orthodox cancer treatments do that!

## Aspects of Issel's Treatment

- Coley's mixed bacterial vaccine opens blockades in the body matrix (all solid, semi-solid and fluid connective tissues), stimulates the production of the body's own interferons, interleukins, colony stimulating factors, tumor necrosis factor and other potent disease fighters.

- Issels' autologous vaccine and biologicals work in a very complex way to "jump-start" the immune system. They are prepared from the patient's own blood and body fluids which represent his/her own unique internal environment. The preparation follows procedures that favor the development of antigenic peptides and other immunogenic compounds in the fight against cancer and other immune disorders.

- Extracorporeal photopheresis (exposure of blood to UV light, outside the body, which is then returned IV) with the dendritic cell vaccine, (FDA approved for cutaneous T cell lymphoma due to the research by Richard L. Edelson, Yale University,) works in the following way:

- Via the photopheresis apparatus pathologic immune complexes can be removed from the blood and a certain quantity of blood is exposed to a controlled amount of ultraviolet energy, which has an enormous immune boosting effect. During this procedure dendritic cells can be collected and separately cultured to maturity and re-infunded into the patient's vein.

- Dendritic cells are responsible for identifying pathogens (viruses, fungi, bacteria, malignant cells) and presenting their identifying markers, antigens, to key lymphocytes that then multiply and attack the disease.

- Photopheresis induces monocytes to transform into dendritic cells, thereby greatly increasing their numbers. By centrifuging blood in a cell separator and passing the white cells through the ultraviolet light chamber, millions of monocytes are converted into dendritic cells. By culturing them with growth factors, these cells can learn to ingest and process pathogens that formerly eluded the immune system. Thus, when they are re-introduced to the body, they awaken sleeping immunities.

- Nutritional immunotherapy, blood oxygenation, glandulars, bontanicals, enzyme therapy aid cellular metabolism, tissue and organ function.

The Issels Treatment has a long and successful track record in cancer immunotherapy history. Even so, take care. Clinics delivering the therapy now are not necessarily as scrupulous as Issels was.

[Falk MH, Issels RD. Hyperthermia in oncology. *International Journal of Hyperthermia* 2001; 17(1):1–18.]


# 10.3 Ukrain

Ukrain was first developed in 1978 by Dr. Wassyl J. Nowicky, director of the Ukrain Anti-Cancer Institute of Vienna. It is a mixture of Greater Celandine (*Chelidonium major*) and an old and long-established cytotoxic drug, thiotepa. The idea is that the combination of the two makes treatment effective at far lower doses than the usual toxic amounts of thiotepa.

The plant *Chelidonium major* has been known for centuries in Russia as a cure for cancer. It contains alkaloids with known anti-cancer activity. In this respect it is worth remembering the periwinkle plant (Vinca major), which has given us two modern cytotoxic drugs, vinblastine and vincristine.

Ukrain has been tested at the US National Institute for Cancer against over 60 lines of human cancer cells and found that in every case it arrested growth 100%. It seems that Ukrain causes a drop in utilization of oxygen. Normal cells are able to recover within a few minutes but for cancer cells this change is irreversible. They literally suffocate to death. Animal studies show that Ukrain is also a powerful stimulant of the immune system.

Unfortunately, Ukrain is not available in mainstream medicine and holistic doctors who use it are few and far between, unless you want to travel to Eastern Europe.

# 10.4 Amygdalin (Laetrile)

I was half inclined to put this in the no-no section, along with other treatments that are a waste of time. I see no valid evidence that this treatment works at all. Everybody who raves about it was doing some other therapy at the same time. You cannot measure real effects that way.

Amygdalin is NOT the reason that the Hunzas saw little or no cancer; their natural diet assured that, as with many other races with simple lives but ate no apricots. *Cancer Is Not An Apricot Deficiency* was the title of one of my take-downs of this prennial therapy!

Amygdalin is a chemical cyanide-like substance found in apricot and other kernels, apple seeds, lima beans, clover, and sorghum. In fact there are two types of lactrile: a patented product, Laetrile®, which is semi-synthetic, and laetrile/amygdalin manufactured in Mexico, which is made from crushed apricot pits.

Laetrile is used world wide against cancer, except in the USA, where it is not approved by the FDA. They say it doesn't work and you may begin to suspect a political angle to this strange limitation of choice. While ever employees of major drug companies sit on the FDA board, no-one sensible would trust the objectivity of FDA views.

Once again the Internet has swept into the niche market and there are countless websites to sell you laetrile at a hefty price (considering it is only crushed nuts). Many clinics have sprung up, especially over the US border into Mexico, to service patients who hope that laetrile will work for them. But does it do any good?

As I said, the evidence is scant... Amygdalin was first isolated in 1830 by two French chemists and was used as an anticancer agent in Russia as early as 1845. Its first recorded use in the United States as a treatment for cancer occurred in the early 1920s but it was judged too toxic and studies ceased.

In the 1950s, a supposedly non-toxic intravenous form of amygdalin was patented as Laetrile® and in the 1970s the patented and natural forms enjoyed a vogue. But as the National Institutes for Cancer points out on its laetrile web page (http://www.nci.nih.gov/cancer_information) no unequivocal evidence has yet been forthcoming.

Perhaps the best that has been shown is that benzaldehyde, which is made from laetrile in the body, does have success against cancer cells. Also, by using the antibody/enzyme trick described above to carry amygdalin right to the tumor target cells (the "smart bomb"), its killing effect was 36 times greater than for amygdalin alone.

Finally, amygdalin was shown to sensitize some cancer cells to radiation, which would in theory help someone who had opted for radiotherapy.

You must examine the evidence and make up your own mind. Remember one study showed that laetrile made patients worse (but only one). Laetrile should only be administered by a knowledgeable physician and there are few. It can be prescribed orally or by intravenous infusion.

Side effects of laetrile therapy are those of cyanide poisoning: nausea and vomiting, headache, dizziness, bluish discoloration of the skin due to oxygen-deprivation, liver damage, abnormally low blood pressure), difficulty walking due to damaged nerves, fever, mental confusion, coma, and eventually death. Surprisingly, the oral form is much more toxic than the IV route, so don't suppose that the products you are being offered on the Internet are the safest way to take it.

Foods claimed to contain amygdalin (some with only tiny traces) are notable for being good fresh sources of vitamins, minerals and anti-oxidants. I doubt amygdalin has anything to do with it.

These include: Apple seeds, alfalfa sprouts, apricot kernels, bamboo shoots, barley, beet tops, bitter almond, blackberries, boysenberries, brewer's yeast, brown rice, buckwheat, cashews, cherry kernels, cranberries, currants, fava beans, flax seeds, garbanzo beans, gooseberries, huckleberries, lentils, lima beans, linseed meat, loganberries, macadamia nuts, millet, millet seed, peach kernels, pecans, plum kernels, quince, raspberries, sorghum cane syrup, spinach, sprouts (alfalfa, lentil, mung bean, buckwheat, garbanzo), strawberries, walnuts, watercress, yams.

I would say eat well, fresh food and lots of antioxidants, and it's unlikely you'll get any more therapeutic benefit by paying for expensive laetrile.

# More On Laetrile!

This article blogged by me provoked a lot of response. It's amazing how many people want to defend this Laetrile (amygdalin) hokum.

One colleague even quoted research by Dr. Kanematsu Sugiura, the scientist who performed the requested tests at the Memorial Sloan-Kettering Cancer Center. He claimed that laetrile inhibited secondary tumors in mice, though it did not destroy the primary tumors. He repeated the experiment several times with the same results (he says).

However, three other researchers were unable to confirm Sugiura's results. While these uncontrolled and inconclusive results were considered too preliminary to publish, they were leaked to laetrile advocates, resulting in significant public uproar that here was an amazing new cancer "cure" being "suppressed".

From that day forward, I don't think anybody in alternative medicine (except me!) followed along with the science. It was a proven deal, that laetrile worked.

Well, it wasn't. What's more, the basic requirements of science were not met. There has to be reproducibility. If others can't copy what you did, chances are, you are WRONG.

But in this story it's even odder because Sugiura disproved himself; he was unable to duplicate his own results.

MSKCC researchers conducted a further controlled experiment in which they injected some mice with laetrile (as Sugiura had done) and others with placebo. Sugiura, who was unaware of which mice had received laetrile, performed the pathologic analysis. In this controlled, blinded follow-up, Sugiura himself was unable to tell which mice had received laetrile and which had placebo.

Subsequently, laetrile was tested on 14 tumor systems without evidence of effectiveness. Given this collection of results, MSKCC concluded that "laetrile showed no beneficial effects."

The Sloan-Kettering press release was, unfortunately, somewhat flawed and this has led to the widespread belief that there was some kind of cover up. Ralph Moss believes there was. I do not believe so.

Why?

Because no other decent science has ever been able to show amygdalin works. What is more It is highly toxic and does not deserve its false reputation of being safe. Amygdalin releases cyanide and there are reported cases of cyanide toxicity among people who overdose on apricot kernels (something the Hunzas never did, by the way). This is exactly like the orthodox approach: something toxic that kills cancer cells. Yes they do die! But only when amygdalin is taken in sufficient quantity to put the patient at risk too.

That's exactly the same as chemotherapy! Think about it...

## It's Just Chemo In Disguise!

Laetrile is laevo-mandelonitrile-beta-glucuronoside and is NOT the same as amygdalin. That's another perpetuated myth. I marvel that people dedicated to holistic treatments, who wouldn't take chemotherapy from a doctor, will take chemotherapy in the form of laetrile. It doesn't make sense!

The humbug started with Dr. Ernst T. Krebs. He is clearly what we British call a "chancer" or perhaps charlatan. During the influenza pandemic of 1918, he apparently became convinced that an old Indian remedy made from parsley was effective against the flu. He set up the Balsamea Company in San Francisco to market his nostrum as Syrup Leptinol, which he claimed was effective against asthma, whooping cough, tuberculosis and pneumonia as well.

During the early 1920s, supplies of Syrup Leptinol were seized by the FDA on charges that these claims were false and fraudulent. See, even if it did work (I'm sure it didn't), Krebs didn't seem too bothered with science, just turning a dollar.

During the 1940s, Krebs was at it again, promoting Mutagen, an enzyme mixture containing chymotrypsin, which he claimed was effective against cancer. No evidence was produced.

He and his son also patented and promoted "pangamic acid" (later called "vitamin B15"), which they claimed was effective against heart disease, cancer, and several other serious ailments. There is no vitamin B15. Krebs, Sr., died in 1970 at the age of 94.

Ernst Krebs, Jr. has often been referred to as "Dr. Krebs" although he has no accredited doctoral degree. He attended Hahnemann Medical College in Philadelphia from 1938 to 1941, but was expelled after repeating his freshman year and failing his sophomore year. After taking courses in five different colleges and achieving low or failing grades in his science courses, he finally received a bachelor of arts degree from the University of Illinois in 1942. In 1973, after giving a 1-hour lecture on Laetrile, he obtained a "Doctor of Science" degree from American Christian College, a small, now-defunct Bible college in Tulsa, Oklahoma. The school, founded by evangelist Billy James Hargis, had no science department and lacked authority from Oklahoma to grant any doctoral degrees.

So the son was such a crappy scholar, he failed to qualify as an MD by any honorable route. Ernst Krebs, Jr. doesn't meet my standards as a medical science leader: more like a phoney, wanting desperately to make dollars and having spotted a market "niche".

[Bruzelius, NJ. The merchants of Laetrile. Boston Sunday Globe, June 17, 1979]

The lack of science is highly revealing.

In 1977, Harold W. Manner, Ph.D., chairman of the biology department at Loyola University in Chicago, achieved considerable notoriety by claiming to have cured mammary cancers in mice with injections of Laetrile and proteolytic enzymes and massive oral doses of vitamin A.

What he actually did was digest the tumors by injecting digestive enzymes in amounts equivalent to injecting a woman with a pint of salt water containing about 1 1/2 ounces of meat tenderizer every other day for six weeks. Not surprisingly, the mice developed abscesses where the enzymes were injected, the tumors were liquefied, and the injected tissue fell off.

No microscopic examinations were conducted and the animals were observed for only a few weeks following treatment, no legitimate assessment of this type of therapy could have been made.

In response to political pressure, the National Cancer Institute did two studies involving Laetrile. The first was a retrospective analysis of patients treated with Laetrile. Letters were written to 385,000 physicians in the United States as well as 70,000 other health professionals requesting case reports of cancer patients who were thought to have benefited from using Laetrile. In addition, the various pro-Laetrile groups were asked to provide information concerning any such patients.

Although it had been estimated that at least 70,000 Americans had used Laetrile—only 93 cases were submitted for evaluation. To me, the fact that there were only 93 cases out of tens of thousands speaks volumes. It doesn't work! Otherwise they would have produced at least 2,000- 3,000 successes.

Twenty-six of the 93 reports lacked adequate documentation to permit any evaluation. The remaining 68 cases were "blinded" and submitted to an expert panel for review, along with data from 68 similar patients who had received chemotherapy. The panel felt that two of the Laetrile-treated cases demonstrated complete remission of disease, four displayed partial remission, and the remaining 62 cases had exhibited no measurable response.

I think that 2 cases out of over 50,000 is *proof positive that laetrile doesn't work*.

A 2006 systematic review by the Cochrane Collaboration concluded: "The claim that laetrile has beneficial effects for cancer patients is not supported by data from controlled clinical trials. This systematic review has clearly identified the need for randomised or controlled clinical trials assessing the effectiveness of laetrile or amygdalin for cancer treatment.

The Cochrane database project is a not-for-profit international cooperation, designed to combine medical science databases from over 100 countries.

[Milazzo S, Ernst E, Lejeune S, Schmidt K (2006). Milazzo, Stefania. ed. "Laetrile treatment for cancer". Cochrane Database Syst Rev (2): CD005476. doi:10.1002/14651858.CD005476.pub2. PMID 16625640.]

# But What About Those Cases Who Recovered?

I get letters from cancer victims who claim they were cured and therefore laetrile works.

Sadly, this proves nothing. While I'm glad for any story of recovery, it is wrong morally and scientifically to hijack the story and claim that laetrile was the real cause. As I revealed on page 9, the "Norway Study" published in 2010 showed that if just left alone a significant number of people recover naturally from cancer.

You have to prove that what you were doing was not one of these lucky outcomes. You would also have to prove that the patient did nothing else at the same time. If anyone changes their diet and takes laetrile, I know for sure which one would produce the cure: diet. It's PROVEN, over and over.

So I'm sorry to prick any bubbles. Don't write me that YOU recovered. I'm glad for you. It doesn't prove laetrile works; it only proves you have a good immune system!

Anyway, it's time to draw a line under laetrile, I think.

# 10.5 Antineoplastons and Burzynski

Sometimes it's hard to separate personality cult from science. Undoubtedly, Stanislaw Burzynski MD, PhD. enjoys a lot of the former. But what about the latter?

In May 1977 Burzynski founded the Burzynski Clinic in West Houston, Texas where he has since treated over 8,000 patients. He founded the Burzynski Research Institute in 1984, where he continues research on antineoplastons. Burzynski is the author or co-author of more than 250 publications, including 66 scientific publications. He holds many US patents for his treatments and inventions.

Antineoplastons are a group of synthetic compounds that were originally isolated from human blood and urine by Burzynski. He has reported using antineoplastons to successfully treat patients with a variety of cancers. In typical response, the FDA wants to see him jailed for life.

In 1991, the National Cancer Institute (NCI) conducted a review to evaluate the clinical responses in a group of patients treated with antineoplastons at the Burzynski Research Institute in Houston.

The medical records of seven brain tumor patients who were thought to have benefited from treatment with antineoplastons were reviewed by NCI. This did not constitute a clinical trial but, rather, was a retrospective review of medical records, for their "best case series." The reviewers of this series found evidence of antitumor activity, and NCI proposed that formal clinical trials be conducted to further evaluate the response rate and toxicity of antineoplastons in adults with advanced brain tumors.

Investigators at several cancer centers developed protocols for two phase II clinical trials with review and input from NCI and Dr. Burzynski. These NCI-sponsored studies began in 1993 at the Memorial Sloan-Kettering Cancer Center, the Mayo Clinic, and the Warren Grant Magnuson Clinical Center at the National Institutes of Health. Patient enrollment in these studies was slow, and by August 1995 only nine patients had entered the trials. Attempts to reach a consensus on proposed changes to increase accrual could not be reached by Dr. Burzynski, NCI staff, and investigators, and on August 18, 1995, the studies were closed prior to completion.

At present, the Burzynski Research Institute is conducting trials using antineoplastons for a variety of cancers. Information about these trials is available from the Cancer Information Service or on the NCI's Cancer.gov Web site at http://www.cancer.gov/clinical_trials on the Internet.

In Jan 2009 The Food and Drug Administration (FDA) reached an agreement with the Burzynski Research Institute, Inc., for the design of a phase III trial of antineoplaston therapy for the treatment of diffuse intrinsic brainstem glioma, a rare but highly aggressive form of childhood brain cancer.

You can surf Internet and watch the emotive 2010 movie *Burzynski* directed by Eric Merola. It documents Burzynski's efforts to gain FDA approval for the therapy. Now there's a second part: *Burzynski Part II: Cancer is Serious Business.*

# Antineoplastons

Dr. Burzynski first discovered new peptides (short amino acid chains) in human blood in the late 1960s during his doctoral work in biochemistry at the Medical Academy in Lublin, Poland.

He found that these peptides, while present in healthy humans, were almost non-existent in the blood of patients with advanced cancer, so it was natural to theorize that returning them to the bloodstream of cancer patients might fight the disease.

Initial studies in the U.S. in the 1970s showed the peptides exhibit anti-cancer activity in vitro (i.e. in a test tube) with little to no toxic side effects on healthy cells.

He was also able to reproduce the peptides synthetically while creating several different versions based on the varying types. The most common and widely studied are intravenous A10 and AS2-1, which can be delivered orally or through an IV.

He named the peptides antineoplastons (ANP), drawn from the word *neoplast*, meaning cancer cell. Cancers are also known as neoplasms.

Dr. Burzynski's research is based on the notion that cancer is caused biochemically, by "increased activity of oncogenes and decreased expression of tumor suppressor genes." I think many doctors would agree with him there; at least it's certainly part of the mechanism.

"Antineoplastons work as molecular switches," Dr. Burzynski wrote in a 2006 paper. They regulate two different genes, p53 and p21. p53 is particularly well-known and has been described as "the guardian of the genome" because of its role in conserving stability by preventing genome mutation. [Read, A. P.; Strachan, T.. Human molecular genetics 2. New York: WIley; 1999. ISBN 0-471-33061-2. Chapter 18: Cancer Genetics] p21 is an anti-proliferator, which essentially reminds cells to die.

Safety of antineoplastons was confirmed by Japanese researchers in 1995. They also concluded that A-10 and AS2-1 are "less toxic than conventional chemotherapeutics." In addition, they reported "disappearance or measureable shrinkage of the tumor" with significantly longer survival rates. [http://www.ncbi.nlm.nih.gov/pubmed/8667595]

However, safety studies aren't meant to prove efficacy.

## Efficacy

In 2014, Dr. Burzynski published the results of 14 clinical trials begun in the 1990s. Many of them spanned over ten years. At first glance, the results don't seem that impressive, but there are a few things to keep in mind:

The people Dr. Burzynski works with all have rare forms of brain cancer. They're usually incurable or at the very least difficult to treat. These are "last chance" patients. Barring any miraculous remissions, these patients would have had a 0% survival rate.

Plus, patients are legally required to have "failed" chemo, surgery, or radiation before being allowed into the trial. They'd been living with their disease for some time while going through other—often toxic—side effects.

So, in the cases of incurable, inoperable, advanced stage cancer, anything is better than 0%. One study followed children with recurrent high-grade glioma. Out of the 15, two had a complete response, two had a partial response (50% decrease or higher), and three achieved stable disease. One patient survived 10 years after treatment. [http://www.burzynskimovie.com/images/burzynsk/JCT_BT-06.pdf]

According to the authors, "4 out of 15 patients is a sufficient number of successful cases to show adequate antitumor activity for initiating phase III testing."

Another study of 17 children with DIPG, two cases were deemed implossible to evaluate; there was one complete response, four partial responses, two with stabilized disease, and eight who developed progressive disease. Again, still frustratingly close to the mark but not out-and-out success. [http://www.ncbi.nlm.nih.gov/pmc/articles/PMC4223571/]

A phase II study published in Cancer and Clinical Oncology in March 2015 was performed on recently diagnosed adults with anaplastic astrocytoma, a rare and nasty cancer with ten-year survival rates between 4% and 17% and low quality of life for patients who elect conventional treatment.

Of the patients in the trial, four were cured, five achieved stable disease, and nine experienced progressive disease. Those who survived had a high quality of life, and no chronic toxicity. [http://www.ccsenet.org/journal/index.php/cco/article/view/42461/24998]

**This is impressive, considering the starting condition of these unfortunate patients. However... and this HAS to be said... remember in section 1.4, I told you some cancers will resolve, no matter what, even if the patient is at death's door.**

So, I still cannot give a wholesome endorsement. You must choose. There are lots of simple, inexpensive and proven alternatives and Burzinski is very expensive ($7,000 to $9,500 per month). Not that I am suggesting it's a rip off; these things cost money. Only that it is a major cost to be factored into your decision.

# 10.6 Insulin Potentiated Therapy

Insulin Potentiation Therapy (IPT) is a controversial alternative cancer therapy (aren't they all?) that uses insulin as an adjunct agent to potentiate the effect of chemotherapy and other medications. That makes it a bit of a hybrid, somewhere between total chemotherapy and natural methods.

This technique was originally developed in Mexico by Dr. Donato Perez Garcia in the 1930's. His son, Donato Perez Garcia Bellon, M.D., and his grandson, Donato Perez Garcia, Jr., M.D, followed Dr. Garcia in this work. Mind if you read about the late Stephen G. Ayre, M.D; you'd practically think he was the leading rescrcher in this method.

I have already referred to the fact that cancer cells seem to have an excessive demand for sugar, because of the low energy glycolysis metabolism (section 3.0). So the administration of insulin, which dramatically lowers blood sugar levels, should in theory weaken cancer cells and make them more vulnerable to attack.

Garcia reasoned that adminstering insulin, followed immediately (within minutes) by chemotherapy, should allow a lower—and therefore safer—dose of chemotherapy to be used.

It's rather like the idea that a company of drunken soldiers could be overcome by a much smaller opposing force than would be required if the company were fit and sober!

In addition, insulin is also believed to increase the permeability of cell membranes, increasing the intracellular concentration and cytotoxic effect of anticancer drugs. That's what it does for glucose, sure; I'm not so sure about the science backing the fact that insulin affects cell membranes in respect of all substances.

But according to practitioners of IPT, a dose as little as one tenth of the normal chemo dose will be effective in this context.

Unfortunately, no real clinical trials have been performed to validate these claims. Moreover there is more than a theoretical risk that concurrent use of insulin and chemo drugs could actually potentiate the toxic effects of chemotherapy on healthy cells. I think it would be rash to ignore the possibility.

My main assessment is to wonder why anyone wants to dabble in low-dose chemotherapy. Given that we know that it is absolutely impossible to kill all cancer cells, as oncologists believe (or at least claim) they do, why should a poor man's version of the same thing have any more effect?

Cytotoxic therapy (killing cells) is a fool's illusion and I think. We are better to concentrate our ingenuity on aiding Nature and stimulating the immune response, as in many of the techniques I have described already in this work.

If you like the sound of the clinical context and want to try it, the best I can say is it won't harm you as fast as chemotherapy, so there is plenty of time to change your mind, without having lost all your defence soldiers!

Some people, of course, swear by it.

I am switching to an impassioned plea to feature this therapy from Carol Roujansky. Here is her story:

### 2 months to Remission, Almost 2 years in Continued, Great Health!

I have been a Reiki Master for the past 20 years, so my diagnosis of cancer came as a complete shock. How could this be happening to me?! Further, I'd been involved in meditation and self growth processes in an international community since 1970 and thought I had been eating a healthy diet. Nutrition and correct supplementation were always foremost for me. So, you see, this diagnosis can appear suddenly for anyone.

My official diagnosis was Uterine Cancer, Grade 2, Stage 4.

On March 30, 2007 I had a 5 hour operation followed by a 13 day hospital stay. At this point I would say that I was entering the "dark night of the soul." My usual optimistic nature was severely daunted and the recovery so hard that I remember saying that I wouldn't have wished it on my worst enemy.

Fortunately, I had a HUGE support group of family, friends and clients. The hospital room was full of people visiting and giving me not only support, but lots of Reiki Sessions (including distance healing, continually, from my well trained students), Jin Shin from another friend, and lots of prayers and up close and distance support in every way. The same continued while at home during the stabilizing period after the hospital and long after.

But following the operation and despite all the support, my spirit was still in a very low place.

Then a crucial and amazing turning point occurred after a visit to a local Tibetan Healer. I "thought" nothing much had occurred, but the next day during my daily walk by the local marina I felt my old indomitable, strong, optimistic spirit bounce back into my body. Yahoo!!! I was back and could now proceed to the next step.

Prior to the operation I did a huge amount of research into all the myriad paths for follow up care as well as extensive diet and supplementation. Finally I was ready to move forward. I vehemently rejected the traditional chemo that was being offered me. There was no way that I would put all those chemicals into my body, killing everything in its path.

Instead I made another wonderful and totally life saving choice, "Insulin Potentiation Therapy" also known as "IPT". I'm in love with the whole IPT process and am one of the few patients who are actively sharing their experiences with the world. Please feel free to contact me and to pass my name to others in need. I have boundless enthusiasm in helping people understand this method, and to help them through the entire course of their treatment with support, if they like. Sharing this healing process with others is a great joy for me!

IPT helped the final stages of my recovery very quickly and easily. The most side effects were feeling a little tired that night and the next morning. After 9 IPT treatments, I tested in remission and have been testing clear for almost two years now!

Crucial to my very quick recovery were many elements, including a great support system, prayer, optimism, creativity in the form of writing about my experiences, exercise, enthusiasm and lots of Reiki. A strong and clear supplementation system fell into place and I adhere to that today. High dose Vitamin C infusions were a big part of my healing program, and I maintain those even now once a month for maintenance.

There is one more crucial factor and that was/is a total overhaul of my diet. Totally removing any and all allergenic foods such as wheat, dairy, sugar, soy, corn, alcohol, coffee have been imperative.

Please feel free to contact me at any time: premcarolreiki@yahoo.com (619-422-4775). Please reference this article in the message area when you contact me. I will be happy to call you back and share more details with you in person.

Many Blessings, Gratitude, Health, Love and Support,

Carol Roujansky, Reiki Master

# 10.7 Chlorine Dioxide Protocol

The MMS (Magic Minerals Solution) protocol was developed by Jim Humble, a gold miner and metallurgist, on an expedition into the jungles of Central America, looking for gold. It was a response to a need to help a member of his expedition who came down with malaria, more than two days away, through heavy jungle, from the next mine. After many years of experience, Humble always carried stabilized oxygen with him on such expeditions, to make local water safe to drink. Facing the possibility of a quick loss of life, he gave it to the stricken man. To everyone's amazement, he was well within a few hours. That seemed like a miracle, but Humble wanted to better understand what had just happened.

Over the course of several years, Jim Humble figured out that what made stabilized oxygen so effective in some malaria cases, was not the oxygen at all, but the trace amounts of chlorine dioxide it contained. Further research led him to come up with a way to produce hundreds, if not thousands more units of chlorine dioxide than what is found in stabilized oxygen. This is through using a higher concentration of sodium chlorite (28% vs. 3% for stabilized oxygen), in conjunction with an activator. The proof of the efficacy of this simple protocol lies in unsubstantiated claims that it has helped over 75,000 people in several African nations—including Uganda and Malawi—rid themselves, primarily of malaria, but also hepatitis, cancer, and AIDS.

Ahem... AIDS?

Anyone can be overloaded with toxins. Most people probably are but won't admit it or, more likely, don't know it. Others would prefer to think they're not. If your health is not perfect, you're habitually low on energy, have trouble keeping your weight down or your blood pressure in the normal range, or constantly dealing with inflammation or pain, or if you have cancer, and indeed you have any medical condition that is adversely affecting your health, then there are likely to be toxins—heavy metal, virus, bacteria, fungus, or parasites—playing a part.

Mainstream medicine will typically respond by loading you up with additional pollutants, many of which indiscriminately kill healthy tissue while going after "the bad guys" to deal with the symptoms. Not so with chlorine dioxide. It only acts on anything harmful. Miracle or not, the effects can be amazing!

There is nothing new about chlorine dioxide. It has been used to sterilise medical equipment for decades and food preparation areas, and it would appear that no germ of any sort, be it a virus, a bacterium, a parasite or a fungus, can tolerate its devastating effects. Because its effects are so rapid, no germ has ever had time or been able to develop a resistance to it. It is like a human being trying to develop a resistance to a hand grenade. It just isn't possible.

Chlorine dioxide and chlorine are not the same. Chlorine is a chemical element. In ionic form, chlorine is part of common salt and other compounds, and is necessary to most forms of life, including human. A powerful oxidizing agent, it is the most abundant dissolved ion in ocean water, and readily combines with nearly every other element, including sodium to form salt crystals, and magnesium, as magnesium chloride.

Chlorine dioxide is a chemical compound that consists of one chlorine ion bound to two ions of oxygen. It's a powerful oxidizing agent meaning that it will snatch electrons from "electron donors." In doing so it denatures chemicals and kills living forms easily. This is important because relative to chlorine dioxide, all pathogens are electron donors.

Chlorine dioxide is extremely volatile. You might call it "hot tempered," but in a very beneficial way. This volatility is a key factor in chlorine dioxide's effectiveness as a pathogen destroyer.

The compound is literally explosive, so much so that it's not safe to transport in any quantity. Therefore, it is common practice to generate chlorine dioxide "on site" at the point of use. You will mix your own, as explained later.

Chlorine dioxide is approved by the Environmental Protection Agency in safely removing pathogens and contaminates like anthrax. So you know it must be effective. However, the concentrations used in such applications can vary from 500 to over 6,000 parts per million (ppm), which would quickly kill a human.

Using the MMS protocol you will produce chlorine dioxide around 1 ppm. You will carry the MMS solution, a precursor which is safe to transport. You make chlorine dioxide right in the cup or glass, just before you swallow it, by adding lemon juice or citric acid.

The MMS solution is 25% sodium chlorite in distilled water. You can produce chlorine dioxide with a single drop, when an "activator" of vinegar, lemon juice, or a 10% solution of citric acid is added. Citric acid is recommended because of its simplicity. The natural pH of sodium chlorite is 13. Adding vinegar, lemon juice, or citric acid creates about 3 mg of unstable but still harmless chlorine dioxide.

## No Resistance

Chlorine dioxide's extreme volatility prevents pathogens from developing a resistance, mainly because when they make contact the pathogens are zapped instantly. Yet (this is the real miracle): healthy cells and beneficial bacteria seem to be unaffected.

As I said in section 3.0, oxygen is pretty effective at killing cancer cells. But chlorine dixiode attacks them much more brutally than plain oxygen, ripping cancer cells or pathogens apart - literally vaporizing them, in the equivalent of a small chemical explosion in our tissues!

Throughout the body, anywhere chlorine dioxide ions, transported via red blood cells, come into contact with pathogens, the pathogens give up their electrons and cease to exist. The chlorine dioxide-armed cells only "detonate" on contact with pathogens, which include harmful bacteria, viruses, funguses, toxins, heavy metals, and parasites. All of these will have pH values that are out of the body's range of good health. They will also have a positive ionic charge.

But healthy cells and organisms (pH 7 and above and with a negative charge) remain untouched.

Chlorine dioxide ions will also oxidize diseased cells... anything that is acidic, with a positive ionic charge.

## What Happens If The Chlorine Dioxide Encounters Nothing?

If the chlorine dioxide ions encounter no pathogens or other poisons, they deteriorate into table salt and in some instances, hypochlorous acid, which the body can also use.

This compound also kills pathogens and even cancerous cells. Hypochlorous acid is so important that its diminished presence in the body is described medically by the term 'myeloperoxidase deficiency'. Many people are afflicted by this condition. The immune system needs a great deal more hypochlorous acid when disease is present. Facilitated by the MMS solution, chlorine dioxide delivers it in quantity.

In other words, if you are totally healthy and have nothing in your body that is at an acidic level below 7, there are no ill effects from taking chlorine dioxide at the appropriate dose. However, your stores of hypochlorous acid will be increased.

That's good!

# 10.7a Side Effects vs. "Healing Crisis"

When swallowed, 2 or 3 mg of free chlorine dioxide are in the solution at the time. However, the body is supplied with chlorine dioxide in a "timed release" manner lasting about 12 hours. Be aware, that before you feel better, it is likely you will feel ill in one way or another.

The nauseating feeling that you may possibly experience, especially if you take too big a dose, is likely the result of chlorine dioxide encountering and destroying a large number of pathogens. We all have pathogens; most of us have lots. Since they build up over time in various organs of the body, they generally affect our health slowly and cumulatively. We don't notice.

But if chlorine dioxide takes them out too suddenly, the result will be a dramatic reaction. All sorts of waste and debris will be released too fast. We call that a healing crisis or sometimes a "Herxeimer reaction".

It can be unpleasant but all you do is stop the medication. When you feel OK again, restart at a much lower dose—just one drop each day if necessary. And then build up again.

Remember, if there is nothing for chlorine dioxide to encounter, it deteriorates into constituents that are totally non-toxic. Nothing poisonous is left behind to build up, as is the case with many medical protocols. Medical treatments currently provide you no way of removing the poisons when they don't work.

Chlorine dioxide, on the other hand, lasts long enough to do its job, and then the amount that does not interact with pathogens or cancer cells becomes nothing more than micro amounts of salt and water. The chlorine dioxide has just a few minutes to do its job, and then it no longer exists.

# 10.7b The MMS Procedure

All you need is your bottle of MMS, a clean, empty, dry glass, an eyedropper and the activator citric acid.

Always activate the MMS drops with one of the food acids, **either lemon juice drops, or limejuice drops,** or citric acid solution drops, the citric acid drops being the simplest.

Always add 5 drops of citric acid or the juice to each 1 drop of MMS, mix in an empty dry glass and wait at least 3 minutes, maximum 10 minutes, then add 1/3 to 2/3 glass of water and drink it.

Repeat this dose in between one and two hours, ideally doing all of this after your evening meal, possibly starting about ¾ hour after you have eaten, as it can sometimes make some people sleepy, apart from which your body does most of its detoxifying during the night.

Start modestly with as little as 1 drop of MMS plus 5 drops of citric acid on your first day (never forget to wait at least 3 minutes for the mixture to react to create chlorine dioxide, which will turn yellow and smell of chlorine, and repeat the dose in one to two hours). Take your time and do not rush. You could stay on this low dose for a few days, and then increase the number (2 and 10, 3 and 15, etc) on subsequent days.

There is no point in going higher than 15 drops (+ 75 drops activator). You'll see this dose urged on websites all over the Net. But really it's rare to need 15 drops for a result.

How do you know when to stop? Your body will tell you when you've reached the optimum dosage for you, and, if in doubt, drop the next dose. Clearing may be a bit uncomfortable, but it need not be intolerable. You may feel like you've been through a battle, and, in a sense, you have.

This gentle approach applies to any chronic condition, and especially if you want to clean up your body. However, if you develop an acute medical condition such as dengue fever or malaria, for example, start straight in at at least 5 drops of MMS to 25 drops of citric acid, although you could possibly start at 8 drops of MMS to 40 drops of citric acid, and don't forget to repeat the dose in between one and two hours. With any luck you will feel remarkably better by the next day. If you are not quite symptom free, repeat the same the next day, increasing the dose by about one third. In an acute situation, you can take three doses a day, each one repeated one to two hours later.

Antidote. If you develop any symptoms you don't like, assume it is the chlorine dioxide working too hard within you. To clear these symptoms, either take a few doses of ½ teaspoonful of sodium bicarbonate in a glass of water or a few grammes of vitamin C in water. Don't take both (one is acid and one alkali, neither will work!) Then either don't take a dose of MMS for 24 hours or drop the next dose and gradually work back up again.

Dangers: Of course you will hear a lot about the supposed dangers of MMS. Critics insist it is "industrial bleach" which is nonsense. It's a tiny fraction of the strength.

The FDA and other regulatory bodies around the world have come down hard on it and you may have some difficulty obtaining it. At the time of writing, it is freely available on Amazon.com but in disguise.

But taking it, you are on your own. Expect plenty of flack. It'll come to you!

# 10.7 Chlorine Dioxide Protocol

The MMS (Magic Minerals Solution) protocol was developed by Jim Humble, a gold miner and metallurgist, on an expedition into the jungles of Central America, looking for gold. It was a response to a need to help a member of his expedition who came down with malaria, more than two days away, through heavy jungle, from the next mine. After many years of experience, Humble always carried stabilized oxygen with him on such expeditions, to make local water safe to drink. Facing the possibility of a quick loss of life, he gave it to the stricken man. To everyone's amazement, he was well within a few hours. That seemed like a miracle, but Humble wanted to better understand what had just happened.

Over the course of several years, Jim Humble figured out that what made stabilized oxygen so effective in some malaria cases, was not the oxygen at all, but the trace amounts of chlorine dioxide it contained. Further research led him to come up with a way to produce hundreds, if not thousands more units of chlorine dioxide than what is found in stabilized oxygen. This is through using a higher concentration of sodium chlorite (28% vs. 3% for stabilized oxygen), in conjunction with an activator. The proof of the efficacy of this simple protocol lies in unsubstantiated claims that it has helped over 75,000 people in several African nations including Uganda and Malawi—rid themselves, primarily of malaria, but also hepatitis, cancer, and AIDS.

Ahem... AIDS?

Anyone can be overloaded with toxins. Most people probably are but won't admit it or, more likely, don't know it. Others would prefer to think they're not. If your health is not perfect, you're habitually low on energy, have trouble keeping your weight down or your blood pressure in the normal range, or constantly dealing with inflammation or pain, or if you have cancer, and indeed you have any medical condition that is adversely affecting your health, then there are likely to be toxins—heavy metal, virus, bacteria, fungus, or parasites—playing a part.

Mainstream medicine will typically respond by loading you up with additional pollutants, many of which indiscriminately kill healthy tissue while going after "the bad guys" to deal with the symptoms. Not so with chlorine dioxide. It only acts on anything harmful. Miracle or not, the effects can be amazing!

There is nothing new about chlorine dioxide. It has been used to sterilise medical equipment for decades and food preparation areas, and it would appear that no germ of any sort, be it a virus, a bacterium, a parasite or a fungus, can tolerate its devastating effects. Because its effects are so rapid, no germ has ever had time or been able to develop a resistance to it. It is like a human being trying to develop a resistance to a hand grenade. It just isn't possible.

Chlorine dioxide and chlorine are not the same. Chlorine is a chemical element. In ionic form, chlorine is part of common salt and other compounds, and is necessary to most forms of life, including human. A powerful oxidizing agent, it is the most abundant dissolved ion in ocean water, and readily combines with nearly every other element, including sodium to form salt crystals, and magnesium, as magnesium chloride.

Chlorine dioxide is a chemical compound that consists of one chlorine ion bound to two ions of oxygen. It's a powerful oxidizing agent meaning that it will snatch electrons from "electron donors." In doing so it denatures chemicals and kills living forms easily. This is important because relative to chlorine dioxide, all pathogens are electron donors.

Chlorine dioxide is extremely volatile. You might call it "hot tempered," but in a very beneficial way. This volatility is a key factor in chlorine dioxide's effectiveness as a pathogen destroyer.

The compound is literally explosive, so much so that it's not safe to transport in any quantity. Therefore, it is common practice to generate chlorine dioxide "on site" at the point of use. You will mix your own, as explained later.

Chlorine dioxide is approved by the Environmental Protection Agency in safely removing pathogens and contaminates like anthrax. So you know it must be effective. However, the concentrations used in such applications can vary from 500 to over 6,000 parts per million (ppm), which would quickly kill a human.

Using the MMS protocol you will produce chlorine dioxide around 1 ppm. You will carry the MMS solution, a precursor which is safe to transport. You make chlorine dioxide right in the cup or glass, just before you swallow it, by adding lemon juice or citric acid.

The MMS solution is 25% sodium chlorite in distilled water. You can produce chlorine dioxide with a single drop, when an "activator" of vinegar, lemon juice, or a 10% solution of citric acid is added. Citric acid is recommended because of its simplicity. The natural pH of sodium chlorite is 13. Adding vinegar, lemon juice, or citric acid creates about 3 mg of unstable but still harmless chlorine dioxide.

## No Resistance

Chlorine dioxide's extreme volatility prevents pathogens from developing a resistance, mainly because when they make contact the pathogens are zapped instantly. Yet (this is the real miracle): healthy cells and beneficial bacteria seem to be unaffected.

As I said in section 3.0, oxygen is pretty effective at killing cancer cells. But chlorine dixiode attacks them much more brutally than plain oxygen, ripping cancer cells or pathogens apart - literally vaporizing them, in the equivalent of a small chemical explosion in our tissues!

Throughout the body, anywhere chlorine dioxide ions, transported via red blood cells, come into contact with pathogens, the pathogens give up their electrons and cease to exist. The chlorine dioxide-armed cells only "detonate" on contact with pathogens, which include harmful bacteria, viruses, funguses, toxins, heavy metals, and parasites. All of these will have pH values that are out of the body's range of good health. They will also have a positive ionic charge.

But healthy cells and organisms (pH 7 and above and with a negative charge) remain untouched.

Chlorine dioxide ions will also oxidize diseased cells... anything that is acidic, with a positive ionic charge.

## What Happens If The Chlorine Dioxide Encounters Nothing?

If the chlorine dioxide ions encounter no pathogens or other poisons, they deteriorate into table salt and in some instances, hypochlorous acid, which the body can also use.

This compound also kills pathogens and even cancerous cells. Hypochlorous acid is so important that its diminished presence in the body is described medically by the term 'myeloperoxidase deficiency'. Many people are afflicted by this condition. The immune system needs a great deal more hypochlorous acid when disease is present. Facilitated by the MMS solution, chlorine dioxide delivers it in quantity.

In other words, if you are totally healthy and have nothing in your body that is at an acidic level below 7, there are no ill effects from taking chlorine dioxide at the appropriate dose. However, your stores of hypochlorous acid will be increased.

That's good!

# 10.7a Side Effects vs. "Healing Crisis"

When swallowed, 2 or 3 mg of free chlorine dioxide are in the solution at the time. However, the body is supplied with chlorine dioxide in a "timed release" manner lasting about 12 hours. Be aware, that before you feel better, it is likely you will feel ill in one way or another.

The nauseating feeling that you may possibly experience, especially if you take too big a dose, is likely the result of chlorine dioxide encountering and destroying a large number of pathogens. We all have pathogens; most of us have lots. Since they build up over time in various organs of the body, they generally affect our health slowly and cumulatively. We don't notice.

But if chlorine dioxide takes them out too suddenly, the result will be a dramatic reaction. All sorts of waste and debris will be released too fast. We call that a healing crisis or sometimes a "Herxeimer reaction".

It can be unpleasant but all you do is stop the medication. When you feel OK again, restart at a much lower dose—just one drop each day if necessary. And then build up again.

Remember, if there is nothing for chlorine dioxide to encounter, it deteriorates into constituents that are totally non-toxic. Nothing poisonous is left behind to build up, as is the case with many medical protocols. Medical treatments currently provide you no way of removing the poisons when they don't work.

Chlorine dioxide, on the other hand, lasts long enough to do its job, and then the amount that does not interact with pathogens or cancer cells becomes nothing more than micro amounts of salt and water. The chlorine dioxide has just a few minutes to do its job, and then it no longer exists.

# 10.7b The MMS Procedure

All you need is your bottle of MMS, a clean, empty, dry glass, an eyedropper and the activator citric acid.

Always activate the MMS drops with one of the food acids, **either lemon juice drops, or limejuice drops,** or citric acid solution drops, the citric acid drops being the simplest.

Always add 5 drops of citric acid or the juice to each 1 drop of MMS, mix in an empty dry glass and wait at least 3 minutes, maximum 10 minutes, then add 1/3 to 2/3 glass of water and drink it.

Repeat this dose in between one and two hours, ideally doing all of this after your evening meal, possibly starting about ¾ hour after you have eaten, as it can sometimes make some people sleepy, apart from which your body does most of its detoxifying during the night.

Start modestly with as little as 1 drop of MMS plus 5 drops of citric acid on your first day (never forget to wait at least 3 minutes for the mixture to react to create chlorine dioxide, which will turn yellow and smell of chlorine, and repeat the dose in one to two hours). Take your time and do not rush. You could stay on this low dose for a few days, and then increase the number (2 and 10, 3 and 15, etc) on subsequent days.

There is no point in going higher than 15 drops (+ 75 drops activator). You'll see this dose urged on websites all over the Net. But really it's rare to need 15 drops for a result.

How do you know when to stop? Your body will tell you when you've reached the optimum dosage for you, and, if in doubt, drop the next dose. Clearing may be a bit uncomfortable, but it need not be intolerable. You may feel like you've been through a battle, and, in a sense, you have.

This gentle approach applies to any chronic condition, and especially if you want to clean up your body. However, if you develop an acute medical condition such as dengue fever or malaria, for example, start straight in at at least 5 drops of MMS to 25 drops of citric acid, although you could possibly start at 8 drops of MMS to 40 drops of citric acid, and don't forget to repeat the dose in between one and two hours. With any luck you will feel remarkably better by the next day. If you are not quite symptom free, repeat the same the next day, increasing the dose by about one third. In an acute situation, you can take three doses a day, each one repeated one to two hours later.

Antidote. If you develop any symptoms you don't like, assume it is the chlorine dioxide working too hard within you. To clear these symptoms, either take a few doses of ½ teaspoonful of sodium bicarbonate in a glass of water or a few grammes of vitamin C in water. Don't take both (one is acid and one alkali, neither will work!)

Then either don't take a dose of MMS for 24 hours or drop the next dose and gradually work back up again.

Dangers: Of course you will hear a lot about the supposed dangers of MMS. Critics insist it is "industrial bleach" which is nonsense. It's a tiny fraction of the strength.

The FDA and other regulatory bodies around the world have come down hard on it and you may have some difficulty obtaining it. At the time of writing, it is freely available on Amazon.com but in disguise.

But taking it, you are on your own. Expect plenty of flack. It'll come to you!

# 10.8 Low Dose Naltrexone

A growing body of research over the past 20 years indicates that your body's secretion of endorphins; your internal, natural morphine-like opioids (opioid just means "like opium") play an important, if not central, role in the workings of your immune system.

You will know that endorphins are the "feel good" chemicals which our bodies produce on board and which light up the brain, so we feel happy and calm. It's as if we had taken opium or morphine, but only in tiny doses and without the terrible side effects or addiction problems of these drugs.

That's nice.

So logically, if we are happy and serene, our immune system is in correspondingly optimum working order and protects us to the best of its ability. And that's what we find: laboratory evidence indicates overwhelmingly that opioids alter the development, differentiation, and function of immune cells, and that both innate and adaptive systems are affected.

Bone marrow progenitor cells, macrophages, natural killer cells, immature thymocytes and T cells, and B cells are all involved. Don't worry too much if you don't know what these all are—but we need 'em!

Now the immune system, we know, protects us from cancer. So here, at last, is a decent scientific model to explain why cancer is largely a disease of stress and unhappiness. Remember the quote from Galen I shared with you in section 2.14 (cancer only strikes unhappy people)?

It makes sense then that we might try and tackle cancer by increasing or modulating what are called opioid-receptors.

That's where a drug called naltrexone comes in.

Naltrexone is a powerful antagonist of opioids. It blocks opioid receptors and so signals don't get through. It's used for things like treating a heroin overdose (blocks the heroin) or treating alcoholism.

At first, it might seem counter-intuitive to use something which opposes opioids. But wait!

Enter **low-dose naltrexone** (LDN). Here the story changes. Low dose naltrexone, where the drug is used in doses approximately one-tenth those used for drug/alcohol rehabilitation purposes, is being used by some practitioners as an "off-label" experimental treatment for certain immunologically-related disorders. These include HIV/AIDS, multiple sclerosis (in particular, the primary progressive variant), Parkinson's disease, cancer, fibromyalgia, autoimmune diseases such as rheumatoid arthritis or ankylosing spondylitis, Crohn's disease, ulcerative colitis, Hashimoto's thyroiditis, and central nervous system disorders.

It is difficult for many to believe that one drug can accomplish so many tasks and this book does NOT endorse all those uses. But LDN does not treat symptoms as most drugs do. It actually works way "upstream" to modulate the basic mechanisms that result in the disease state.

It is believed to up-regulate vital elements of your immune system by increasing your body's production of metenkephalin and your natural endorphins, hence improving your immune function.

Dr. Burton M. Berkson, of the Integrative Medical Center Of New Mexico in Las Cruces has published two studies on IV LDN coupled with alpha lipoic acid (ALA) for the treatment of cancer.

The first, on the reversal of pancreatic cancer was published in 2006, and the other, on the reversal of B cell lymphomas, came out in 2007. This is certainly promising. [Berkson, October 2008 LDN conference at the USC Medical Center]

# LDN Protocol

Typically, LDN is taken at bedtime, which blocks your opioid receptors for a few hours in the middle of the night.

LDN can be prescribed by your doctor, and should be prepared by a reliable compounding pharmacy.

Naltrexone is a prescription drug, so your physician would have to give you a prescription after deciding that LDN appears appropriate for you.

Naltrexone in the large 50mg size, originally manufactured by DuPont under the brand name ReVia, is now sold by Mallinckrodt as Depade and by Barr Laboratories under the generic name naltrexone.

LDN prescriptions are being filled by hundreds of local pharmacies, as well as by some mail-order pharmacies, around the US (this could change at any time). Some pharmacists have been grinding up the 50mg tablets of naltrexone to prepare the 4.5mg capsules of LDN; others use naltrexone, purchased as a pure powder, from a primary manufacturer.

Remember, the trials I mentioned were based on IV adminstration. The oral might not compare at all. But given the extreme low toxicity of ALA and LDN, it's worth a try.

For a more complete list of past and current research, please see the lowdosenaltrexone.org website.

You can also read a book: *The Promise of Low Dose Naltrexone Potential Benefits in Cancer, Autoimmune, Neurological and Infectious Disorders*. By Elaine Moore, co-author SammyJo Wilkinson Foreword by Dr. Yash Agrawal, MD, PhD.

A gentle word of warning: LDN can also reverse the effects of sexual satiety, meaning you want more sex, lots more! It can induce early morning erections in patients who suffer from erectile dysfunction (ED).

# 10.9 Dimethyl Sulfoxide

Here's an amazing substance that was once hailed on mainstream TV ("60 Minutes") as a miracle and the NY Times said, in a lead editorial published April 3, 1965, that "DMSO is... the closest thing to a wonder produced in the 1960s." Yet DMSO is now largely forgotten, since it is not hyped by Big Pharma, the way they do for drugs.

DMSO is an organic, sulfur-rich substance found in the woody part of trees. It was first discovered by a Russian researcher Alexander Zaytsev in 1866. It absorbs easily and a drop placed on the skin will be sucked in almost instantly. Over 12,000 modern papers have studied its amazing properties.

Among other properties, DMSO is a tremendous pain reliever. But it also has a real part to play In fighting cancer the "chemical route". It seems to protect the body from the ravages of chemo agents, notably cyclophosphamide, and at the same time can persuade many types of cancer cells to start behaving more normally. It relieves pain noticeably and helps the patients normalize the sickly feeling so obvious with cancer.

DMSO performs best with the lymphoma group of cancers. Note that it doesn't actually kill tumor cells, so much as turn them back to well-behaved counterparts.

Several studies of this group of compounds, called polar solvents, have shown this tendency to be very pronounced. This could be called tumor maturation therapy, since it turns wild, uncontrolled "young" or undifferentiated cells into sensible citizens of the body.

A particularly interesting 1968 study showed that DMSO combined with a dye (hematoxylin) went straight for cancer cells. The dye was carried in too. Yet the surrounding tissues were not stained. If this study shows nothing else, it is that DMSO surges into cancer cells! The potential for carrying agents into tumors remains largely unexplored.

[E. J. Tucker, M.D., F.A.C.S., and A. Carrizo, M.D. *International Surgery*, June 1968, Vol 49, No. 6, page 516-527]

Why doesn't the FDA approve it? Well at first they admitted this was such a versatile substance with so many applications, they simply didn't have enough staff to evaluate it. Quite likely too, they cannot cope with the idea of a compound sold commercially as a solvent can also have drug status.

But you know the FDA is not there for your protection but to protect the drug industry. Such a cheap, safe adjuvant to therapy simply cannot be released to the public. So they complain about lack of safety reports (there are hundreds of good papers) and lack of patient experience (there are over 100,000 patient success reports of safety, which the FDA commissioners simply ignore). They claims there are eye dangers; there are none.

DMSO is used in the rest of the world quite ethically by doctors. No problem. Toxicity: less than aspirin, if used properly. The supposed changes in eye function were alterations in refractive index (not opacity), seen only in pigs, dogs and rabbits. Yet the FDA makes a big deal out this.

No eye changes have ever been seen in humans, despite worldwide use of DMSO. In Portland, Oregon. Dr Jacob and Edward Rosenbaum MD, Clinical Professor of Medicine and Head of the Department of Rheumatology at the University of Oregon Medical School, had 32 patients examined by an ophthalmologist and then treated with DMSO, 30 grams daily for between three and nineteen months. They were then reviewed by the ophthalmologist. None of them showed the characteristic lens changes seen in animals.

DMSO is used topically, in medication and intravenously. The only FDA-approved use of DMSO is for interstitial cystitis, a type of bladder inflammation. It's a strange thing but DMSO is suddenly safe if it's used for that purpose only!

Dosage of DMSO varies by body weight. The IV route is best but it has measurable benefits even taken orally.

# 10.10 Hydrazine Sulfate

*"Hydrazine sulfate, a drug that costs about a dollar a day, reverses the devastating weight loss called cachexia that kills most cancer patients. This simple chemical, developed in 1969 by Dr. Joseph Gold, director or the Syracuse Cancer Institute, works in half of all the patients who take it. Yet more than two million cancer patients starve to death yearly because the National Cancer Institute (NCI) continues its 20-year suppression of this life-saving drug. Meanwhile, doctors at the Petrov Institute of Oncology in St. Petersburg treating 1,000 patients with hydazine sulfate report long-term survival even in those with lymphatic cancer, the type that killed Jacqueline Onassis."*

**Dr Julian Whitaker, M.D.**

*"True to an apparent mission of preventing effective cancer cures from being discovered, NCI worked skillfully to discredit hydrazine sulfate and to keep any knowledge from the general public."*

**John Diamond**

*"NCI's actions with respect to hydrazine sulfate, characterized by intimidation, coercion, steadfast opposition, and possibly clinical trial-rigging, are truly one of the most shameful, scandalous medical undertakings in this country's history, depriving vast numbers of people of their health, happiness, and lives."*

*Dr Joseph Gold*

*"The most remarkable anticancer agent I have come across in my 45 years experience in cancer."*

**Dean Burk, MD. at the time head of cell chemistry research at the NCI in the 1970's**

Dr. Joseph Gold reported in the 1970s that hydrazine sulfate inhibited the growth of cancers in rats, including melanoma, lymphoma and leukemia. Hydrazine sulfate inhibits anaerobic glycolysis, the metabolic process which mainly feeds cancer cells. In a large Leningrad study, involving over 700 patients with many types of cancer, the patients thrived better. However the tumor regressed in only 10% of cases. This theme of being better nourished, despite the on-board cancer, recurs through most studies and appears to be one of the main benefits of hydrazine sulfate.

Despite assertions to the contrary by official bodies and vested interest groups, there have been many clinical trials of hydrazine sulfate published in peer-reviewed medical journals which circulate worldwide, including ten years of randomized clinical trials performed by Harbor-UCLA Medical Center from 1981-1990. Yet spin doctors at the National Cancer Institute continue to blatantly lie and claim "hydrazine sulfate has shown no anticancer activity in randomized clinical trials."

The truth is that every single, informed-consent, controlled clinical trial of hydrazine sulfate, performed in accordance with internationally accepted criteria and standards of scientific conduct—without exception—has indicated efficacy and safety of the drug.

The only contrary results have been the National Cancer Institute's own sponsored trials of hydrazine sulfate in which incompatible agents (medications) were used with the test drug. It must be stressed that no legitimate researcher on this planet would ever knowingly use an incompatible agent—or one even suspected of incompatibility—in the trial of a test drug. Use of an incompatible agent in a drug test, which acts to cause a negative study, can only mean that the NCI researchers deliberately sabotaged the trial. Does that sound too crazy to believe? Get this...

The drug's discoverer, Dr. Joseph Gold, had found that HS could provoke very dangerous effects if patients were taking other drugs, especially tranquilizers. Several warnings were given to NCI before it began its test. The warnings were explicit. *Patients could die if they were taking tranquilizers at the same time as HS.*

It turned out that none of the NCI patients were warned about this. In fact it emerged that 94% of those patients were in fact on tranquilizers.

Barry Tice, an investigator for the US General Accounting Office (GAO), looked into the NCI trial of hydrazine sulfate after it was over. He called Dr. Gold and told him he had found a "smoking gun." There was an internal NCI memo which showed that NCI was well aware of the problems involved in the drug combinations.

But the GAO did not back up Tice, its own investigator. The final GAO report on the NCI clinical trials of hydrazine sulfate simply accused NCI of sloppy bookkeeping.

In the June 1995 issue of the *Journal of Clinical Oncology*, a letter from the NCI was published. The letter stated that NCI had omitted mentioning, in its own published account of its cancer study, that 94% of the patients had been on tranquilizers. But, because this letter did NOT mention how dangerous that situation was, it looked like NCI was simply admitting to a technical and unimportant mistake. A clerical error.

So what did happen to the patients in the NCI hydrazine sulfate study?

We don't know. The results have been suppressed. But NCI concluded that hydrazine sulfate was ineffective.

The drug, hydrazine sulfate, a cheap, widely available, unpatentable competitor for chemotherapy dollars, was eliminated. No profit there.

Penthouse Publisher

There is more to this incredible story. Penthouse publisher Bob Guccione's wife, Kathy Keeton, who was the founder of Longevity, a magazine that was part of the Guccione empire, was diagnosed with "galloping breast cancer" in 1995. She was given 6 weeks to live.

She refused chemotherapy and became a VERY high-profile case of a person taking hydrazine sulfate instead.

She also chose radiation to reduce one of her many tumors—a growth around her bile duct. Dr. Gold said the dose of radiation should be small, because hydrazine sulfate would enhance the effect of the radiation. But the radiologist gave her the full dose instead, burned her liver and caused later scarring.

Despite that, Keeton recovered. In fact, a year after her predicted death date, her cancer was in full remission. The hydrazine sulfate was a remarkable success.

Guccione ran ads in Penthouse, asking for families of the dead victims in the NCI experiment to come forward and join a class-action suit against NCI. Guccione estimated there had been 600 victims in the NCI clinical test.

In October 1997, Kathy Keeton went into a major and well-respected NY hospital for surgery. From all accounts, this operation had nothing to do with cancer. Complications occurred. She died (shades of Joan Rivers).

Of course, in its crass ignorance, most of America assumed Keeton had succumbed to cancer. Further "proof" that hydrazine sulfate did not work.

Predictably, the FDA got into the act. On April 23, 1998, the federal agency raided a distributor of hydrazine sulfate, Great Lakes Metabolics, in Rochester, Minnesota. In 2000, the FDA shut down the company that supplied hydrazine sulfate to Great Lakes, and Great Lakes went out of business.

In 1996, when hydrazine sulfate (HS) was still very much in the public spotlight, Dr. Gold stated he received 20 phone calls in one day from doctors at Sloan Kettering. These doctors wanted to obtain HS on the sly for their patients. Gold stated that roughly 2/3 of the patients were from the doctors' families. And yet six of these slime-ball doctors had refused to give HS to other patients at Sloan Kettering.

I can tell you more about integrity at the Sloane-Kettering:

In September 1973, Sloan Kettering (SK), perceived as the most prestigious cancer center in the world, started an HS study on terminal patients. The lead physician, Dr. Manuel Ochoa, had agreed to give each patient 60 mg a day for 3 days and then 60 mg 3 times a day after that. But Dr. Gold learned Ochoa was changing the protocol drastically. He was giving 1 mg the first day, then 2 mg the next day, and so on, building up to a top of 30 mg--except in some cases he actually gave patients 120-190 mg a day, which are brutal overdoses.

In 1975 SK announced HS was worthless. Ochoa was never indicted, as he should have been, for attempted murder.

By 1978, the FDA was cracking down on HS. 5,000 patients in the US were on the medicine. The FDA falsely stated that HS "caused bone marrow toxicity". It doesn't. *But in fact bone marrow toxicity is one of the most explicit and well-known side effect of chemo drugs, which are fully approved by the FDA! (hair loss is the other)*

*This is the evil state of cancer science, in the USA especially, and elsewhere.*

### Supplies

Hydrazine Sulfate can be obtained from compounding pharmacists, without a prescription. Dr Gold's protocol is as follows:

1- 3 days, take one 60 mgm capsule (before breakfast); days 4- 6 take one capsule before breakfast and one before dinner; from then on take 3 capsules a day, morning, noon and evening, before food. Continue for 6 weeks then take a break for a further 2 weeks. Then resume.

If you want to take it, you must avoid certain other medications, alcohol and some foods (cheese in particular).

# 10.11 Coffee Enemas For Liver Stimulation

*In as much as detoxification of the body is of the greatest importance, especially in the beginning, it is absolutely necessary to administer frequent enemas, day and night (on the average, we give coffee enemas every four hours, day and night, and even more frequently against severe pain, nausea, general nervous tension and depression)...Some patients take enemas every two hours, or even more frequently, during the first days of the treatment. More advanced cases are severely intoxicated and the absorption of the tumor masses, glands, etc., intoxicates them even more. Many years ago I lost several patients by coma hepaticum, since I did not know, and therefore neglected, the vital importance of frequent and regularly continued elimination of poisonous substances, with the help of juices, enemas, etc.*

**Dr Max Gerson, M.D. (A Cancer Therapy)**

You don't have to be on the Gerson program to benefit from a coffee enema; indeed, you don't even have to have cancer!

Coffee contains substances called chloretics which increase toxin excretion via the bile. The coffee enema is probably the only pharmaceutically active chloretic compound that may be safely administered several times a day without toxic effects. Severe coffee allergics may be unable to benefit from this. It was recognized by Gerson that coffee enemas are effective in stimulating the liver enzymes called the glutathione-S-transferase system, which is vital for detoxification. Increased activity of these enzymes confers powerful antioxidant properties, good for breaking down carcinogenic substances. The chloretics open the bile ducts (like opening the drains) and then the glutathione-S-transferase system throws out all the unwanted junk and poisons.

**Note:** Drinking coffee does not confer this undoubted benefit!

A coffee enema is administered as follows.

1. Add 3 teaspoonsful of fresh ground organic coffee (not instant or decaffeinated) to 2 pints (1.3 litres) of distilled water (available from the pharmacy). Boil for 5 minutes, to drive off the oils. Then cover it and simmer for a further 15 minutes.

2. Strain through gauze or a typical plastic coffee filter and allow to cool to body temperature. Put this in the enema bag. Hang the bag at about standing head height.

3. Then lie down. Lubricate and insert the nozzle, several inches (well beyond the rectal canal). Open the stop cock and allow the liquid to drain very slowly into your intestines. Relax and breath slowly while this takes place.

4. Try to take the whole bag and retain for around 15 minutes. If you feel spasms or unpleasant symptoms, close the stop cock or if there isn't one, simply lower the bag to the floor to stop the flow. Wait for half a minute and then try again.

5. Immediate symptoms of headache, fever, nausea, intestinal spasms and drowsiness generally indicate the flushing of toxins. Increase the frequency if this happens. If you wake with a headache and drowsiness, this could mean withdrawal symptoms. Try an extra enema last thing at night.

6. IMPORTANT: After the last enema at night you need to inject via your rectum about 50mls. of cold-pressed sunflower seed oil, flaxseed oil or similar, to line your intestines and protect the mucus membranes for next day.

7. Keep all equipment clean but sterility is not required.

# Section 11

## Electromagnetic Factors in Cancer

After presenting a rather effective lecture on cancer...the windshield was shot out of my car on the road back to San Francisco. The next night the glass window in the tail gate was shot out (300 miles removed from the first shooting). The police said, 'maybe someone is trying to tell you something'. The late Arthur Harris, M.D. was threatened by two men with assassination if he continued to use laetrile. Since that time we have de-centralised the work so that, if any two of us are shot out of the saddle, it will have only a slight negative effect on the program.

**Dr. Krebs**

# 11.1 Children Are Especially At Risk

Alarming research indicates that children and teenagers are five times more likely to get brain cancer if they use cell phones. The study is raising fears that today's young people may suffer an epidemic of the disease in later life.

The Swedish research was reported tat the first international conference on cell phones and health. It came from a further analysis of data from one of the biggest studies carried out on the cell phone/cancer link, headed by Professor Lennart Hardell. Professor Hardell told the conference that "people who started mobile phone use before the age of 20" had more than five-fold increase in glioma, a cancer of the glial cells that support the central nervous system.

The risk to young people from household cordless phones was almost as great. Cordless phones caused a fourfold increase in risk.

Young cell phone users are five times more likely to get acoustic neuromas, disabling tumors of the auditory nerve that often cause deafness.

Multiple studies have shown that children absorb more MWR than adults. One found that that the brain tissue of children absorbed about two times more MWR than that of adults, and other studies have reported that the bone marrow of children absorbs 10 times more MWR than that of adults.

However, not a single U.S. health agency is warning about the extra risks to children. Which is ironic, since American kids have the most WiFi gadgets.

"Belgium, France, India, and other technologically sophisticated governments are passing laws and/or issuing warnings about children's use of wireless devices," the review authors write.

They write that MWR exposure limits have remained unchanged for 19 years. They also note that smartphone makers specify the minimum distance from the body that their products must be kept so that legal limits for exposure to MWR aren't exceeded. For laptop computers and tablets, the minimum distance from the body is 20 cm (about 7.8 inches).

**But our concern here is cancer.**

Evidence is beginning to mount alarmingly that microwave radiation from cellphones is a cause of malignant disease. Already studies have been produced showing significant increases in problems like leukaemia and brain tumors.

I found a compelling double-blind medical study carried out in India in 2005 and published in the Indian Journal of Human Genetics

> [Ghandi, G. "Genetic Damage in Mobile Phone Users: Some Preliminary Findings," Indian J Hum Genetics, 2005, 11:99-104.]

The study analyzed micronucleated cell damage in blood and buccal (mouth) tissues of people who use their cell phone 1- 15 hours a day. The control group had never used cell phones at any time. DNA samples were coded and scored blind in strict protocol.

The test results of the "Indian study" are very significant. The non- cell phone users had an average of only 4% of their cells with DNA damage. The persistent mobile phone users showed an average of 39.75% cell DNA damage. The blood of one 24-year-old male revealed 63% micronucleated cells. He had used a cell phone for 1-2 hours per day for two years.

The hundreds of types of human cancers have one thing in common—they all begin at the cellular level when DNA genetic material in one or more cells becomes damaged. This damage can be passed from parents, or caused by the effects of an environmental carcinogen. "… Genetic mutations in one single cell are sufficient to lead to cancer," says Dr. Henry Lai, awell-knownscientist at the University of Washington, who has years of genetic and bioenergetics research to his credit ["Evidence for Genotoxic Effects (RFR and ELF Genotoxicity)" Dr. Henry Lai, Department of Bioengineering, University of Washington, Prepared for the BioInitiative Working Group, July 2007, see BioInitiative Report].

**Here's another:**
Prof Rony Seger, a cancer researcher at the Weizmann Institute of Science in Rehovot, Israel, and colleagues exposed rat and human cells to electromagnetic radiation at a similar frequency to that emitted by mobiles. The power of the signal was around 1/10th of that from a mobile.

After just five minutes the researchers identified the production of extracellular signal-regulated kinases (ERK1/2) – natural chemicals that stimulate cell division and growth.

Cancers develop when the body is unable to prevent excessive growth and division of cells in the wrong place.

Prof Seger said: "The real significance of our findings is that cells are not inert to non-thermal mobile phone radiation.

"We used radiation power levels that were around 1/10th of those produced by a normal mobile. The changes we observed were clearly not caused by heating."

I can't emphasize enough that there are far too many studies showing this kind of result to ignore the problem. Scientists who say there is no problem are being shockingly dishonest. They, of course, are paid by the telecommunication companies to blow smoke in everyone's eyes.

# 11.2 What Can You Do?

The first thing you have to do is to establish the scale a problem in your environment and there are various ways you can do this using hand-held field detection meters, which you can buy most places for under $100 each. The one I use is called a Trifield Meter 100XE and retails on Amazon for about $140. You have the possibility of measuring the magnetic field (a gauss meter) or the electrical field (volts per square metre or Teslas) or a third kind of interference field I shall describe shortly (RF).  There are other devices, of course. Good ones are so easy that even a non-technical person can use one; usually there is a failsafe display that simply goes "red for danger"

If there is a problem, you may need to get specialist help to correct it.

Take your meter everywhere in the home—and also your office and other hang outs. There are many sources of exposure:

- microwave oven
- WiFi phones around the home
- Television
- Computer
- Games consoles

In the old days cathode ray tubes were a significant source of intense radiation including soft x-rays. But today's plasma screens are equally hazardous in a different way, producing dangerous transient spikes which I shall discuss shortly.

One of the worst hazards I used to find was a person's sleeping place. Often the night stand is a place where people have a radio and alarm clock, maybe teamaker and a telephone which may or may not be WiFi. Then there are electric blankets and waterbeds which may add their own magnetic fields. Even the metal springs of a mattress may become charged up in the home field, so that they carry a continuous magnetic flux.

Couple this with the fact that rooms are typically wired with a ring main running right round the room and which with oscillating current will generate an intense magnetic field within the ring and you have a formula for danger. It's unfortunate that we spend maybe a third of our time lying in this hazardous bedroom field.

For over 30 years I have been advocating the fitting of what is called an EMF demands switch. This is a device which shuts down electrical supply to the whole house at night when the last equipment and last light are switched off (except for the refrigerator and freezer, of course). Only when someone throws a switch to call for light does the device allow the resupply of mains electricity. But you can go through the night without being surrounded by an electromagnetic field.

# 11.3 Dirty Electricity

I'd also like to describe a newly recognized hazard from electromagnetic fields and mains electricity, thanks to the work of engineer Dave Stetzer and Dr Magda Havas. It has been christened "dirty electricity" and it affects most homes. Dirty electricity takes two forms: transient spikes at high frequencies and leakages of current to ground.

Let's talk about transient spikes first. Most people know computers and sensitive equipment need to be protected from sudden high frequencies spikes in the electrical system ("surges"). They're very damaging but frequently occur in mains supply electricity. Indeed neighbor houses and even industry nearby could be creating dangerous transient spikes in your home, even if you are clean. So we fit surge protectors, if we are wise, in the power supply to sensitive equipment.

The thing is that no one has taken these transients seriously as a human health hazard until now. Yet they are unquestionably harmful. It brings down the immune system and that is the LAST thing you want in your situation.

So you do need to act.

The aforementioned Dave Stetzer produces a useful meter with which you test your home for dirty electricity. If the readings are reasonable or within the normal range you probably don't have a problem.

If the meter shows you do have a problem, you need to fit some protective filters. Stetzer Electrical supplies these too. You keep adding filters till the meter shows the readings are back in the safe zone. Then you can relax.

For Stetzer-Graham supplies, see the link later in this section.

The other kind of "dirty electricity" problem is due to the fact that electrical utility companies insist on dumping too much current to earth. They do this because their power lines are hopelessly out of date and simply can't cope with the huge electrical burden of modern technical and electronic way of life.

But instead of upgrading their systems, they choose to send more of the return current into the ground (way beyond what is allowed by law in some locales). The result is that some places do not have a neutral earth as we understand it but the ground is already highly charged. In fact this can be dangerous and a person standing on the floor with their feet and touching a water pipe might receive a significant electrical charge. Clearly this makes a nonsense of earthing your electrical equipment to the water pipe. The water pipe may be bringing current into your home instead of taking it away!

Well, this is not strictly radiation and not a proven cancer problem. But there is no question that it is a biological burden that your body can well do without if you're battling a dangerous disease.

OK, these are the things that you can do:

Get TriField Meter, or a gauss meter and an electrical field meter and test your home thoroughly, paying particular attention to the bedroom where you sleep and also to any favorite chair such as the place you watch TV or where you sit working at your computer. You need to fix anything you find.

Buy or borrow a Stetzer meter and test your home transients. If you're having a problem you need to search for the cause of the problem and remedy as much as you can. Sources of high-frequency dangerous transients include electronic equipment, plasma TVs, computers, loose wiring and especially dimmer switches. Remove or fix as much as you can find. Then further reduce the load by fitting Stetzer filters. Ignore any scientific ruckus that you come across on the net, trust me you need them.

# 11.4 Now, Cell Phones

So how important is this EMF radiation thing to cancer patients (cell phones and the like)?

I've been writing since the 1980s about the dangerous effects of electromagnetic radiation fields on human biology. For the first 10 years I was a voice in the wilderness but, today, recognition of this problem has spread to such an extent that only those completely out of touch would not be aware of the controversy and concern.

There is very special emphasis on the potential hazard of microwave radiation from cell phones, since we carry these close to our person, often within a few inches of vital organs, such as the heart, brain and gonads.

Electromagnetic radiation from mobile phones—both the radiation from the handsets and from the tower-based antennas carrying the signals—has been conclusively linked to development of brain tumors, genetic damage, and other exposure-related conditions. [Sue Kovach: http://www.lifeextension.com/magazine/2007/8/report_cellphone_radiation/Page-01]

What exasperates most sensible people is that, despite the evidence, communication companies like T-Mobile and AT and T run a well-oiled media machine to deliberately and wickedly spread disinformation and mislead the unwary public about the dangers of cellphones and antennas.

Laws are enacted to protect the industry and the average citizen is denied any right to safety and personal representation. Politicans, as we know, are corrupt and slick liars. But it's not just them...

The media and news anchors always support the communications industry and trumpet safety, without even mentioning the true science that concerns us all. Some media people, of course, are just ignorant, stupid or gullible. That's still irresponsible. But many, we must know, are corrupt and being paid to lie.

For example, a Danish epidemiological study announced to great fanfare the inaccurate conclusion that cell phone use is completely safe. [Schuz J, Jacobsen R, Olsen JH, Boice JD Jr, McLaughlin JK, Johansen C. Cellular telephone use and cancer risk: update of a nationwide Danish cohort. *J Natl Cancer Inst.* 2006 Dec 6;98(23):1707-13]

In other words, it's a fix!

George Carlo, PhD, JD, (not my favorite activist) is an epidemiologist and medical scientist who, from 1993 to 1999, headed the first telecommunications industry-backed studies into the dangers of cell phone use. That program remains the largest in the history of the issue. But he ran afoul of the very industry that hired him when his work revealed preventable health hazards associated with cell phone use and he decided to speak out.

True to form, the history of the argument deflects from the real science and becomes a campaign of smearing and discrediting Carlo and other's like him.

This is some of the story:

# Cell Phones Reach the Market without Safety Testing

The cellular phone industry was born in the early 1980s, when communications technology that had been developed for the Department of Defense was put into commerce by companies focusing on profits. This group, with big ideas but limited resources, pressured government regulatory agencies—particularly the Food and Drug Administration (FDA)—to allow cell phones to be sold without pre-market testing.

The rationale for this, known as the "low power exclusion," distinguished cell phones from dangerous microwave emitters, based on the amount of power used to push the microwaves. At that time, the only health effect that was recognized was the so-called thermal effect: the power to heat human tissue. Cell phones didn't fry you, like a microwave oven, therefore they are safe... kind of mentality. As a result, cell phones were exempted from any type of regulatory oversight, an exemption that continues today.

An eager public grabbed up the cell phones, but according to Dr. George Carlo, "Those phones were slowly prompting a host of health problems."

Today, more than half the world's population are cell phone users (was 3.6 billion, out of 7.2 billion, as of Sep 2014). More people have a cell phone than have a toilet.

So these phones are here to stay; no question. The problem is, how can we protect ourselves? Or indeed: *can we protect ourselves?*

One thing is clear, aaccording to the "other science" story: The amount of time spent on the phone is irrelevant, as the danger mechanism is triggered within seconds. And researchers say *if there is a safe level of exposure to EMR, it's so low that we can't detect it*.

Very worrying.

First step: if you live in the USA, immediately go to the website www.antenna-search.com and enter your address. The data that returns will tell you how many antenna are within 3.0 miles of your home. **You will be horrified!**

I did it for myself on Sep 24th, 2015, and there are 44 microwave towers and 141 antennas near my home.

It's a complicated issue but there is some evidence that melatonin and vitamins C and E rotect us from this kind of radiation. Better get started with these, if you are not already taking them.

# Children are especially at risk

Alarming research indicates that children and teenagers are five times more likely to get brain cancer if they use cell phones. The study is raising fears that today's young people may suffer an epidemic of the disease in later life.

The Swedish research was reported tat the first international conference on cell phones and health. It came from a further analysis of data from one of the biggest studies carried out on the cell phone/cancer link, headed by Professor Lennart Hardell. Professor Hardell told the conference that "people who started mobile phone use before the age of 20" had more than five-fold increase in glioma, a cancer of the glial cells that support the central nervous system.

The risk to young people from household cordless phones was almost as great. Cordless phones caused a fourfold increase in risk.

Young cell phone users are five times more likely to get acoustic neuromas, disabling tumors of the auditory nerve that often cause deafness.

Multiple studies have shown that children absorb more MWR than adults. One found that that the brain tissue of children absorbed about two times more MWR than that of adults, and other studies have reported that the bone marrow of children absorbs 10 times more MWR than that of adults.

However, not a single U.S. health agency is warning about the extra risks to children. Which is ironic, since American kids have the most WiFi gadgets.

"Belgium, France, India, and other technologically sophisticated governments are passing laws and/or issuing warnings about children's use of wireless devices," the review authors write.

They write that MWR exposure limits have remained unchanged for 19 years. They also note that smartphone makers specify the minimum distance from the body that their products must be kept so that legal limits for exposure to MWR aren't exceeded. For laptop computers and tablets, the minimum distance from the body is 20 cm (about 7.8 inches).

**But our concern here is cancer.**

Evidence is beginning to mount alarmingly that microwave radiation from cellphones is a cause of malignant disease. Already studies have been produced showing significant increases in problems like leukaemia and brain tumors.

I found a compelling double-blind medical study carried out in India in 2005 and published in the Indian Journal of Human Genetics

[Ghandi, G. "Genetic Damage in Mobile Phone Users: Some Preliminary Findings," Indian J Hum Genetics, 2005, 11:99-104.]

The study analyzed micronucleated cell damage in blood and buccal (mouth) tissues of people who use their cell phone 1- 15 hours a day. The control group had never used cell phones at any time. DNA samples were coded and scored blind in strict protocol.

The test results of the "Indian study" are very significant. The non- cell phone users had an average of only 4% of their cells with DNA damage. The persistent mobile phone users showed an average of 39.75% cell DNA damage. The blood of one 24-year-old male revealed 63% micronucleated cells. He had used a cell phone for 1-2 hours per day for two years.

The hundreds of types of human cancers have one thing in common—they all begin at the cellular level when DNA genetic material in one or more cells becomes damaged. This damage can be passed from parents, or caused by the effects of an environmental carcinogen. "... Genetic mutations in one single cell are sufficient to lead to cancer," says Dr. Henry Lai, awell-knownscientist at the University of Washington, who has years of genetic and bioenergetics research to his credit ["Evidence for Genotoxic Effects (RFR and ELF Genotoxicity)" Dr. Henry Lai, Department of Bioengineering, University of Washington, Prepared for the BioInitiative Working Group, July 2007, see BioInitiative Report].

**Here's another:**
Prof Rony Seger, a cancer researcher at the Weizmann Institute of Science in Rehovot, Israel, and colleagues exposed rat and human cells to electromagnetic radiation at a similar frequency to that emitted by mobiles. The power of the signal was around 1/10th of that from a mobile.

After just five minutes the researchers identified the production of extracellular signal-regulated kinases (ERK1/2) – natural chemicals that stimulate cell division and growth.

Cancers develop when the body is unable to prevent excessive growth and division of cells in the wrong place.

Prof Seger said: "The real significance of our findings is that cells are not inert to non-thermal mobile phone radiation.

"We used radiation power levels that were around 1/10th of those produced by a normal mobile. The changes we observed were clearly not caused by heating."

I can't emphasize enough that there are far too many studies showing this kind of result to ignore the problem. Scientists who say there is no problem are being shockingly dishonest. They, of course, are paid by the telecommunication companies to blow smoke in everyone's eyes.

# Using A Field Meter

The first thing you have to do is to establish the scale a problem in your environment and there are various ways you can do this using hand-held field detection meters, which you can buy most places for under $100 each. The one I use is called a Trifield Meter 100XE and retails on Amazon for about $140. You have the possibility of measuring the magnetic field (a gauss meter) or the electrical field (volts per square metre or Teslas) or a third kind of interference field I shall describe shortly (RF). There are other devices, of course. Good ones are so easy that even a non-technical person can use one; usually there is a failsafe display that simply goes "red for danger"

If there is a problem, you may need to get specialist help to correct it.

Take your meter everywhere in the home—and also your office and other hang outs. There are many sources of exposure:
- microwave oven
- WiFi phones around the home
- Television

- Computer

- Games consoles

In the old days cathode ray tubes were a significant source of intense radiation including soft x-rays. But today's plasma screens are equally hazardous in a different way, producing dangerous transient spikes which I shall discuss shortly.

One of the worst hazards I used to find was a person's sleeping place. Often the night stand is a place where people have a radio and alarm clock, maybe teamaker and a telephone which may or may not be WiFi. Then there are electric blankets and waterbeds which may add their own magnetic fields. Even the metal springs of a mattress may become charged up in the home field, so that they carry a continuous magnetic flux.

Couple this with the fact that rooms are typically wired with a ring main running right round the room and which with oscillating current will generate an intense magnetic field within the ring and you have a formula for danger. It's unfortunate that we spend maybe a third of our time lying in this hazardous bedroom field.

For over 30 years I have been advocating the fitting of what is called an EMF demands switch. This is a device which shuts down electrical supply to the whole house at night when the last equipment and last light are switched off (except for the refrigerator and freezer, of course). Only when someone throws a switch to call for light does the device allow the resupply of mains electricity. But you can go through the night without being surrounded by an electromagnetic field.

# 11.5 Saxton Burr

This section should be read in conjunction with my book *Medicine Beyond*: www.alternative-doctor.com/medicinebeyond/

Those of you who have read *Medicine Beyond* will know of the amazing discoveries of Harold Saxton Burr and Georges Lakhovsky, decades before their time.

In the 1920s and 30s Professor Harold Saxton Burr at Yale began to experiment with electrical recordings of living energy fields of trees and subsequently humans. Trees were particularly suitable, since they could be left wired up for long periods. Burr was fascinated to note changes brought about by sunlight and darkness, cycles of the moon, sunspots and seasonal changes.

Studying humans, he and his colleague Dr Leonard Ravitz noticed that human emotions affected this field. Voltages would be high when the patient was feeling good and would drop when he or she was below par. Burr foresaw the fascinating possibility that '...psychiatrists of the future will be able to measure the intensity of grief, anger or love electrically as easily as we now measure temperature or noise levels today. 'Heartbreak', hate or love, in other words, may one day be measurable in millivolts'.

Burr and colleagues also discovered a voltage rise just before ovulation, which drops just as the egg is released. Healing wounds also change voltage. But most remarkable of all, there are voltage changes due to malignant tissue and Burr was eventually able to predict, from reversal of the polarity across the abdominal wall, when a woman would in the future develop cancer of the cervix. This anticipates later prognostic work with electro dermal screening described here (section 14).

What Burr and his colleagues were measuring was simply voltage potential. But he himself points out that changes can be measured at a distance from the affected organ or even outside the body, holding the electrodes above the skin, showing it is therefore a true field effect. He called it the 'Field of Life' or L Field for short.

I highly recommend Saxton Burr's book "Blueprint For Immortality". Be sure to get yourself a copy.

# 11.6 Georges Lakhovsky

Lakhovsky was an investigative genius, born in 1869 and his seminal book *The Secret Of Life* was published in 1925. That puts him ahead of Saxton Burr but the reader will soon readily appreciate that progressively he belongs here in the sequence, since his visionary ideas look far forward into the world of modern bio physics.

George Lakhovsky was a Russian engineer who became a naturalized French citizen and was ultimately awarded the Legion of Honour for his scientific technical services during the First World War. He had to flee his adopted country before the Nazis and died in New York in 1942.

Like those who went before him, Lakhovsky had to endure much calumny and ridicule. As one of his supporters remarked: 'The publication of *The Secret Of Life* resulted in causing great annoyance to the custodians of infallible doctrines who made up with carping verbiage what they lacked in clarity of vision'. As Lakhovsky himself put it: 'I have been attacked by physicists ignorant of biology and by biologists ignorant of physics who consequently can neither understand my theories nor judge my experiments'. [Keith Scott-Mumby, *Medicine Beyond*, Mother Whale Inc, Reno, 2015, p.116]

This extraordinary man of diverse talents showed that recorded sunspot activity parallelled magnetic disturbances and auroras on Earth. He also established a correlation between sunspot activity and good wine vintage years.

I have eslewhere called attention to Lakhovsky's observation that geological terrain seemed to have a potentially dangerous connection with cancer causation (see section 11.7)

Lakhovsky foresaw that one day it may be possible to project images of cancer tumors as an energy disturbance onto a TV screen; today we have MRI and CAT scanners.

But it is Lakhovsky's ideas about biological radiation fields that interest us here. His fundamental scientific principle was that every living thing emits radiation and this has important health implications. According to Lakhovsky the nucleus of a living cell may be compared to an electrical oscillating circuit. This nucleus consists of tubular filaments, chromosomes and mitochondria, made of insulating membranes but filled by an electrically conductive intra cellular fluid. These filaments have capacitance and inductance properties and are therefore capable of working like radio transmitters and receivers.

In Lakhovsky's model, life and disease is a matter of a 'war of radiations' between the body's cells and microbes. If the radiations of the microbe or cancer win, disease and death will result. If the cell's own energy transmission wins, then health is preserved. We have arrived at a very advanced and quite defensible energetic view of disease. Lakhovsky himself went on to conduct very many experiments in this vein. The results he got were little short of startling for his time and so one may presume there is a lot to be derived from his theories.

For many years, Lakhovsky had a great interest in the mechanism of cancer formation. That in itself was unusual in his time. There was no 'War Aginast Cancer' media circus running then and a leading London surgeon of the day pointed out that funding of cancer research did not even amount to one penny per person in the British Isles!

There were many hypotheses advanced as to the causation of cancer at that time, including heredity, infection by viruses, local trauma, pollution and nutritional deficiency. It seems certain that all these factors may play a part. But Lakhovsky was convinced that oscillatory disequilibrium, that is cellular radiation energy disturbance, was the predominant factor in the onset of malignancy.

The problem was, how to reverse it.

Our bodies consist of around 100,000,000,000,000 (a hundred trillion) cells and hardly any two oscillate exactly alike. This is partly due to differing tissues but also variation through time in the status of each individual cell. The impact of extraneous radiation would also produce modulations, such as the resonance effect. Finding a standardized harmonizing frequency would seem to be a Sisyphean task.

With brilliance and ingenuity, Lakhovsky invented his celebrated Multiple Wave Oscillator, generating a field in which every cell could find its own frequency and vibrate in resonance. The practical successes he began having in hospitals soon confirmed the validity of his theory.

Numerous cases recovered and were documented by excited doctors. He was careful to avoid talking in terms of a cancer 'cure'. However he did unequivocally cure a number of cases; all the others showed variable but marked degrees of improvement.

If any reader would like to follow one of his simple experiments on plant cancer, this is not difficult to perform and will provide a fascinating home workshop on the properties of biological radiation. In this experiment Lakhovsky purposely dispensed with the oscillator and relied instead on the presence of ambient radiations.

He took a series of Geranium plants inoculated with the *Bacterium tumefaciens* (=tumor making bacterium) which causes cancer like growths on the plants: 'A month later, when the tumors had developed, I took one of the plants at random which I surrounded with a copper spiral consisting of copper and measuring 30 cm. in diameter, its two extremities, not joined together, being fixed into an ebonite support (a rigid plastic tube, such as a spent ballpen stem, would suffice perfectly well). An oscillator of this kind has a fundamental wavelength of about 2 metres, or 150 megaHerz, and picks up the oscillating energy of innumerable radiations in the atmosphere.

"I then let the experiment follow its natural course during several weeks. After a fortnight, I examined my plants. I was astonished to find that all my geraniums or the stalks bearing the tumors were dead and dried up with the exception of the geranium surrounded by the copper spiral, which has since grown to twice the height of the untreated healthy plants'.

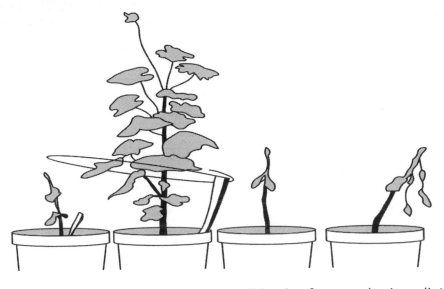

The oscillator was picking up and damping all kinds of atmospheric radiations. He bewails that, even in his day, so many radio transmitters were springing up that 'there is no detectable gap in the gamut of these waves'. Consider the health problem implied by this, when today we have a million times the intensity of blanket radiations that he experienced.

## 11.6a Lakhovsky's Multiwave Oscillator

By the 1920s, Lakhovsky had clinics all over Europe, delivering his electromagnetic oscillatory, or "vibrational" therapy.

Lakhovsky's method was so successful he was approached by several hospitals in New York hoping to test his apparatus experimentally. Remarkable results were obtained from a seven-week clinical trial performed at a major New York City hospital and that of a prominent Brooklyn urologist in the summer of 1941.

What seemed like a promising development in the use of the MWO in America quickly faded after Lakhovsky unexpectedly died in New York in 1942 (age 73). *A car struck and killed him in a most mysterious manner.* His equipment was removed from the hospital and patients were told that the therapy was no longer available.

Nobody intelligent could believe this was just one of those things. The murderous hand of Maurice Fishbein (the AMA) and Big Pharma is all over this story. The pharmaceutical companies and doctors figured out they could make a lot of money "treating" people, not making them well, and then getting someone else to pay for it. They continue to ruthlessly discredit valuable therapies that threaten their profits.

However, in the countries not under the sway of Big Pharma, like the former Soviet Union, electromagnetic field therapy did not die out, but was further developed and is still widely deployed throughout hospitals. Their scientists learned that when magnetic fields are pulsed, their effect was considerably enhanced. It covered the innate vibration of a wider range of cells and tissues, Lakhovsky would probably have said.

Enter Nikola Tesla, another modern individual to be recognized for manipulating electromagnetic fields for health purposes. His methods and patents in the early 1900s for the Tesla coil were also used for electromagnetic medical devices.

These devices were often large round solenoid coils of wire that would surround the patient while they would stand or lie on a bed. They were energized directly from the 50 or 60 Hz sine wave electrical system. The patient would usually experience an immediate relief in pain.

Tesla's methods for electrotherapy were originally embraced by electricians who wanted to commercialize electricity. However electro-therapeutic devices eventually fell out of favor with doctors when educators in western medical schools chose to only educate medical students in the use of pharmaceuticals and surgery (a result of the infamous Flexner Report 1910).

In addition, a concerted effort by the pharmaceutical industry to discredit electromagnetic therapy caused it to be branded as "quackery" and electrical medical devices were only to be considered for diagnostic purposes such as X-ray. Tesla's advances were quickly forgotten.

Although electromagnetic therapy has become widely adopted in Western Europe, its use was restricted to animals in North America. Veterinarians became the first health professionals to use PEMF therapy, for healing things like broken legs in race horses. Professional sports doctors then decided to experiment with veterinarian devices off label on professional athletes which ultimately led to legally licensed devices for human use in the United States—but under strict stipulations that it was not to be used for non-union bone fractures, except under a medical prescription from a licensed doctor.

Based on a 2007 clinical trial, in which patients with either chronic generalized pain from fibromyalgia (FM) or chronic localized musculoskeletal or inflammatory pain were exposed to a PEMF (400 microT) through a portable device fitted to their head during twice-daily 40 min treatments over seven days, Thomas et al. conclude, "PEMF may be a novel, safe and effective therapeutic tool." [Pain Res Manag. 2007 Winter;12(4):249-58]

# 11.7 Pulsed Electromagnetic Field Therapy (PEMF)

By the 1920s, Lakhovsky had clinics all over Europe, delivering his electromagnetic oscillatory, or "vibrational" therapy.

Lakhovsky's method was so successful he was approached by several hospitals in New York hoping to test his apparatus experimentally. Remarkable results were obtained from a seven-week clinical trial performed at a major New York City hospital and that of a prominent Brooklyn urologist in the summer of 1941.

What seemed like a promising development in the use of the MWO in America quickly faded after Lakhovsky unexpectedly died in New York in 1942 (age 73). *A car struck and killed him in a most mysterious manner.* His equipment was removed from the hospital and patients were told that the therapy was no longer available.

Nobody intelligent could believe this was just one of those things. The murderous hand of Maurice Fishbein (the AMA) and Big Pharma is all over this story. The pharmaceutical companies and doctors figured out they could make a lot of money "treating" people, not making them well, and then getting someone else to pay for it. They continue to ruthlessly discredit valuable therapies that threaten their profits.

However, in the countries not under the sway of Big Pharma, like the former Soviet Union, electromagnetic field therapy did not die out, but was further developed and is still widely deployed throughout hospitals. Their scientists learned that when magnetic fields are pulsed, their effect was considerably enhanced. It covered the innate vibration of a wider range of cells and tissues, Lakhovsky would probably have said.

Enter Nikola Tesla, another modern individual to be recognized for manipulating electromagnetic fields for health purposes. His methods and patents in the early 1900s for the Tesla coil were also used for electromagnetic medical devices.

These devices were often large round solenoid coils of wire that would surround the patient while they would stand or lie on a bed. They were energized directly from the 50 or 60 Hz sine wave electrical system. The patient would usually experience an immediate relief in pain.

Tesla's methods for electrotherapy were originally embraced by electricians who wanted to commercialize electricity. However electro-therapeutic devices eventually fell out of favor with doctors when educators in western medical schools chose to only educate medical students in the use of pharmaceuticals and surgery (a result of the infamous Flexner Report 1910).

In addition, a concerted effort by the pharmaceutical industry to discredit electromagnetic therapy caused it to be branded as "quackery" and electrical medical devices were only to be considered for diagnostic purposes such as X-ray. Tesla's advances were quickly forgotten.

Although electromagnetic therapy has become widely adopted in Western Europe, its use was restricted to animals in North America. Veterinarians became the first health professionals to use PEMF therapy, for healing things like broken legs in race horses. Professional sports doctors then decided to experiment with veterinarian devices off label on professional athletes which ultimately led to legally licensed devices for human use in the United States—but under strict stipulations that it was not to be used for non-union bone fractures, except under a medical prescription from a licensed doctor.

Based on a 2007 clinical trial, in which patients with either chronic generalized pain from fibromyalgia (FM) or chronic localized musculoskeletal or inflammatory pain were exposed to a PEMF (400 microT) through a portable device fitted to their head during twice-daily 40 min treatments over seven days, Thomas et al. conclude, "PEMF may be a novel, safe and effective therapeutic tool." [Pain Res Manag. 2007 Winter;12(4):249-58]

## General Health Benefits

The whole of my book "Medicine Beyond" (www.alternative-doctor.com/medicinebeyond/) is about the existence of thrilling life energies, which inform and empower our cells and tissues. Atoms, molecules, cells and organs, all have different and unique characteristic oscillatory rates. Indeed, that is why cyclotron resonance devices (and dowsers) can detect specific tissues and disease processes.

Lakhovsky tells us that not only do all living cells produce and radiate their own oscillations, but they also receive and respond to oscillations imposed upon them from outside sources. Indeed, that's why cell phones, microwave radiation and so forth, are so inherently dangerous.

But why not give the cells a dose of healthy, "juicing up" vibrations, the sort that living organisms like? Typically these are low frequency oscillations or ELFs, as they are called (extremely low frequencies). It is possible to enliven body tissues and healthy physiological mechanisms and structures by using pulsed electromagnetic fields.

A lot of people have caught onto this idea and it's working out just fine in practice, with or without the approval of regulatory bodies. As usual, where in one territory you are told it's illegal and maybe even dangerous, in other parts of the world it's everyday medicine from properly trained, certified and ethical MDs and practitioners.

Wherever you live, you need to know about this up-and-coming therapy.

# 11.7a PEMF Improves The Blood

In 2013 I was in London, speaking at a conference on cancer alternatives, when I met Dr. Med. Henning Saupe from Kassel, Germany. We didn't really agree over Laetrile therapy but—as gentlemen doctors—we agreed to differ!

But I was impressed by Dr. Saupe's demonstration of the value of PEMF therapy in energizing blood; specifically, in the power of PEMF to free up red blood cells that stick together and create a viscosity problem.

What took place was remarkable, not just as a treatment for a cancer patient but I would argue for anyone, in any state of health. Especially, I would laud it as a treatment against any sort of aging, decay, metabolic slowdown or vascular insufficiency (the last covers most things due to aging!)

A sample of blood was taken and examined under dark field microscopy (which allows you to see living blood, instead of dead and stained specimens). What you see (image 1) is lots of red blood cells, stuck and jammed together in ropes called "rouleaux" (like a pile of coins on its side). This is a bad formation that signifies sickness and means that red blood cells cannot flow freely through tiny capillaries and so deliver their "load" of oxygen efficiently. The blood is sludged, to use an everyday word.

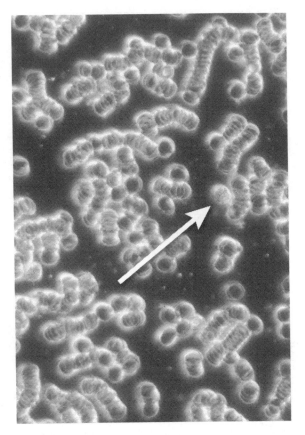

Also, (arrowed) you will see a slightly different cell; that's a white blood cell. But it's quite as small as the red blood cells (it should be much larger, double or treble the size) and it is also very hemmed in and can't function.

Finally, pathology number three, if you look closely you will see the blood plasma, the background fluid, is filled with fibers, rather like carpet shedding its pile. That's very bad; those are fibrinogen threads and when present in large quantities like this acts like a buried landmine that will explode at the least thing and cause instant clotting.

The more fibrinogen is present in the blood, the more likely a coronary thrombosis (myocardial infarction) or a stroke. Meantime, the fibers too add to the bloods overall viscosity or sludging. The rule is: the less viscosity, the better (providing the clotting mechanism is intact).

This sluggish blood was reflected in the patient, who said she was tired and had no energy.

It's important to remember that very little chemical substance which might be tried as a treatment of cancer (vitamin C, polyphenols, enzymes or Artemisin or any other holistic therapy), would have any effect in such a state. Not even Otto Warburg's oxygen in high concentration could bind to these cells and mobilize the blood!

What followed was 15 minutes of PEMF therapy, directed towards the patient's pelvis, chest, thyroid, pancreas and liver. And then another blood sample was taken (image 2). The changes that are evident are just amazing.

In such a short time the red cells have separated and are flowing smoothly and sweetly. When they bump into each other, they soon separate; in other words they do not stick together.

Also, the white cell is no longer trapped but disengaged and, most remarkable of all, it's more than doubled in size! Plus you can't see the fibers any more; the blood plasma is swept "clean".

This is of enormous importance to cancer patients, those fighting virtually any disease and those who resist aging. As Georges Lakhovsky taught us, our life is the energy in our cells. They vibrate and if that oscillatory rate drops to the levels shown by this lady, then blood perfusion in impaired and cancer is almost inevitable. Conversely, if we energize our cells with this kind of energy medicine treatment, the cells regain their gusto, move around and function as they should. Wow!

This is not to call it a cancer "cure". Indeed, it is different from many alternative therapies in that it is not aimed at the cancer at all; it's aimed at the blood support system and general cellular energies. Nevertheless, if you have fully understood what I have written here, you will likely judge this to be a must-have approach, in addition to anything else you may be employing against your cancer (and, yes, even in conjunction with chemotherapy and radiotherapy).

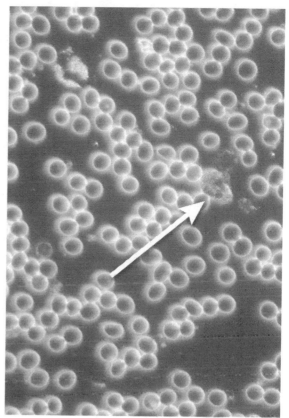

Personally, I relish this against aging. As a confirmed "Boomer", I want to live a lot longer; the party we've always promised ourselves has only just begun! With PEMF to jolly up my tissues and keep them clean and refreshed, I expect to go on dancing a lot longer yet. Care to join me?

The device used in this amazing demonstration, by the way, was the PMT-100

[Markov, Marko S. "Expanding Use of Pulsed Electromagnetic Field Therapies." Electromagnetic Biology & Medicine 26.3 (2007): 257–274. Academic Search Complete. EBSCO. Web. 10 June 2010]

# 11.8 The Rife Machine

Now it's time to look at what could be the greatest and most exact and workable cancer cure of all time: the discoveries of Royal Raymond Rife in the 1930s.

Royal Raymond Rife was unarguably a brilliant technician. He was hired by Henry Timken, an industrial magnate, and under Timken's sponsorship produced the most technologically advanced speedboat marine engine of the day (1915), generating 2700 HP.

Rife went on with Timken's support to develop microscopes and almost perfected the art, producing compounded quartz prisms in a glycerine bath, which gave resolutions of up to 50,000 diameters; this was at a time when the best commercial laboratory microscopes could give only up to 2,000 diameters. Rife's Universal Microscope was without doubt the greatest optical instrument ever designed; no-one can seriously question this aspect of Rife's work.

It's what he *saw* that started the acrimony and disputation.

He illuminated the microorganism (usually a virus or bacteria) with two different wavelengths of the same ultraviolet light frequency, which resonated with the spectral signature of the microbe. These two wavelengths produced interference where they merged. This interference was, in effect, a third, longer wave, which fell into the visible portion of the electromagnetic spectrum.

So when viewed, the organism would appear to light up in a blaze at a certain characteristic frequency.

Rife likened this effect to using light like this as the equivalent of a chemical stain in conventional microbiology.

This new technique gave Rife a unique advantage and enabled him to see things nobody had ever seen before with ordinary microscopes.

Rife became the first human being to actually see a live virus, and until quite recently, his microscope was the only one which was able to view live viruses. Even more amazingly, he saw that when a Tubercle bacillus was destroyed, it split into many smaller living particles, which he called TB viruses (this was not naivete; a virus at that time was just considered to be a filterable bacterium).

These altered forms we call pleomorphism and it is bitterly disputed, even today, that such a thing can take place. Of course none of the experts who deny its existence have ever looked through a Rife microscope!

But Rife also saw something else, something startling, something that shouldn't be there!

# 11.8a Bacillus X

Rife saw curious tiny little living virus-size organisms in the blood of cancer patients. They were too small to be bacteria but were not viruses. He found they gave off a distinctive purple-red emanation when viewed in the microscope. He named this entity bacillus X, or "BX" and claimed to have verified its existence in every instance of carcinoma he examined.

At that time virus causation of cancer was unheard of (today it's looking like most cancers could be caused by viruses). On our present model, BX was cancer trouble just waiting to happen.

He injected rats with the organelles and created cancers. These were then used to obtain more organelles and pass the disease on to the next rat and so. In fact Rife was able to convert from cancer to the organelle and back 104 times. Cancer, he concluded, was transferred by something smaller than a bacterium.

But few were prepared to believe Rife. Despite widespread media of the day claiming that "The cure for cancer has been found", the idea of a cancer virus or cancer bacterium was too far beyond the boundaries of knowledge at the time (1932).

# 11.8b Lethal Rays

Rife discovered that if you play a resonant electromagnetic frequency to an organism it will oscillate or vibrate with it, until it bursts, like the singer's trick of singing the specific note of a drinking glass and make it shatter.

This killing disruption was called *electroporation*, and led to the cell's immediate malfunction and death. The "kill frequency" Rife termed the mortal oscillatory rate or MOR. As well as bacteria and viruses, it worked against cancer cells. It was 100% effective. He had found, at last, the cure for cancer!

Now, this is critical: Rife stated quite clearly that you need the MOR killer frequency of the rod form of the bacillus and the viral form or the "BX" (cancer) organism simultaneously, to get any effect.

This feature is missing from all subsequent me-too "Rife machines".

The MORs for the BX (cancer) and BY (sarcoma) forms of malignancy were listed by Rife as follows:

    1,604,000
    11,780,000
    17,033,663

Fortunately, perhaps surprisingly, normal healthy human cells were completely unharmed by these lethal waves.

By 1935 Rife was ready to begin experiments using his "ray" machine on humans with cancer and TB. Out of 16 terminally ill patients, 14 were pronounced clinically cured after 70 days; the other 2 subsequently recovered after the end of the trial. In other words a 100% success rate on patients in the worst possible condition. This result is outstanding and passes into medical history as a truly great achievement. More shame on those who still refute it, over 70 years later.

This "ray" method was truly a breakthrough.

In his career Rife won 14 government awards in recognition of scientific achievements and was honored with a medical degree at the University of Heidelberg in Germany. Yet today his name is often viewed as synonymous with quackery and "Rife machines" are illegal in his home country (though not, of course, elsewhere in the world). That's how far Rife's star has fallen and has yet to be resurrected.

Much has been written about the final destruction of the Rife microscope and his frequency machines. We have accounts claiming the FDA burst into his office at gun point and smashed all his equipment. The stories of raids are more likely distortions of actions taken against Life Lab Inc, a later company making copycat frequency machines, with Rife as a titular research head but without any real involvement.

It's true that Morris Fishbein, editor of the Journal of the AMA tried to buy into Rife's company Beam Ray and became very maliciously vindictive when he was not allowed to. As a result of his actions doctors using the device were "visited" by the AMA and told to send it back, or face loss of their license (incidentally, Fishbein and the AMA used the same tactics against Harry Hoxsey, who developed a successful herbal cancer cure).

But Rife's own colleagues probably did him nearly as much damage by producing machines which did not stick to the proper specifications and failed to work consistently. It was even speculated that one of his key engineers, Phillip Hoyland, was sabotaging the program because he desired to grab the action for himself.

Regardless of all this, I think the final demise of the machine was much simpler to explain and far less dramatic.

Rife came to the market with his machine in the 1930s. It cost $7,000 which in those days was a very considerable investment, even for an MD. No matter, he sold a number of them.

But also in the 1930s, by a twist of fate, sulfonamide antibiotics swept over the horizon, followed rapidly by penicillin, and this new class of drugs soon overran the therapeutic picture at a fast gallop. When it was possible to knock out virtually any pathogen with a drug costing just a few dollars, quickly, safely and simply (according to perceptions of the day), who would want to invest in a costly machine that was inconveniently large, expensive to run and difficult to operate?

It was the same bad luck with his advanced microscopes. They were the very best of the day, precise and advanced, but very costly.

Unfortunately for Rife, the electron microscope was also just around the corner (1931) and optical microscopes, no matter how powerful, were doomed to be eclipsed. Of course electron microscopes can only ever look at dead tissue; but that's the fashion in so-called science. Nobody, it seems, wants to do anything so corny as look at real living organisms!

There is another factor little talked about, which is that the authentic Rife machines were super-regenerative RF transmitters. Without going into the technical details, that meant they ultimately fell foul of Federal Communications Commission regulations.

Remember, by this time radio stations were springing up all over the US and the FCC developed strict guidelines as to who was allowed to broadcast, where, when and at what frequencies. Rife machines were really doomed by this one factor alone.

Rife was simply a man out of his time. He died in 1971, frustrated and sad, a broken man, an alcoholic.

Most of his knowledge has passed into history and most claims for authentic "Rife machines" are bogus. You can tell any of these knock off fakes because they use disease "codes", instead of displaying a frequency.

Typical machines today use pads in contact with the patient and Rife himself roundly condemned this approach. Without an RF carrier frequency the audio frequencies will only go through the connective tissue and not the cell.

And of course they don't work. But you see them touted at every health fair and exhibition.

# 11.8c The Rife Code Breakthrough

Since the first edition of this book, an important new breakthrough has been made.

As I hinted, Phillip Hoyland was a treacherous employee of Rife and did him untold harm. It has emerged he took advantage of Rife's ignorance of electronics and substituted the published frequencies with "codes" derived from an algorithm which he used secretly. Whether it was just to sabotage Rife, perhaps being paid by Fishbein or the AMA, or whether Hoyland was intending to steal the effective frequencies for himself may never be known. He took his algorithm and the codes to the grave with him.

However, the code has been cracked just in the last year before writing this! We now understand how to much more closely replicate what Rife really did.

He was using audio-range frequencies on a "carrier wave" or radio RF in the megahertz band (3.8 MHz). 90% of modern knock-offs use only the audio-frequencies. What they are selling is NOT RIfe technology.

Correct machines are now being manufactured and I know where to get them. Unfortunately, manufacturers and sellers are running scared, since the FDA recently clamped down hard and sent one seller to jail for life (just for trying to help sick people).

Outside the USA, of course, you're good to go!

## There's more!

I see that another related "breakthrough" was reported in 2007. John Kanzius from Eerie PA claims to have hit on the idea of using radio waves to kill cancer. It sounds remarkably like Rife's method.

Kanzius' idea, in fact, is a little different from Rife's. He proposes sending immunologically tagged nanoparticles to the tumor site (well within current medical science capabilities) and then, by bombarding the site with radio frequencies, to heat up the tumor and "fry" it (actually another type of hyperthermia: see also section 9).

Kanzius' idea takes advantage of what Rife found, which is that normal human tissue is transparent to radio frequencies and, in the suggested doses at least, is unharmed by it. In any case the risk of radiation sickness from RF is less than with radiotherapy and far less of a problem than dying of cancer.

I think it will work and work well. It's in trial now. The real question is "Will the cancer industry allow it?"

They might, because they can patent and charge fortunes for the nanoparticle technology. But I predict very few doctors will see this as the real vindication of Rife's genius.

This section is taken from my book "Medicine Beyond", which you can get here:

http://www.alternative-doctor.com/medicinebeyond

# 11.8d Rife Gone Mainstream!

And now there is yet another twist to this fascinating story!

Conventional scientists now talk about "electrochemotherapy", in which doses of a chemo drug, such as bleomycin or cisplatin are driven into the cancer cells by high-frequency pulsed electro-magnetic waves.

What happens is that the electric pulses upset the cell physiology and cause the cell membranes to become temporarily leaky or permeable. The effect is called "electroporation" and was exactly what Rife discovered, except that in his research the effect was so strong that the cell walls literally burst and the cell contents spilled out, killing it (see "irreversible electroporation" below).

Let me quote a study published in the prestigious conventional *British Journal Of Cancer*: "Electrochemotherapy enhances the effectiveness of chemotherapeutic agents by administering the drug in combination with short intense electric pulses…. applied to tumours percutaneously after intravenous or intratumour administration of bleomycin.

The tumours were measured and the response to the treatment evaluated 30 days after the treatment. Objective responses were obtained in 233 (85.3%) of the 273 evaluable tumours that were treated…. The application of electric pulses to the patients was safe and well tolerated."

[Cancer. 1998 Jun;77(12):2336-42].

Over 85% response rate? That's remarkable.

In fact on PubMed, the US government database of medical studies, I found 280 articles on the topic of electrochemotherapy. One fairly recent paper (2008) was entitled "Electrochemotherapy: An Emerging Cancer Treatment"

[Int J Hyperthermia. 2008 May;24(3):263-73]

So there is great progress. Of course other drugs and perhaps vaccines can also be administered and driven into cells with this technique. It has even been speculated that electroporation may allow delivery of modified genes in fighting disease.

[Mol Biotechnol. 2009 Jan;41(1):69-82]

Electrochemotherapy is not *exactly* the same as Rife's work. But what if you drop out the chemo and concentrate just on the radiation aspect?

# 11.8e Irreversible Electroporation

In my researches I found that Rife technology abounds in orthodox science and medicine! That's right. Of course they don't call it Rife technology: it's known as irreversible electroporation. It's electrochemotherapy moved on and without giving the drugs.

The actual mechanism of cell death in Rife's method is called "irreversible electroporation". A paper from the Department of Bioengineering, Graduate Group in Biophysics, University of California at Berkeley, tells us more:

> Certain electrical fields when applied across a cell can have as a sole effect the permeabilization of the cell membrane, presumable through the formation of nanoscale defects in the cell membrane. Sometimes this process leads to cell death, primarily when the electrical fields cause permanent permeabilization of the membrane and the consequent loss of cell homeostasis, in a process known as irreversible electroporation. This is an unusual mode of cell death that is not understood yet. While the phenomenon of irreversible electroporation may have been known for centuries it has become only recently rigorously considered in medicine for various applications of tissue ablation.

[Technol Cancer Res Treat. 2007 Aug;6(4):255-60.]

Permeabilization is a ridiculous word, even in this context; it simply means "making permeable" (in other words, leaky!) Porous is the familiar word; hence: electroporation.

Ablation is a medical term for destroying (tissues).

Irreversible is just a way of saying dead, finito, done!

To those who know the full story, it seems kind of ironic that the FDA would approve a Rife-type device. Yet that is precisely what happened in April 2011, when an FDA panel backed a novel, noninvasive device that uses an electrical field designed to blast apart cancer cells, as a potential treatment for brain cancer.

The device, called the NovoTTF (for tumor treating fields), was designed by a private firm, NovoCure Ltd., which has operations in Israel and the U.S. It is being developed for use in patients with glioblastoma, a common form of brain cancer, initially for use after standard treatments fail.

NovoCure's device is designed to disrupt the division of cancer cells in the brain using alternating electrical fields delivered by means of insulated electrodes applied to the surface of the scalp.

The portable device uses electric fields to disrupt the division of cancer cells that allows tumors to grow and spread. The electric fields have little effect on healthy cells because they divide at a much slower rate, if at all, compared with cancer cells.

The FDA approved the device specifically for a tumor type known as glioblastoma, the most aggressive form of brain cancer. Five-year survival for the disease is just 2% for patients over 45 years old, according to the American Cancer Society.

If it proves out, then we may see approval extended to a wide variety of cancerous situations; not just the hopeless glioblastoma cases.

The panel of non-FDA medical experts voted 7 to 3 in favor of a question that asked whether the benefits of the device outweighed the risks. Two panel members abstained from voting. The panel unanimously said the product was safe, but split on whether the product is effective.

Unfortunately, in a 237-patient trial, this device did not produce the miracle recoveries we would like to see. In fact survival for those using the device was about on a par with those taking chemo (about 6 months). But at least their quality of life was better.

In a European study, patients fared better and the therapy produced double the normal survival time. The FDA, of course, couldn't care less about studies on non-Americans (since they can't control the outcomes!)

Brain tumors are notoriously aggressive and difficult to treat; glioblastoma is the worst of all. Only time will tell whether, with tweaks, modern electroporation devices can start to get the amazing results that Rife did.

The NovoTTF is now re-named as the Optune™. Novocure has not released the frequencies that they use. Their website (www.optune.com) is now claiming "a large clinical study has shown that the Optune is as effective as chemotherapy in treating recurrent glioblastoma."

I have prepared a revolutionary report on this new aspect of cancer therapy, that is destined to become part of the orthodox medical canon. You can get a copy here:

http://www.alternative-doctor.com/downloads/ElectroChemotherapy.pdf


## Irreversible Electroporation In The News

Just as I am revizing this book, irreversible electroporation is in the news again.

This time it's been shown effective against tricky pancreatic cancer. This one is bad news because it grows silently within and is usually only discovered too late, when it has invaded the liver and other tissue and become inoperable. By 2020, this cancer is expected to be second only to lung cancer as a cause of cancer-related death, according to the *Pancreatic Cancer Action Network*.

Survival rates are pretty poor. Average is as little as 6 weeks from diagnosis. But now they can be significantly extended. OK, gone is better! But increased survival without having to lose your hair and barf up several times a day is a big improvement on the previous picture.

Surgeons have learned to use short electrical bursts to kill cancerous cells in delicate areas without destroying noncancerous tissue nearby, such as nerves. The electrical bursts make permanent holes, or pores, in the cells, eventually killing them, the researchers said.

In other words, irreversible electroporation!

The people in the current study, published in the Sep 2015 *Annals of Surgery*, all had a pancreatic tumor that had extended into nearby organs, making complete surgical removal impossible. The zapping technique is intended to corral the cancer cells and extend the patient's survival.

All of the 200 adults with stage 3 pancreatic cancer included in the current study underwent electrical IRE treatment after completing chemotherapy.

About half of the patients in the study experienced complications. But any side effects were directly related to the surgical procedure and not the electroporation procedure.

The average survival was two years, the study found. The study authors followed some patients for as long as seven years.

It doesn't work for stage 4, where the cancer has spread widely, so they have not yet learned to make it body-wide, as Rife did. It will come, eventually.

# 11.9 GEMM Therapy And Seckiner Gorgun

While we are on the topic of EMF devices and electroporation as a cancer treatment, do not forget the work of the late Suleyman Seckiner Gorgun in Turkey. He is a largely unknown modern equivalent of Rife and, it has to be said, he carried out far more scientific proofs of his method than Rife ever did.

Gorgun was born in Istanbul on 12th of May, 1950 and graduated in medicine in Pakistan.

In 1972 he began working on cell cultures at the Marine Biology Laboratory in Izmir, Turkey, to observe the effects of external electromagnetic fields on cells. He developed what was first called the "Method of Gorgun" but later became known as GEMM therapy (Italian: *Generatore Elettro Magnetico Modulato*), a therapeutic device generating specially modulated, low power (0.25 watt) radio waves.

In 1974 he had fine tuned his method and went to Germany to present the outcomes to Prof E. Shaumlöffel at Marburg University. There was significant regression of the tumors on mice inoculated with cancer, using the device.

In 1979 Gorgun went to Thailand to continue his research on the biological effects of electromagnetic waves at the Thailand National Cancer Institute. The Institute's Chief of Research Laboratory Petcharin Srivatanakul's report states the following :

"Dr. Seckiner Gorgun and Mr. Erol Banko from Turkey came to demonstrate the effect of microwaves on lymphoblastoid cell lines, i.e. P3H3 and P3HR1 cells at Research Division, National Cancer Institute, Thailand. After treatment with microwaves for 2-5 hours at the frequency range between 1 Hertz to 50 MegaHertz, some experiments showed that almost all of the cells are dead, as well quantity of the cells are markedly decreased." (*sic*)

Outcomes of the research were submitted at the 6th Balkan Medical Congress in Ankara in 1979 under the title "Sur le Traitement du Cancer par Controle de la Mitose".

In 1982 Dr. Gorgun went to France to work with the renowned French Immunologist Prof. Raymond Pautrizel at the University of Bordeaux to demonstrate the effects of his treatment on Trypanosoma and Plasmodium parasites, which also proved susceptible to RF terminal electroporation.

In 1988, after some controversy in Italy, a Turin Court declared that the GEMM Therapy was safe and let Dr. Gorgun to continue to work on his system. The expert designated by the court Prof Mario Maritano states in his comprehensive report that the system is not only safe but also beneficial.

## 11.9a Procedure

Therapy sessions are carried out daily, generally lasting around 30 minutes through antennas directed towards the patients lying in therapy beds.

Depending on the type and stage of the disease & the condition of the patient, the therapy may last anywhere from a few weeks to several months.

GEMM Therapy is very safe. It is CE certified. It uses a power of only 0.25 watts. Compared to X-rays or gamma rays used in conventional radiotherapy, radio waves have at least a billion times less energy and have no direct destructive effect on normal, healthy issues.

## 11.9b Gorgun's Model

GEMM Therapy shares what may now be the traditional few of EMF radiation as a means of destroying cancer cells. But he went further with our understanding of what happens (remember, Rife was not medically trained and knew very little medical science).

Gorgun focused on molecular communication. In this sense Gorgun is closely aligned with  the writings of Georges Lakhovsky and his theory of molecular and cellular frequencies.

Gorgun's own theories are a little unclear, in that he believes that he is stimulating good cellular mechanisms, which are favored over those of malignant cells. That may be, but it is clear from published studies that he ended up with a bunch of dead cancer cells! So irreversible electroporation is still at the heart of his method.

In other words, GEMM's therapeutic waves are at the target protein's precisely calculated specific resonant frequency, in order to give signals to stop, modify or reverse the malfunctioning processes.signals

## 11.9c Cellular Resonance In More detail

A typical human cell consists of 10,000 different proteins where all biological processes within a cell, tissue or organism depend on selective interactions between them and their targets such as other proteins, DNA regulatory segments or small molecules.

Proteins are linear sequences of 20 different amino acids, and their unique three-dimensional structure transcribed and translated from the DNA determines their biological function.

So what is it that enabled the tens of thousands of different kinds of molecules in the organism to recognize their specific targets?

## The Classic Lock and Key Model

The classical "lock and key" or its modified "induced fit" models assumes that in the extremely crowded environment of the cell (where there are billions of molecules) by random collisions those molecules that have complementary shapes lock onto to each other so the appropriate biochemical reactions can take place.

This random collision approach is also supposed to explain how enzymes can recognize their respective substrates; how antibodies in the immune system can grab onto specific foreign invaders and disarm them; and how proteins can dock with different partner proteins or latch onto specific nucleic acids to control gene expression etc.

Well, that's what everyone is taught. And the theory is NONSENSE. If you have read my book "Medicine Beyond", you will know I draw extensively on the late Jacques Benveniste's work (the Memory Of Water man). Benveniste pointed out that the "lock and key" model was totally untenable and would require thousands of years, statistically, for any two related molecules to actually collide.

He realized that molecules were actually signaling their presence to their key receptors using resonance magnetic frequencies. This are virtually instantaneous and act across distance; in other words no actual contact of molecules an receptors is required.

You can get a copy of "Medicine Beyond" here:

http://www.alternative-doctor.com/medicinebeyond

## Resonant Recognition Model

Now that Benveniste is no longer with us, Prof. Irena Cosic holds the chair. She is currently Head of the School of Electrical and Computer Engineering in RMIT in Melbourne. She teaches and writes on bioelectromagnetism and has published a research book and over 120 publications, including book chapters, journal, and conference papers.

Prof Cosic showed in her extensive research that all protein sequences with the same common biological function have common characteristic frequency component that is related to the protein's biological function.

Furthermore, it was shown that the proteins and their targets have the same characteristic frequency in common that can be used for recognition and interaction between the particular protein and its target at a distance (as Benveniste suggested).

Thus, protein interactions can be considered as resonant energy transfer between the interacting molecules and by applying an electromagnetic field, it is possible to program, predict, design and modify proteins and their bioactivity.

GEMM is based on the principle of applying the precisely determined electromagnetic fields to the target proteins at the selected resonant frequency to regulate the malfunctioning biological process in a controlled fashion.

A comprehensive description of the method and its effects on neoplastic cells is provided in Dr Gorgun's article "Studies on the Interaction Between Electromagnetic Fields and Living Matter Neoplastic Cell Culture" which appeared at the *Journal of Frontier Perspectives*

[ISSN: 1062-4767., Volume: 7., Number: 2., Fall, 1998].

# Section 12
## Geopathic Stress

Dr Johnson died in 1944. The suspicion exists that he was silenced...However two federal inspectors did examine his hospital record in the late 1950's. They concluded it was likely that he was poisoned.

**Barry Lynes**

# 12.1 Geopathic Stress Crossings Or "Grids"

In addition to geophysical influences such as streams and rock strata, there have been defined a number of grids detectable only to dowsers. The Hartmann Net (described by Dr Ernst Hartmann) consists of a grid of north-to-south lines, crossed by east-to-west, alternatively charged positive and negative. The grid lines are 2-3 m (6-9ft) apart and some 15-20 cm (6-8in).

The Curry Grid (described by Manfred Curry) runs diagonal to the Hartmann Net at approximately 3 ½ m (7ft) apart and 80cm (2 ½ ft) wide, but unlike the Hartmann Net it doesn't vary. There are the same positive and negative bands and, where positive intersects with positive or negative with negative, these are particularly dangerous spots known as nodes. If these fall over underground water, they are said to be even more dangerous.

This idea of invisible "grids" may not be too fanciful. Again, in *Medicine Beyond*, I described how Polynesian islanders were able to navigate accurately over vast ocean distances because there were able to see a grid of lights under the sea.

It may be just a metaphor but it worked for them and modern dowsers keep finding it (I could feel the Curry Grid crossing, when directed by Käthe Bachler).

# 12.2 Diseases

Probably any disease can result when the body is put under any kind of stress. Geopathic disturbance is just another kind of stress. For some patients in critical condition, it may be the "last straw" phenomenon, that pushes them over the edge into a disease.

Probably the most common single finding on a geopathically stressed individual is that he or she is resistant to other forms of treatment. Either there will be partial success followed by a relapse, or treatment will fail completely until the individual is removed from the source of stress.

The sleeping place is particularly important; most of the trouble seems to come when the bed lies on a dangerous spot, and although there are theories about protective devices such as amulets, iron bars outside the house, etc., there is little doubt that Käthe Bachler's advice is best: simply move from the danger zone.

# 12.3 The Architectural Movement

Safe siting of houses and buildings is now no longer the province of the Chinese 'dragon men', as traditional *Feng Sui* dowsers were called ('dragon's breath' being a Chinese name for good influences). Western architects have begun to take the matter very seriously.

The Ecological Design Association is a consortium of architects interested in furthering knowledge about geopathic stress. Gaia Environments Ltd is a commercial organization with the same end in view. Safe House is a UK mail-order firm dealing in products for an ecologically better way of life.

# Section 13

## Miscellaneous Health Factors

Over the next three years, Krebiozin was destroyed. But to destroy Krebiozin you first had to destroy Andrew Ivy. How do you destroy the most influential, respected scientist in the United States? You get friends in the media. You get rid of his academic affiliations. You start a whisper campaign. And next thing you know, nobody wants to know the man.

It took about five years, then they brought him up on a trial of fraud. It was at that point the longest medical trial in the United States' history. At the end of it, the jury found Ivy and the Durovic brothers innocent. Not only that, but they found the FDA irresponsible. And the jury actually made a statement, which is rare, about the contempt that the FDA had for honesty in what it did at trial.

**Gary Null**

# 13.1 Keep Moving for Health

OK, next up comes what could easily be chosen as my FOURTH pillar of health (remember the previous 3 pillars, section 2).

I'm talking about exercise and movement. There is no question that physical activity is built into our nature and is part of the healthy human experience. We are active and extremely mobile bipeds. It's what we are supposed to do.

Nature thinks of us constantly on the move, nomadic, hunter-gatherers, eating here and there, moving on a little, repeating the process and so on. Endlessly moving about the plains. The key word is MOVING.

Unfortunately for modern Man, we are living very far from this natural ideal and, in doing so, we are undermining the health and vitality of our metabolism and tissues. We live almost entirely sedentary lives. We burn too few calories.

There a surprise sting in the tail from that: because we need fewer calories we tend to eat less. That means our intake of fresh vital food is way below what it should be. These days you read a lot about antioxidants in food, resveratrol, protective cancer-fighting flavonoids and so on. All very well; and these foods do keep the natural hunter-gatherer free of cancer (it's unknown, in fact, among stone age peoples).

**But the amounts we get in our diet today are relatively worthless**—just not enough to protect us. We'd need to eat nearly twice what we do to gain many of the wonderful health benefits of fresh food you keep reading about.

That said, if you change your diet and eat heavily towards anti-oxidant and nutrient-rich fresh food, it certainly will help.

But there is another side to the equation, which nobody seems to be talking about: you must participate in significant levels of activity to be really healthy, to eat well and yet not bloat out with obesity.

How much? Well, I recently wrote a paper for my subscribers on the Victorian diet. Now I know everyone thinks Victorians ate terribly and were sick and malnourished. True part of the time. But that sad state of affairs only came about late in the 19th century, with the introduction of manufactured food (like tin cans), and adulteration foods with white lead (bread) and red mercury (curry powder), plus all the other hideous practices.

But there was a time when mid-Victorians, around 1850, were healthier than us, and lived just as long once past childhood, and *cancer was almost unknown*. Specialist doctors of the day described it as "rare". Moreover those who got cancer far outlived today's victims and suffered less.

What's the difference between them and us? The Victorians walked 10- 20 miles a day on average (little public transport in 1850) and ate over 4,000 daily calories, yet were still not obese, due to that level of exercize.

Because of their huge calorie requirements they took in huge amounts of antioxidants and other nutrients. **Even poor people, who ate a little meat only once a week, ate far better than today's typical Americans!** It's ironical to say we just don't eat enough. But as a one-time Professor of Nutrition I can tell you we are just not getting the amounts we need, even when we are getting the right quality of food.

## So you have a choice

You can eat better; that's one route. But you can also exercise far more and so take in more valuable foodstuffs, without getting overweight. I'm not suggesting you do 10 miles a day (that would be ideal). But I do believe we should all spend at least 4- 5 hours a week engaged in physical activity. Walking is the very least you should do; cycling is better; swimming or tennis is better still; workouts in the gym are not as good; neither is lengthy vigorous running, because that releases masses of free-radicals in the body.

# 13.1a White Cells On Parade

There is another surprise benefit to exercise: it releases a shower of white cells into the peripheral blood. I pointed this out in my 1994 book (*Food Allergy And Environmental Illness*) and it's as true today as it was then. Studies show it.

We all know that white cell activity means a busy immune system, with attitude. That's a scary story for cancer cells! So there are few things you can do that are more valuable than generate white cells. Exercise is a simple guaranteed way to do that.

Just to rub the message in, a study headed by Dr. Kathleen Wolin ScD showed what the researchers called "robust" evidence (that means pretty convincing) – that people who are physically active are 24% less likely to develop colon cancer. That pattern held for men and women, regardless of whether they got their activity on the job or in their spare time.

The study itself was the pooling of 52 other published studies on the same theme. That means 24% is an average; some studies would have shown even greater reduction. Some missed it. But even when you water the percentages down with averages, it still comes out in unmistakable terms.

Wolin's study doesn't prove that physical activity alone prevents colon cancer. Physically active people may have other advantages that lower their colon cancer risk. And colon cancer can still strike active people; many factors affect cancer risk.

But it demonstrates quite clearly that exercise is good and can influence the outcome.

"There is an ever-growing body of evidence that the behavior choices we make affect our cancer risk. Physical activity is at the top of the list of ways that you can reduce your risk of colon cancer," say Wolin, who works in St. Louis at the Siteman Cancer Center at the Barnes-Jewish Hospital and the Washington University School of Medicine.

[*British Journal of Cancer*, Feb. 10, 2009]

# 13.2 Latest! (from WebMD)!

Feb. 26, 2009 -- About a third of common adult cancers may be preventable in the US—and that doesn't even count cancers that could be prevented by not smoking.

This claim is part of report from the World Cancer Research Fund (WCRF) and its sister organization, the American Institute for Cancer Research (AICR).

In the new report, the WCRF and AICR estimate that in the US, eating a nutritious diet, being physically active, and keeping body fat under control may prevent:

    38% of breast cancers

    45% of colorectal cancers

    36% of lung cancers

    39% of pancreatic cancers

    47% of stomach cancers

    69% of esophageal cancers

    63% of cancers of the mouth, pharynx, or larynx

    70% of endometrial cancers

    24% of kidney cancers

    21% of gallbladder cancers

    15% of liver cancers

    11% of prostate cancers

Diet, physical activity, and limited body fat could prevent 34% of those 12 cancers overall in the US, and 24% of all cancers, according to the report.

Those estimates are all about the big picture—the effect on the overall population—not an individual's chance of developing cancer.

The WCRF/AICR report also includes tips for governments, industries, school, media, and other institutions worldwide to promote healthy lifestyles. Among those recommendations:

- New developments should be designed to encourage walking and cycling.

- Government and school cafeterias should provide healthy foods and drinks.

- Food and drink industries should price healthy fare competitively with other products and stop promoting sugary drinks and unhealthy foods to kids.

- Workplaces should have policies and environments that are supportive of breastfeeding.

- Media should promote cancer prevention and flag misleading cancer claims.

That guidance is in line with the American Cancer Society's recommendation for community action, notes Colleen Doyle, the American Cancer Society's director of nutrition and physical activity. "Reversing the obesity epidemic will require bold action and multiple strategies, including policy changes at national, state, and local levels that make it easier for people to eat better and be more active," Doyle says in an ACS official statement.

The WCRF/AICR, which has previously published cancer prevention tips for individuals, stresses that cancer prevention means trimming the odds of developing cancer, not totally eliminating cancer.

Well, I say it can go a long way to prevent it altogether. And if you get cancer, better get physically active before the disease limits you. That way you can go a long way to reversing it too...

# 13.3 Sleep and Inflammation

I have already convinced the reader, I hope, of the power of inflammation to start up cancer, disrupt the immune system and prolong or block any healing process, including the battle against cancer.

One of the powerful things that deep, restful sleep does for us is lower levels of inflammation. People who sleep poorly or do not get enough sleep have higher levels of inflammation, a risk factor for heart disease and stroke, and something that stokes up the fires on the side of cancer.

Acute sleep deprivation leads to an increased production of inflammatory hormones, cytokines and changes in blood vessel function.

[Meier-Ewert HK, et al. Effect of sleep loss on C-reactive protein, an inflammatory marker of cardiovascular risk. J Am Coll Cardiol 2004;43(4):678-83]

Gene Damage: Professor Derk-Jan Dijk and his colleagues at Surrey University, UK, found that volunteers who got less than six hours of sleep each night over the course of a week had changes to 711 genes linked to inflammation, the ability to fight disease, and stress. These changes might have an impact on obesity, diabetes, heart disease, brain function and, of course, cancer (not mentioned by Dijk).

The findings appeared in the journal PNAS, 2014. [Mistimed sleep disrupts circadian regulation of the human transcriptome. *Proceedings of the National Academy of Sciences*, January 2014 DOI: 10.1073/pnas.1316335111]

Quite simply, deep restful sleep is the best healing there is. It's been known for millennia and I doubt this pole position will ever change. It works!

That means you cannot afford to go into sleep deprivation mode, if you are addressing cancer.

## 13.3a Stages Of Sleep

Usually sleepers pass through five stages of sleep each night: 1, 2, 3, 4 and REM (rapid eye movement) sleep. These stages progress cyclically from 1 through REM then begin again with stage 1. A complete sleep cycle takes an average of 90 to 110 minutes. The early sleep cycles each night have relatively short REM sleeps and long periods of deep sleep but later in the night, REM periods lengthen and deep sleep time decreases.

*Thus the deepest and most valuable sleeptime is when you first go to bed.* Remember that.

Stage 1 is light sleep where you drift in and out of sleep and can be awakened easily. In this stage, the eyes move slowly and muscle activity slows. During this stage, many people experience sudden muscle contractions preceded by a sensation of falling. 5 – 10 minutes.

In stage 2, eye movement stops and brain waves become slower with only an occasional burst of rapid brain waves. When a person enters stage 3, extremely slow brain waves called delta waves are interspersed with smaller, faster waves.

In stage 4, the brain produces delta waves almost exclusively. It's the deepest level of all.

Stages 3 and 4 are referred to as deep sleep or "delta sleep" (delta brainwaves), and it is very difficult to wake someone from them. In deep sleep, there is no eye movement or muscle activity.

(In 2008 the sleep profession in the US eliminated the use of stage 4. Stages 3 and 4 are now considered stage 3. They are out of step with the rest of the world.)

Slow wave sleep comes mostly in the first half of the night, REM in the second half. Waking may occur after REM. If the waking period is long enough, the person may remember it the next morning.

In the REM period, breathing becomes more rapid, irregular and shallow, eyes jerk rapidly and limb muscles are temporarily paralyzed. This is the time when most dreams occur, and, if awoken during REM sleep, a person can usually remember the dreams. Most people experience three to five intervals of REM sleep each night.

Infants spend almost 50% of their time in REM sleep. Adults spend nearly half of sleep time in stage 2, about 20% in REM and the other 30% is divided between the other three stages. Older adults spend progressively less time in REM sleep.

## 13.3b Ways To Induce Sleep

Take a walk before bed

Cease all strong brain activity at least an hour before you want to sleep (turn off computers, TV, smartphones and tablets!)

Remove all fixed electrical appliances from around your bed

If your sleep is very disrupted, be sure to get a dowser to check for geopathic stress (section 12.1)

Consider multi-media sensory stimulus devices, like the Kasina, which take you down to sleep by inducing theta frequencies.

# Section 14

## Electro-Dermal Screening May Help

Medicine in our country has been on a crusade over the last 100 years to wipe out every other form of medicine. One of the things they did that was unique was they lobbied to make words legal only for them to use. Today in the US, only a medical doctor can diagnose a disease, prescribe something, and cure you. Nobody else can say "diagnose", "prescribe" and "cure". That means that nobody can cure you but a medical doctor....I can't say "Chaparral is the cure for a tumor"....

**Dr Richard Shulze, ND**

# 14.1 Disease Origins Database

Next, as I think of it, comes Dr. Kildare meets Chinese traditional medicine in cyberspace. The doctor calls up a comprehensive database of disease entities and possible cures. On my own system there are over 25,000 entries. This is fairly typical for systems of this type.

By highlighting an entry and pressing the return key, the doctor can access the energy signal named there on the screen. This can then compare it with what is coming from the disease zone; he does this by touching Spleen 2 with the probe, where he found the biggest drop. He no longer looks for pathological drops but is probing to see if there is a resonance. This is shown by a reading at or very close to the balance reading of 50. This means a 'yes' from the body.

This system is called "electro-dermal screening" or EDS for short. Such devices are constantly evolving and the modern ones simply read the patient's energetic field. Actual physical contact with electrodes is not necessary.

# 14.2 Causal Chains

With this entirely new perspective on disease it is possible to start seeing the onset of pathology in a different way. It becomes obvious there is no one cause for a disease. Even TB is not caused by the tubercle bacillus (if it was, we would all have it). TB is caused by a series of weakening effects, mainly malnutrition and emotional shock (remember those dramatic Victorian novels!).

The LAST link in the chain is the tubercle bacillus grows, unopposed by a health immune system. That is one way that conventional medicine errs. To just look at the last step is to ignore all the other stages in the cascade or what I call a tumbledown, leading to cancer and other illnesses.

The all-important question, naturally, is where did this sequence start? If we can find this and correct it, that will open the door to a new therapeutic plan—one that works where other measures have failed. It can seem like lateral thinking gone mad sometimes. But there is always a curious understandable logic behind the events, once they are put into the right sequence.

The skilled EDS specialist looks at cancer as the final results of many disease pathways. We are used to thinking of it as a tissue ageing process, where toxins and pathogens have accumulated to such an extent that the body defences can no longer cope. We try to undo the ill-effects of years of negative health, thread by thread.

You'll be able to read much more about these new theories in my book "*Medicine Beyond*". (www.alternative-doctor.com/medicinebeyond)

# 14.3 Focus (Plural Foci)

A very worrying concern and challenging management problem we find in EDS is the toxic focus. It is quite clear to the unprejudiced observer that foci can generate problems far from where they are found. There is compelling evidence that toxic and infective matter can travel along nerve channels, as well as in the more obvious blood route (all this is described and explained in greater detail in *Medicine Beyond*).

I become worried if I think of the bigger implications.

A focus may also pose dangers by initiating pathological changes locally, that is without spreading to a remote site. Professor of Neurology in Stockholm Dr Patrick Stortebecker makes it clear that a peri-apical osteitis is a very typical finding in close proximity to a jaw cancer.

# 14.4 Cancer Triggers

After years of study, it becomes clear that certain recurrent themes show up in the origins of cancer. These are:

1. Early immune shocks (childhood disease and vaccinations)

2. Geopathic stress, centerd especially around the patient's bed or daytime chair

3. Degenerative toxic focus, most commonly in the teeth or jaws but also often in the tonsils or pelvic abdominal areas

4. Unresolved emotional trauma.

5. Miasmic influences, from parent to child, passed through the generations

6. Radiation and/or electromagnetic exposure

7. Personal chemical pollution with toxins such as nickel, cadmium, mercury, aflatoxins (from moulds and fungi), pesticides, benzene, toluene, xylene, formaldehyde, isopropyl alcohol and 'autotoxins', chiefly from the patient's own intestines.

All these conditions are considered elsewhere in this manual.

EDS specialists make no attempts to treat the cancer directly, only to treat the contributory causes. If he or she is going to survive the intruder, the patient will need a fortified immune system that is capable of closing down the attack. This can only be achieved by detoxing, removing coincidental and distracting pathology, pumping up nutrition and taking remedies known to stimulate immunity.

Of course this cannot all be done with homeopathy. I myself give intravenous drips containing high-key nutritional supplements, especially high-dose vitamin C which is a proven safe cytotoxic agent.

Suitable complex homeopathic remedies that would be considered and tested by any good EDS specialist are:

- Viscum (Mistletoe) in various combinations. Iscador or Viscum compositum (see section 8.1).

- Echinacea compounds, alternating as immune boosters.

- Glyoxal (very powerful and for intermittent use only)

- Causticum

- Carcinominum (nosode)

- Phytolacca, Conium and Thuja.

- Drainage remedies, eg. lymphomyosot (HEEL), galium

- Detoxing compounds (Berberis, Nux vom, etc)

- Defense remedies eg. Tonsilla comp., Discus comp. (HEEL)

- Miasms, individually or composite, as in Psorino-HEEL.

- Specific tumor nosodes, bronchus, uterus, cervical cancer etc.

Dental and other foci will need to be eliminated (section 15). In truth, it comes back to my old saw that all good health measures are anti-cancer measures.

# 14.5 Let Me Finish With A Word Of Warning

These EDS systems are very "operator sensitive", by which I mean the operators ability and knowledge influence the outcomes (unlike blood work or x-rays, which are absolutely objective).

This is not a problem if the operator is good and is honest about the shortcomings. But I know from experience many medically-untrained operators of these devices make outrageous claims about the accuracy of what they are finding.

The newer versions, such as the EPFX/QXCI, are absurdly difficult to use and some practitioners simply cannot get it to work. It's no different than dowsing.

Having said that, some owners of these devices show uncanny skills. But in all I find it impossible to support a device that works some of the time and not at others, or for some operators and not others.

**Just remember, it depends on the operator more than the machine and you won't be fooled!**

# Section 15

## Killer Dental Dangers

We are being run by rich trash without regard for the truth or reality.

**James Watson**
1962 Nobel Laureate,
discoverer of DNA double-helix

# 15.1 Toxic Dentistry

It is not really stretching the human mind too far to suggest that most dentistry is, by nature, quite toxic. Modern methods rely heavily on materials such as metals, plastics and polymers, ceramics and prosthetic structures of many kinds.

Unfortunately, EDS practitioners (previous section) are discovering that most of this foreign material is stressful to the body. It can be a considerable drain on the immune system and therefore a major contributory cause of fatigue and chronic ill health. In this new context we can only urge people even more emphatically to try to prevent dental problems from starting up. Good diet and adequate teeth hygiene may, even in this day of antibiotics, still be a key life-saver.

# 15.2 I do not exaggerate

They say that a dentist doesn't kill his patients. I can only add my weight to the view of many other EAV practitioners, which is that they certainly do! It's just that they and the medical profession are not aware of the connection and so miss the significance of the danger.

It is possible to reduce the damage by taking sensible anti-tox procedures before, during and after a dental program. EAV tests show that this at least minimizes the impact of high-tech dentistry. Such elementary measures would include vitamin C, charcoal (to absorb toxins), homeopathic support and immune drainage remedies, such as Heel's lymphomyosot or Pascoe's Pascotox.

# 15.3 Galvanic Fields And Energetic Disturbance

Slightly more bizarre is the phenomenon of electrical fields around certain teeth and the effects these produce. I remember well the first time I saw Hal Huggin's slides of teeth cut open to show the scorch marks, where electrical current had been running for many years. Teeth can work like little batteries. This is quite logical: there are two or more metals and a saltwater fluid medium (saliva). This is how Allessandro Volta's original batteries were made; the battery of your motorcar is essentially the same thing.

The trouble starts from the fact that electrical currents actually leech the mercury out of the teeth, because of an effect called electrolysis. This is why patients sometimes complain of a constant metallic taste in the mouth, made worse by hot fluids and salty food (more electrolysis).

If that isn't scary enough, then the reader should know that electrolysis is capable of releasing deadly mercury vapour. This goes straight to the brain tissue where it is highly invasive and toxic.

But the problem is even more complicated. The currents generated by amalgams can be quite considerable and these are being formed very close to brain tissue, which operates at far lower potentials (a few millivolts). I have seen momentary spikes of up to one volt when testing teeth for the battery effect; this is enough to light a small torch battery.

Remember the brain is really only a few millimetres from the upper jaw bone where the roots of the teeth lie, just the other side of the thin cranial bone and the meninges. Thus there is potential for mental dysfunction and this is often found in clinical practice, by asking the appropriate questions.

# 15.4 Energetic Fields

EAV practitioners are finding teeth foci as a common cause of energetic disturbance. The problem is immensely more complicated than it at first might seem.

Several key acupuncture meridians cross the line of teeth as they pass over the face. An abcess or 'transmitting focus' can actually create pathological results anywhere along the line of that meridian. That includes cancer.

These are reconnected again with secondary organs and sites. Thus problems with a front incisor tooth may impact on the kidneys, since this meridian passes through the incisors. But the kidneys, in turn are related to the knee joints. If I see a patient with incisor problems or a bridge in this location I can surprise them by asking about the arthritis in his or her knees. Try it yourself!

Sometimes the consequences of these interconnections are very surprising and virtually beggar explanation but should make us very wary indeed about the effects of dentistry.

Let me tell you the amazing story about dental foci I quoted in *Medicine Beyond*. It concerns the research work of a brilliant holistic dentist, Weston Price (he gave his name to the Weston Price Foundation)

# 15.5 Root Canal Fillings

We have here a topic where conventional medicine, decades ago, stood right where alternative innovative dentists stand today. The story is a fascinating one and begins in the first decade of this century with one Dr. Frank Billings. His research published in 1914 showed that 95% of all focal infections in the body came from the teeth and tonsils. Billing's work in turn was found by Weston Price, a leading dentist of his day. Price was an advocate of healthy natural lifestyle and keynote nutrition; in every way he was a great thinker and a pioneer of values that we cherish today.

Price had a woman patient for whom he had done a root canal filling. She subsequently developed bad arthritis; it was so severe that she had become bedridden most of the time and her hands were so badly swollen she could barely feed herself.

Price was honest enough to ask the question that no dentist cares to ask: could he have made her ill systemically by propagating generalized infection, as Billings had shown? He removed the root canal filled tooth, carefully and aseptically, to see what would happen. The woman promptly recovered.

From this case forward, Price became very interested in the problem of root canal fillings. He had considerable success in helping patients and published his results widely. There are copious papers by him in the medical and dental literature, most of it from the early 1920s.

It is important to recognize the Price was a leading conventional dentist of the day, not a crank. His views were listened to and, for a time, it became the fashion among doctors to recommend extracting teeth with root canal fillings as a cure for arthritis.

In fact it progressed to widespread tooth extractions, root canals or not, which was not what Price originally taught. Unfortunately, many cases did not recover as expected. The patient not only continued to suffer the arthritis but was now without any teeth. The approach became unpopular and was eventually discontinued.

As a result, Price's views were discredited and lost sight of. It was one of those cases where the pendulum swung too far in a particular direction. Price was right, of course, but there needed to be some way of choosing patients who would benefit from removing root canal fillings.

EDS gives us the means. It is now a common aspect of EDS diagnosis to consider the safety and validity of root canal fillings. They may not be a problem. If the person is fit and strong, with a good immune system, the situation can continue unchanged for many years. But if at some time in the future he or she undergoes too much stress or suffers from a major illness, the resistance may be compromised and the dangers of root canals become manifest and dangerous.

The problem is that, although root canal work looks fine on x-ray, and it might appear that there is a perfect occlusion of the former root canal down the heart of the tooth, microscopic examination reveal a different story. Tooth dentine, which is hard and screeches like rock when the dentist attacks it with his drill, is really composed of numerous tiny tubules. It is said there are 3 miles of end-to-end tubules in every tooth; they are supposed to conduct nutrients to keep the tooth alive and healthy. When bacteria gain access to the tooth, they lurk in these tubules. Filling the root canal does not flush the pathogens out of this domain. In fact the bacteria are then trapped in a closed off space and inevitably cause trouble.

Pathogens have to go somewhere when they multiply. They can migrate through what are called lateral tubules and escape into the periodontal membrane and subsequently into the bony tissue of the jaw. From there they migrate around the body.

As biological dentist and author of Root Canal Cover Up George Meinig puts it 'These bacteria are kind of like people, if they get to like Seattle or Reno or someplace they decide that's where they are going to have their home. Well, the bacteria travelling round the body, they may get to the liver, the kidneys or the heart or eyes or some other tissue and they set up an infection in that area. This is why the degenerative diseases occur from the teeth'.

# 15.6 Transmitting Teeth

Now we come to the part that is definitely weird. Everything so far is at least logical, if rather unnerving. It makes sense. From here it makes no real sense, except in the insubstantial quantum domain or as we would once have said, 'the etheric'.

What Weston Price did in the 1920s was to take infected and pathogenic root canal filled teeth and surgically stitch them into rabbits for observation. It is one of those situations like Benjamin Franklin sending up a kite into a thunder storm; a mixture of perverse genius and intuition that leads to some important scientific insight.

What Weston Price found was that the rabbits became ill with the same diseases as the patients, or if not exactly the same diseases, then the same organ was attacked in some way. If the human had nephritis (cured after tooth extraction), then the rabbit got nephritis; if the human had cancer, heart disease or arthritis, that was what the rabbit got.

Eye problems were particularly striking; if the human had only mild eye trouble, the rabbit would react so severely as to go blind in two or three days.

The only real conclusion is that the tooth carried some message of disease using an unknown code. Whether it was a quantum field factor or some other means of information transference is simply not known. You would think this absolutely fascinating series of experiments would have scientists racing to investigate the significance of what Price found. Instead, his work was promptly forgotten for over 50 years. So much for the progress of scientific thought.

# 15.7 What You Can Do

You might be worried about what is written here. This could be with good cause, but don't over-react. The first thing to do is make contact with a biological dentist, as they call themselves. These are advanced dentists who appreciate Price's work and freely use homeopathic remedies, nutrition and other natural accompaniments to dental hygiene.

They also willingly interact with EDS practitioners, preferring the body's own signals for guidance.

Read more and become informed about the issues. Everyone should take responsibility for their own health care and this applies equally to dentistry. To leave decisions solely to your dentist, if he or she is of conventional thought mode, is to be subject to yesterday's science and it may do you harm in the long run, as we have seen with the mercury story (there remain dentists who still insist there is no problem with mercury amalgams).

Eat a proper diet which avoids sugars that cause dental decay and feed micro-organisms.

Use co-enzyme Q10 supplements (ubiquinone). This has been shown to have unequivocal benefit for periodontal (gum) disease. More teeth are lost due to gum disease than decay (cavities).

Large doses of vitamin C seem to be very helpful for periodontal disease and toxicity of all kinds. Take large amounts before, during and after any dental program – at least 10 g (21/2 teaspoonsful) daily.

## Resources:

1. Stortebecker P. DENTAL CARIES AS A CAUSE OF NERVOUS DISORDERS, Bio-Probe Inc, Orlando, USA, 1986.

2. G Meinig ROOT CANAL COVER-UP, Bion Publishing, Ojai, California, 1995.

3. Radio interview of the Laura Lee Show, transcript published in the TOWNSEND LETTER for DOCTOR AND PATIENT, August/ September 1996.

Listen to an audio explaining more about dental hazards and how to deal with them here on one of my websites:

http://www.askdoctorkeith.com/dental.htm

# Section 16
## Tests For Cancer Markers!

Cancer is a word, not a sentence.

**John Diamon**

# 16.1 Risk markers are different

Some people have a greater chance of developing certain types of cancer because of mutation or alteration, in specific genes. The presence of such a change is sometimes called a risk marker. Tests for risk markers could help reduce a person's chance of developing a certain cancer. The BRCA1 and BRCA2 gene are examples of this type of marker.

So risk markers can indicate that cancer is more likely to occur; while tumor markers can indicate the actual presence of cancer. That's the difference.

We can use tumor markers in the detection, diagnosis, and management of some types of cancer—and wise alternative physicians know their cancer markers and use them to manage patients, just like their mainstream colleagues.

The most practical use of markers is to check how a patient is responding to treatment. A decrease or return to a normal level may indicate that the cancer is responding to therapy, whereas an increase may indicate that the cancer is not responding. After treatment has ended, tumor marker levels may be used to check for recurrence.

In this context, serial measurements are more important and easier to interpret than one-offs.

The National Academy of Clinical Biochemistry (NACB) publishes *Practice Guidelines and Recommendations for Use of Tumor Markers in the Clinic*, which focuses on the appropriate use of tumor markers for specific cancers. It's more trustworthy than non-profits like the American Cancer Society, which seem to have a clear agenda of denying the public the right to choose alternative therapies if they wish.

# 16.2 Sensitivity and specificity

For a screening test to be helpful, it should have high sensitivity and specificity. Sensitivity refers to the test's ability to identify people who have the disease. Specificity refers to the test's ability to identify people who do not have the disease. Most tumor markers are not sensitive or specific enough to be used for cancer screening.

Cancer researchers are now turning to proteomics (the study of protein shape, function, and patterns of expression) in hopes of developing better cancer screening and treatment options. Proteomics technology is being used to search for proteins that may serve as markers of disease in the earlier stages or to predict the effectiveness of treatment or to tell more accurately the chance of the disease returning after treatment has ended. More information about proteomics can be found at www.cancer.gov/cancertopics

Even commonly used tests may not be completely sensitive or specific. For example, the well-known prostate-specific antigen (PSA) levels are often used to screen men for prostate cancer, but this is controversial.

Elevated PSA levels can be caused by prostate cancer or completely benign conditions, and most men with elevated PSA levels turn out not to have prostate cancer. Moreover, it is not clear if the benefits of PSA screening outweigh the risks of follow-up diagnostic tests and cancer treatments.

Recent estimations have suggested that the PSA test does not actually save lives and should be dropped.

For instance a study published March 2009, funded by the National Cancer Institute in the USA, showed no increase in survival times, which is all that really matters. But just to confuse things, at about the same time, a European study appearing in the same issue of the *New England Journal of Medicine* did show a modest, 20% survival benefit associated with PSA screening in men followed for an average of nine years.

Which one is right? No way to tell.

PAP, that's Prostatic Acid Phosphatase, is another prostate enzyme that's sometimes elevated but is no more valuable as a marker than the common PSA check.

Another tumor marker, CA 125, is sometimes used to screen women who have an increased risk for ovarian cancer. Scientists are studying whether measurement of CA 125, along with other tests and exams, is useful.

So far, CA 125 measurement is not sensitive or specific enough to be used to screen all women for ovarian cancer. So mostly it's used to monitor response to treatment and check for recurrence in women with ovarian cancer.

I see no point in going through a whole series of markers. You'll hear of carbohydrate 19-9 and carcinoembryonic antigen or CEA. Then Carbohydrate 15-3 and 27-29; these last two seem to relate to breast cancer. VEGF Test (vascular-endothelial growth factor). This indicates whether cancer is developing its own blood supply. If we know this, specific treatment can be applied to halt new blood vessel growth. Without a blood supply a fast-growing cancer would soon starve and die. As I remarked elsewhere in the book, shark's cartilage seems to have some benefit in blocking this signaling substance.

Another significant test is TGF-Beta. It stands for transforming growth factor. Cancer cells produce a lot of this chemical, which suppresses the immune system, so it's worth tracking.

Some of the markers are not really specific to cancer but still get used. Tests like pyruvate kinase and lactic acid simply measure metabolism. Tumors, remember, are pretty active metabolically.

You don't need to remember all these names. You can study more about them at cancer.gov. I'm really only mentioning them because of Dr Kobayashi's work in Japan, which I'll come to in a moment.

First, let me tell you about a couple of alternative cancer markers you probably WON'T be told about by your doctor!

# 16.3 Telomerase

The enzyme telomerase produces telomeres, located at the ends of each chromosome. These protect the ends of chromosomes as cells divide. In a normal cell, the telomeres break up and shorten each time the cell divides. After a cell divides 50 to 100 times, the telomeres shorten so much that they can no longer protect the chromosome, and the cell eventually dies. Remember this information, though, comes from scientists who know next to nothing about nutrition!

We now know that cancerous cells seem to be able to switch telomerase back on. In fact cancer cells can keep it going indefinitely, which is why they have this fantastic capability for dividing over and over, seemingly immortal.

Thus telomerase is bad news, which is why we monitor it and why you want to watch it fall on your therapy program. The telomerase test was originally a urine test but has now been developed as a blood test.

Fetal and baby cells contain lots of telomerase, which helps to keep DNA healthy; eventually we all lose it. So the appearance of more telomerase in the blood in later life is highly suggestive of active cancer, since malignant cells contain 10- 20 times normal levels. They can create their own telomerase.

Your practitioner can use the telomerase test to monitor the suppression of cancer activity (or not). However there may be some confusion, due to the fact that simple infections may send levels up. Still, it is useful by making comparisons and, although high levels may be confusing, levels which have dropped to nil are indicative of success against the tumor.

Important points: when first seen, a cancer patient may have quite low telomerase levels in the blood. But that's not necessarily good. It means the cancer cells are cloaking themselves and hiding from the immune system.

Also, when natural treatments are commenced, telomerase levels will often go sky high. This frightens patients. But is actually a good sign, that the cancer cells are being destroyed and broken up, releasing the telomerase.

It might be possible to tame cancer by attacking it in this telomerase weak link.

The trouble is studies in human cancer cells have indicated that disrupting telomerase as a means of halting cancer cell replication or inducing cell suicide would require an almost complete loss of normal telomerase activity.

And this would require either swamping the enzyme with an overwhelming amount of mutant telomerase or finding a sufficiently potent drug to completely inhibit the enzyme.

Nobody can guess the implications if that.

But UCSF researchers report that they were able to slow the growth of human cancer cells - or cause them to commit suicide altogether -- by creating just a miniscule mutation in the telomerase enzyme.

By inserting a tiny mutation in the gene coding for a small but critical portion of the telomerase enzyme caused it to not work, which prompted a dramatic response from cancer cells.

"We were quite surprised at how strong the effect was," says the senior author of the study, Elizabeth Blackburn, UCSF professor of biochemistry and biophysics. "Cancer cells are tough. They usually ignore the signals that tell them to commit suicide. But by spiking the telomerase enzyme with just a little bad telomerase we saw a powerful effect." Blackburn, by the way, in 1985, co-discovered the telomerase enzyme.

# 16.4 Testing Breakthrough For Hidden Cancers

One of the most important things we have been in need of is a way to test for cancers l-o-n-g before there is a tumor. Current medical science cannot detect anything smaller than a pea and even bigger ones often get missed.

Scans are a waste of time and very dangerous. A CT scan delivers as much as 500 times the radiation of a standard X-ray, potentially causing an estimated 1.5 to 2 percent of all cancers in the United States. PET scans are even worse, because the whole body is exposed to radiation. A study of database records of more than 31,400 patients who had a CT scan in 2007 at Brigham and Women's Hospital or Harvard's Dana-Farber Cancer Center found that 15% of the patients had received estimated cumulative radiation doses that were higher than the radiation exposure from 1,000 chest X-rays.

In other words, these "screening" methods are likely to create more cancer than they detect. Using them is nuts, if not criminal!

What's needed is a chemical screening that can tell, early on, that a patient is harboring a cancer; I mean very early on, when treatment is easy and can be accomplished by little more than changes in diet and lifestyle.

Waiting for your orthodox oncology markers to show up is like waiting till you are really in the danger zone. By the time they are elevated, you are in trouble.

What could be better then?

Well, suddenly a whole rash of cancer marker tests have shown up. Dr. Garry Gordon waxes lyrical about the profile of tests carried out by Dr. Kobayashi in Japan (next section). But now there is more choice than ever.

There's the Oncoblot test, the CYP1B1 and Dr. Schandl's "Cancer Profile". Each of these is far superior to the AMAS test of the past which, despite claims, is not highly reliable. It was the best we had for years but that's no longer true.

## ONCOblot® Test

The Oncoblot blood test identifies a specific type of protein in the blood, ENOX2, which exists only on the surface of a malignant cancer cell. The ENOX2 proteins are shed into the circulation and can be detected in the blood. These proteins serve as highly sensitive markers for early detection in both primary and recurrent cancer. It's organ specific, meaning it can often tell with certainty where the cancer is located.

The physician draws the blood and sends it to the lab. Results take approximately 15 business days. The cost is $850.00 at this time. (www.oncoblotlabs.com)

But does it work?

Based on analyses of over 800 Oncoblots covering 26 different kinds of cancers with clinically confirmed diagnoses, 99.3% were positive for cancer based on ENOX2 presence.

Of these, the organ site of the cancer was determined correctly in 96% of the samples; there were no false positives; and less than 1% false negatives.

That's really quite extraordinary.

# PYP1B1

To gasp the potential of this test it's necessary to do a bit of in depth explanation. Let's back up and talk about salvestrols. These are potent plant chemicals and are probably the real reason that raw, healthy plants protect us against cancer, not antioxidants. Resveratrol is the best-known of them.

In a series of papers in *The Journal of Orthomolecular Medicine*, Professor Gerald Potter, Head of Cancer Drug Discovery Group, De Montfort University, Leicester UK, and Professor M.D. Burke and co-workers introduced the concept of salvestrols and gave them the name. Together they developed the PYP1B1 enzyme test.

This is quite an involved story but suffice it to say that salvestrols destroy cancer cells pretty well. They are highly anti-inflammatory and a sort of botanical police force for the body. One of the reasons cancer and degenerative diseases are increasing so much in the West is likely that food processing and manufacture drastically reduces salvestrol levels (they taste rather bitter and are deliberately removed).

The key to investigating the properties of salvestrols is an enzyme called PYP1B1, which does not occur in healthy cells; it's only found in cancer cells, such as breast, colon, lung, esophagus, skin, lymph nodes, brain and testis. Salvestrols are metabolized by PYP1B1 into a metabolite which destroys cancer cells. This is an arrangement which suits us very well.

We can test for the presence of PYP1B1 and, if it's found, infer that a cancer is present. We can then load the system with salvestrols and the PYP1B1 will produce the cytotoxic metabolite and wipe out the cancer. At that point the PYP1B1 will vanish, because only cancer cells have it!

There are NO false positives, the developers claim. If there is PYP1B1, you have cancer. Period.

I expect one day Big Pharma will try to develop a drug to fit into this schematic. But for the moment they remain icily cold towards salvestrol research.

Incidentally, salvestrols are destroyed by fungicides on plants, *and* Laetrile (Amygdalin). It is common knowldge that I do not accept any research that says laetrile is a valid anti-cancer agent (except that cyanide kills all cells; that's hardly helpful). Anyway, here's proof, if needed, amygdalin doesn't work and is potentially destructive, compromising nature's own natural cancer protection.

The results claimed for laetrile (amygdalin) are without exception the results of OTHER actions taken at the same time. No study has ever been carried out investigating only laetrile in humans. (see section 10.4)

So far as I know the PYP1B1 test is not offered publicly at this time.

# Dr. Schandl's CA Profile Testing

Dr. Emil Schandl is certainly a survivor, having lived as a Jew in Nazi Germany, fought in the Hungarian uprising of 1956 and then made it to freedom. He founded American Metabolic Laboratories in Hollywood, Florida.

His test centers around an analysis of 6 key enzymes, each of which alone might not be so accurate but, taken together, give a very good score rate.

For example, 68% of cancer cases show elevated levels of human chorionic gonadotrophin hormone (hCG). Measuring for the enzyme PHI (phosphohexose isomerase, a tumor marker that regulates anaerobic cellular metabolism), levels were elevated in 36 percent of the patients. Add the enzyme GGTP (gamma glutamyl transpeptidase, a sensitive liver enzyme), levels were higher in 39 percent of patients And finally a test for CEA (carcinoembryonic antigen, a general tumor marker, originally designed to monitor colorectal cancers) showed elevated levels in 51 percent of patients.

But looking at these cancer markers together (hCG, PHI, CEA), 221 positives in 240 breast cancer patients (92% accurate) were detected. Of lung-cancer patients, 127 of 129 (97% accurate) were correctly diagnosed. cent) were correctly diagnosed. And with colon-cancer patients, 55 positives out of 59 patients (93% accurate) were correctly identified.

These are great scores.

But Schandl also added 2 more tests which are revealing: thyroid stimulating hormone (I have written in all my books that thyroid hormone is crucial in cancer cases); and DHEA.

He has tested thousands of patients with this profile, with accuracy greater than 90 percent. When a patient is actually being treated for cancer, Schandl's tests can be used to monitor the success (or ineffectiveness) of ongoing cancer therapy.

The current cost is $386.

http://americanmetaboliclaboratories.net

# 16.5 Dr. Kobayashi

I think I should bring you up to date with the remarkable work of Dr. Kobayashi, a Japanese oncologist. He has developed a panel of ten tumor markers coupled with a computerized algorithm that is clearly very useful in the early detection of cancer.

By combining several markers at once and having a computer program seek out the patterns that are suggestive of cancer is a big step forward. I'm sure there will be other work like this in future; but for the moment Kobayashi is out on his own.

He uses three series of markers:

Tumor specific ones; tumor associated markers and simply growth related markers. I'm not going to list them all here.

But suffice it to say he can detect cancers fairly accurately that weigh about a gram or less. That's too small to show up on any conventional screening and too small almost to be detected by the eye at surgery. So he may have something important for us here.

Dr. Kobayashi has not only refined the sensitivity and range of the normal values of these markers, but has weighted their level of importance and inter-relationship as a pattern recognition for 5 tumor stages.

He classifies the results as: Tumor free, two levels of Pre-cancer, Pre-clinical cancer and, five, results suggestive of cancer weighing over 1 gram.

This tumor classification can pretty accurately assess the risk of cancer developing in apparently healthy persons.

The great thing with Kobayashi is that he is a conventional doctor given over the mainly holistic methods.

For example he studied the benefits of fasting for cancer patients—remember everything I said about diet in earlier sections of this manual. Austrian herbal naturopath Rudolph Breuss healed cases of cancer of the larynx, intestines, breast, kidney, and uterus, as well as leukemia, Hodgkin's and other cancers, during the 1970's—just using fasting. (see section 2.2)

Well, Kobyashi followed several immune signaling substances, including one group called the cyclic nucleotides; we know those are powerful and positive regulators of the immune system and help it eliminate cancer cells just as soon as they form. These are found in all living cells. The cyclic nucleotides, according to Kobayashi, were favorably increased by fasting, adoptive immune (sensitized lymphocyte) therapy, and their combination.

Through interpreters, we know that Dr. Kobayashi has kept approximately 15,000 patients cancer-free over an 18 year duration, by implementing primarily natural methods of treatment during stages IV & V.

We now have to wait for this success program to filter through and become gradually adopted. My friend Dr Garry Gordon in Phoenix is working closely with Kobayashi and hopes to bring his methods here to the Western US.

I for one look forward to seeing their impact on conventional thinking.

Don't get this test mixed up with the The Kobayashi Maru in Star Trek, a training exercise designed to test the character of cadets.

# 16.6 More Markers!

Logically, you might think that counting the number of cancer cells in circulation in the blood might be a good way to measure the potential dangers of a cancer. There are some surprising problems with this.

Dr. Hamer (section 2.14) has pointed out that it's very rare indeed to find cancer cells in circulation. From that he has speculated that secondary cancers are not spread via the blood but are new cancers that have arisen, due to the shock of diagnosis.

Whereas, I respect the work of Dr. Hamer, I disagree with him in this. I turn instead to the model of Rife's, whose brilliant microscope (section 11.9) enabled him to see tiny sub-bacterial bodies that he likened to viruses and called the BX organism. Like Rife, I think that this is how cancer is spread to remote tissues. Rife found the BX organism in all cancer patients and was able to kill it with 100% success, using his amazing beam ray machine.

Despite the scarcity of circulating cancer cells, using this phenomenon is a cancer marker is not a lost cause. I found a recent study previewed in a cancer journal *The Lancet Oncology*, Feb. 10, 2009, which stated that checking for changes in the number of circulating tumor cells (CTCs) could help doctors predict advanced cancer patients' survival and response to treatment.

In the years since I wrote that remark, circulating tumor cells (CTCs) and circulating tumor DNA (ctDNA) have come into the limelight. At an international conference ahead of my publication of this book (16/17th November, 2015, Boston, UDA) a number of papers will be read focusing primarily on biofluid-based molecular biomarkers, such CTCs, ctDNA and other protein-based circulating biomarkers. There is much interest in the potential of ctDNA for developing biological fluid-based biopsies (such as using plasma, urine, or other biofluids) and the presenters in this field will bring together the most up-to-date information and current state-of-the-field.

I will add it to my writings, once published.

Suffice it say, for the moment, that circulating tumor cells are pivotal to understand the biology of cancer and its metastasis and hold great promise as specimens to help guide treatment decisions, evaluate disease burden and monitor tumor progression. Due to the scarce amounts of CTCs in blood, their enrichment and characterization represent a major technological challenge. Proprietary processes are now being developed to address this issue. For example, AdnaGen has developed a process which enriches disease specific tumor cells using magnetic particles in an antibody mixture, an approach called immunomagnetic cell enrichment.

[http://www.prnewswire.com/news-releases/qiagen-expands-leadership-in-liquid-biopsies-with-new-circulating-tumor-cell-technology-for-development-of-companion-diagnostics-296474481.html]

There will be more on this (obvious) diagnostic approach in the future. It's been long in coming but current advances in technology make it now a viable approach and, no doubt, it will soon become the number one assay of cancer and treatment progress.

# 16.7 Methylation Marker

Here's another likely advance. It relies on the fact that many cancers appeared to be viral in origin. The first ever virally-caused tumor to be identified was Burkitt's lymphoma. There are probably many other diseases caused by viruses that we haven't yet realized.

Three other common human pathogens are definitely known to cause cancer. These are Epstein-Barr, the human papilloma virus (HPV) and hepatitis B. HPV is strongly linked to cervical tumors, and hepatitis B has been tied to liver cancer. About 15% of all cancer cases worldwide are linked to a viral infection.

But the virus doesn't always cause cancer. Moreover, survival is not a genetic matter, since according to a recent study, those who developed the cancer and those who didn't had identical genomic make up.

What appeared to be different was that when the infected person developed cancer, there was clear evidence of a methylation process. According to the researchers, covert methylation (an enzyme-mediated modification to DNA) may prove to be a type of camouflage to help the virus elude the body's natural defense system.

Therefore, according to the study, measurements of the presence or absence of the methylation process would provide a very good marker for who would and wouldn't develop cancer due to these and presumably other viruses.

The findings were published online in Genome Research, Feb. 9, 2009

Methylation is a phenomenon that we call epigenetics (meaning above and beyond genetics). I learned for myself some 30 years ago that epigenetics is the number one factor influencing genetic outcomes. I saw time and again serious diseases, even genetic disorders, switched off easily by changing environmental factors, such as cleaning up chemicals in the environment and improving diet.

It's clearly the medicine of the future, and you need to look out for breakthroughs of this kind. Eventually pioneer doctors like me, who through the 70s, 80s and 90s claimed that environmental triggers were responsible for over 80% of disease, will be proved correct (in fact, we have already been proved correct, although 80% may be an underestimate).

# 16.8 Instant $3 accurate pancreatic cancer test

Never say America is finished; it's still the land of amazing possibilities.

Where else, I wonder, could a 15 year old kid come up with a successful $3 screening test for deadly pancreatic cancer and get it patented? Because that's what happened....

Jack Andraka, a pupil at a Maryland high school student, came up with a quick basic dip-stick sensor test, using simple diabetic test paper and a $50 meter from Home Depot. He focused specifically on early-stage pancreatic cancer after losing an uncle to the disease.

Pancreatic cancer is so deadly because it's hard to diagnose until it's too late. The median (similar to average) survival time following is only five months from diagnosis. Only 4% of patients make it past the five-year mark, once diagnosed. Chemo, radiation and surgery are ineffective, basically.

A few holistic practitioners, like the late Nick Gonzalez with his Beard enzyme therapy, claim far better than average survival rates, but the fact remains that pancreatic cancer is one of the most deadly because it is so difficult to diagnose early enough to be treatable.

Patients would typically show up after months of "minor" symptoms that the patient tries to ignore, like weight loss, abdominal pain, and chronic itching. Only after months of feeling unwell does the patient finally report for an exam. Jaundice is often the symptom that first alarms the patient.

If the doctor recognizes the symptoms as possible pancreatic cancer, an imaging test is usually needed to confirm the diagnosis. X-rays are no help and these days we do a CT scan, an MRI, or an ultrasound.

If the imaging test shows a mass on the pancreas, most doctors order a biopsy. When the mass is confirmed as pancreatic cancer, it's way too late.

Andraka's test changes all that. It's 168 times faster, 400 times more sensitive, and 100 times more selective than the closest conventional tests being used.

At around $3 it's also 26,000 times less expensive — and it doesn't seem to give false positives or false negatives!

In a single-blinded study of 100 patient samples, Andraka's test gave a 100 percent correct diagnosis of pancreatic cancer.

The science is sophisticated and requires nanotube "cylinders" coated with a specific antibody designed to attach to the protein or virus you're testing for. In this case, they bind to a protein that's associated with pancreatic cancer cells.

A simple electrical meter tells the technician whether there's been a shift in the space between the nanotubes, which only happens when the targeted protein or virus comes into contact with the antibodies on the surface of the nanotubes.

Brilliant!

For his efforts, Jack Andraka won the $75,000 Gordon E. Moore award at the Intel International Science and Engineering Fair.

Obviously, the dollars and suits want his invention (for which he has a patent pending). He'll have to hope the unscrupulous cancer mafia don't invest the millions of dollars to somehow break his patent. Granting the license of a major laboratory that can fight back is probably the only way to prevent that.

He'll get very rich and he deserves it.

Oh, and already Andraka is saying his test can be used for early diagnosis of lung and ovarian cancer as well — two more diseases where early diagnosis plays a major role in survival rates.

Watch out for this one!

[SOURCE: http://www.huffingtonpost.com/2012/05/22/
jack-andraka-15-wins-inte_n_1535741.html]

# 16.9 The Greek Connection

## 16.9a The Greek Cancer "Cure" (Alivizatos)

You may have heard of this test, developed by Dr. Hariton-Tzannis Alivizatos, of Athens, Greece. Make sure you differentiate it from the "other" Greece Test (next section, under the control of Ioannis Papasitoriou). You'll be glad you did!

Dr. Alivizatos uses a blood test that he says can diagnose the location and extent of cancer in a person's body. Dr. Alivizatos closely guards how he conducts this test and what it measures, refusing to share this information with cancer researchers. That puts me on my guard.

Dr. Alivizatos maintains he can interpret the results of this blood test on a numeric scale of 0.1 to IO, without defining the units of the scale or explaining in any way what the scale measures. According to Dr. Alivizatos, a person is free from cancer if the result is 0.1 to 2.5 on the undefined scale; a person has "a tendency toward cancer" if the result is 2.51 to 3.0; a person has cancer if the result is 3.01 to 8.5; and a person has no ability to fight cancer if the result is greater than 8.5.

Fascinating if this is even near accurate.

If you opt for treatment with Alvitos, he injects what he calls a serum. This substance is said to contain a combination of organic substances such as sugars, vitamins, amino acids, and other factors.

Again Alivizatos closely guards the composition of this substance as a secret. Already I am turned off this doctor. Apparently, a surgeon from Seattle, Washington, is reported to have obtained three used syringes containing small amounts of the serum when he presented himself as a cancer patient to Dr. Alivizatos in 1979.

Laboratory analysis at the University of Washington identified the substance in these syringes as pure nicotinic acid (B3).

Patients receive daily injections of the "serum" for six to 30 days. Promotional materials state an injection of this substance "boosts the immune system and helps rid the body of cancer tumors and cells," purportedly without any serious side effects.

Progress is monitored every 6 days by repeating the blood test every six days.

Dr. Alivizatos urges people undergoing the Greek Cancer Cure to follow a diet low in salt and acids, to limit their physical activities, and to avoid certain drugs such as aspirin and laxatives. Promotional ma terials quote the 1989 cost of the treatment and stay in Athens as $4,000 per couple.2

Dr. Alivizatos asserts that he has had success in using his injections to treat can cers of the skin, bone, uterus, stomach, and lymphatic system, as well as noncancerous conditions such as stomach and duodenal ulcers and lupus erythematosus. He claims that he "cures" 80 to 86 percent of people with advanced stages of cancer and up to 90 percent of those with stomach and duo denal ulcers.

What Dr. Alivizatos means by cure, however, is unknown. He presents no data on how many patients he has treated, or any objective evidence of how their cancers or other conditions were diagnosed and confirmed, how their response to treatment was measured, nor how long they survived without evidence of recurring disease.

Although Dr. Alivizatos asks people who seek the Greek Cancer Cure to provide him with medical records from their hometown physicians before and after treatment, he has stated that he keeps no records of his own concerning the patients he treats. That last is the third switch off for me. How can he know his results, if he's not keeping records?

You make up your own mind

Hariton-Tzannis Alivizatos, MD, is a microbiologist who says he developed what he calls the Greek Cancer Cure about 30 years ago. Sometime before 1983, Dr. Alivizatos temporarily lost his license to practice medicine in Greece when he failed to submit the substance he injects intravenously to the government for testing.

He regained his license after submitting this substance for testing but was asked to stop using the substance because it was not effective in treating cancer. In 1983, the Hellenic Medical Association investigated Dr. Alivizatos for medical malpractice and suspended his license for two years. He has now resumed activities. [this is according to the American Cancer Society, who love to dish the dirt on alternative and holistic practitioners who threaten their revenues with a "cure", so you may choose to take it with a pinch of salt]

# 16.9b The Greece Blood Test (Papasotiriou-GNCC)

This is better. Not to be confused with Alivizatos' work: the Greece Cancer Test is administered by Research Genetic Cancer Center International GmbH. The company's headquarters are in Switzerland but the laboratories are in Northern Greece. There are branch offices in the U.S.A., in Central Europe, in the United Kingdom, in Cyprus and Hungary.

The founding figure, Dr. Iaonnis Papasotiriou MD, formerly worked in the department of Experimental Physiology and Biochemistry in the Medical School of Thessaloniki.

The test is based on growing the patient's own circulating tumor cells. We now know that the deadly ability of cancer to spread and start up in remote locations is due to circulating stems cells which carry the malignancy factor. These are circulating tumor cells (CTC's) and cancer stem cells (CSC's) and even what are called CSC-like cells.

You will not be able to order this test directly with the lab. A licensed practitioner must draw the blood. The weak link is that it has to get to Greece very fast, before the stem cells die (2-3 days).

If there are circulatory tumor cells (CTC's) and cancer stem cells (CSC's) present, the strain will be cultivated and isolated. The cultured cancer cells will be tested with over 50 nutraceuticals (including Laetrile!) which have been proven to promote apoptosis (programmed cell death) of cancer cells. The cancer cells are also tested with various chemotherapies, to check which treatment is the most effective for you.

This is therefore a personalized treatment program; what may be effective for one individual may not be for the next person.

## Who Needs The GNCC Test?

- People who want to actively engage in reducing their risk of developing cancer in the future

- People with an increased risk of cancer e.g. due to family history, lifestyle or environmental issues who want the opportunity to engage in a screening program for early detection and diagnosis.

- People with a current diagnosis of cancer who want more information about treatment options for them as an individual – including natural treatments.

Contact: R.G.C.C. Ltd, 115 M. Alexandrou Str., 53070 Filotas-Florinas, Greece

Tel: +30-24630-42264 E-mail: office@rgcc-genlab.com

Note that Dr. Papasotiriou is not shy of the scientific literature. I found a paper by him and his colleagues on PubMed, concerning the value of flow cytometry, among other things. [Case Rep Oncol. 2011 Jan-Apr; 4(1): 44–54

Use this technique with confidence. Be sure not to get it confused with Alivizatos "cure" in Athens. But also please remember the problem of chemo resistance developing in cancerous cells. This may rapidly render the results of the test unreliable or require re-testing, at extra expense.

# 16.10 Doctor Fido Will See You Now!

What, dogs as cancer markers?

I first learned of the ability of dogs to sniff out cancers from a letter published in the prestigious Lancet. It cited a story of a woman whose dog constantly sniffed at a mole on her leg. On one occasion, the dog even tried to bite the lesion off. The constant attention from the dog prompted her to seek medical advice and when the path lab report came back, it was found to be a malignant melanoma!

Since it was caught early, the patient recovered fully from this very dangerous cancer and has remained well, with no sign of recurrence. The dog saved her life.

In another instance, a man aged 66 years developed a patch of eczema on the outer side of his left thigh, which grew slowly over 18 years, to about 1–2 cm in diameter. When dry, the lesion would become scabby, and it caused occasional itching. Various doctors tried treating it with steroids and antifungal creams, without any benefit.

Then a pet Labrador arrived in the home and the dog began to persistently push his nose against his owner's trouser leg, sniffing the skin lesion beneath it. This prompted the patient to return to his family physician for review. An excision biopsy (removal) showed it to be a basal cell carcinoma. After it was gone, the dog showed no further interest in the area, so the animal was definitely reacting because of the pathology.

[Williams H, Pembroke A. *Sniffer dogs in the melanoma clinic?*. Lancet 1989; 1: 734.]

Naturally, the idea of a pet detecting dangerous cancers and saving the owner's life generated a lot of media interest.

Subsequently, a dermatologist in Florida teamed up with a retired police-dog handler with 33 years' experience in training dogs, including service in Vietnam. They used conventional sniffer-dog techniques to train George, a schnauzer, to recognize pathological specimens of malignant melanoma and set him to work on humans.

George was introduced to a patient with several moles thought to be cancer-free. However one mole caused George to go crazy, and excision of the lesion confirmed early malignant disease.

So the idea of dogs being able to sniff out disease, often before any overt pathological changes have taken place, has begun to take hold of the medical community. They'll be looking for ways to make money at it. But what the heck, if a few dogs acquire the skills, I foresee queues of worried people lined up outside the kennels for a walk past!

Better than oncologists by far!

Further investigation has showed that dogs are astonishingly accurate (far more accurate than oncologists with all their paraphernalia). Dogs were 97% successful at detecting lung cancer* and scored an impressive 88% at detecting breast cancer, regardless of attempts to mask the smell through food or cigarettes.

Other scientific studies have documented the abilities of dogs to identify chemicals that are diluted as low as parts per trillion.

Already dogs are used to warn of epileptic seizures, low blood sugar and heart attacks, although whether they are detecting changes in smell or physical behavior is still unknown. Some canines know how to call 911 in an emergency.

Now a new study, led by Michael McCulloch of the Pine Street Foundation in San Anselmo, California, and Tadeusz Jezierski of the Polish Academy of Sciences, Institute of Genetics and Animal Breeding, has been investigating whether dogs can detect cancers only by sniffing the exhaled breath of cancer patients.

In this study, five household dogs were trained within a short 3-week period to detect lung or breast cancer by sniffing the breath of cancer participants. The trial itself consisted of 86 cancer patients (55 with lung cancer and 31 with breast cancer) and a control sample of 83 healthy patients. All cancer patients had recently been diagnosed with cancer through biopsy-confirmed conventional methods such as a mammogram, or CAT scan and had not yet undergone any chemotherapy treatment.

During the study, the dogs were presented with breath samples from the cancer patients and the controls, captured in a special tube. The results of the study showed that dogs can detect breast and lung cancer with sensitivity and specificity between 88% and 97%.

The high accuracy persisted even after results were adjusted to take into account whether the lung cancer patients were currently smokers. Moreover, the study also confirmed that the trained dogs could even detect the early stages of lung cancer, as well as early breast cancer. The researchers concluded that breath analysis by trained dogs has the potential to provide a substantial reduction in the uncertainty currently seen in cancer diagnosis.

# Breath Testing

The presence of chemicals in exhaled breath indicative of disease is itself nothing new. One of the critical tests for the presence of Helicobacter pylori, the stomach bug frequency associated with peptic ulcer (and therefore the "cause" of peptic ulcers to modern reductionist thinking), is the amount of hydrogen in exhaled breath from the patient.

In my book *Diet Wise* I pointed out the value of this breath test in detecting dysbiosis. Inadequate digestion and malabsorption allows a test sugar load to reach the colon and there cause fermentation by bacteria.

Martin Gotteland and colleagues at the Institute of Nutrition and Food Technology in Santiago, Chile have shown conclusively that effective probiotic administration in humans significantly reduces hydrogen gas in excreted breath.


## Where Next?

The next stage is to explore more fully the possible uses of dogs in early detection. Could dogs pick up Ebola, TB or AIDS in travelers returning from high risk areas? We don't know. But we do know that a dog's sense of smell is very complex and has "layers", unlike our ability to focus on just one chemical at a time.

Now a new project focused specifically on detecting ovarian cancer through analysis of exhaled breath has been awarded a federal research grant by the Congressionally Directed Medical Research Program. Epithelial ovarian cancer is the fifth leading cause of cancer death in women. Early diagnosis is the most important step toward reducing morbidity and mortality from epithelial ovarian cancer. If found early, even in the hands of conventional oncologists the (5-year) survival rate is over 90%.

The existing best current method to test for ovarian cancer, a combination of a blood marker called CA-125 and ultrasound of the lower abdomen, is really not an accurate indicator of early-stage disease.

Preliminary tests, under careful double-blinded conditions, showed the ability of trained dogs to distinguish ovarian cancer cases from controls using samples of exhaled breath condensate with accuracy of over 97%. Their hit rate was compared to that of a method involving a super-accurate instrument called a Gas Chromatography/Fourier transform Ion Cyclotron Resonance Mass Spectrometer (GC/FT-ICR MS). I have already explained the principle of cyclotron resonance in the book *Medicine Beyond* and predicted its growing place in modern medicine as a "virtual diagnostic" tool.

Of course if the relevant breath marker chemicals are identified, it may be possible to dispense with the doggies altogether.

But personally I think I'll take the dog for a walk and if it yaps excitedly at a neighbor's gate I might feel inclined to ring the bell and ask if everyone inside is OK!

[March 2006 issue of the *Journal of Integrative Cancer Therapies* published by SAGE Publications;  European Lung Foundation, news release, Aug. 17, 2011]

# Section 17

## Bad Stuff
## To Avoid

Time is shortening. But every day that I challenge this cancer and survive is a victory for me.

**Ingrid Bergman**

# 17.1 The Hulda Reger Clark Problem

## What problem?

Well, in my view, Hulda Reger Clark was a big blot on the alternative cancer scene. I do not mean by that people did not getting well in her care. The problem is her story and claims, which bring discredit on good doctors and healers. She was, I believe, a sham, but even if she was genuine she was seriously misguided and spreading nonsense as fact. Her teachings are very harmful to the common good.

Clark called herself "doctor" and states her degree is in physiology. The Register of Ph.D. Degrees conferred by the University of Minnesota July 1956-June 1966, states that Clark received her degree with a major in zoology and a minor in botany. This is a curious falsehood and makes one wonder about her overall integrity. Presumably she was trying to give herself a phoney medical credibility. That's always a red flag.

I read her book *The Cure For All Cancers years ago*; such a title obviously demanded attention. But after a few pages I promptly tossed it. It's phoney and dishonest.

Clark's "cures" are worse than bogus; they are derisory. She would test a patient using electronic dowsing and say "You have cancer" and then, a few days or few weeks later, test again and say "I've cured you". She provides no documentation, no evidence for either the presence of cancer or the fact that it is subsequently cured (sometimes in as little as a few days!)

The majority of the people described in the 103 case reports did not have any proven clinical cancer. Of those that did, most had received standard medical treatment or their tumors were in their early stages and would likely have recovered anyway. In these cases, Clark pronounced them cured but did not follow what happened after they left her clinic—so she could not possibly know how they got along afterward. In some instances, she counted patients as cured even though she noted that they died within a few weeks after she treated them.

Clark's claim of 100 consecutive cures then becomes the hype of a snake oil salesman, rather than any recognizable science. It's nonsense and somewhat arrogant, in my view. Clearly she does not understand the true nature of electronic dowsing; which is that it can only reflect the operator's beliefs and there is no objectivity whatever.

If the practitioner is good, the dowsing will often come out right. But to believe there is anything to this, other than the dowser's "hunch" is a delusion, as I explained with all similar devices in "Medicine Beyond".

Clark's assertion that all cancers are caused by just 2 agents: iso-propyl alcohol and a parasite called *Fasciolopsis buskii* is quackery and nonsense and at variance with what generations of skilled and careful holistic doctors, far better educated in medicine than she ever was, have found. The causes of cancer are many and complex. Thus there is no one cure, either.

I've never met a single patient who had any success with her "zapper" machine, though doubtless some zealots will attest to its efficacy (she gave away the circuit diagram to a "zapper" in her book, by the way, so charges of financial gain do not weigh).

I believe, based on many more years experience than Clark's, that the results she was getting were from normal, obvious measures that we all recommend, like change of diet and lifestyle. It is erroneous to attribute these to her zapping, even though it somewhat parallels the work Royal Rife (section 11.9).

But my point is that this is still disinformation and is causing people to mis-assign the value of cures.

The curious thing is that she eventually had an army of adoring fans following her. I suppose they have suspended all rational judgment and ignored the nonsense. People who are desperate may do that.

Part of her success, I'm sure, is that what she did could sometimes work—meaning that her high frequency "zapping" of pathogens and possibly cancer cells is plausible, given the knowledge of Rife's research. But I remind you that Rife himself did not believe that the plates/electrodes approach was effective.

Cleaning up parasites, as Clark claims, will only help the immune system and thereby benefit cancer. Improving the diet will also, unarguably, help cancer pateints. That doesn't mean her other theories hold much water, however beguiling they may be to some. Indeed the number one cause of cancer she claimed, *Fasciolopsis buskii* does not occur in the Western world, only in the Far East.

You can have the real secret of cancer cures for less than $50, not $10,000s which Hulda Reger Clark charged.

Read again my 3 pillars (section 2).

I found this post at: http://www.cancerguide.org accessed 2/27/2009

Leandra Smith, a sarcoma patient who unfortunately has since died, visited Hulda Clark's clinic in Tijuana, Mexico and posted a message about what she observed to the CANCER-L mailing list on August 30, 1996, and she also wrote about it some more in a message to me. What follows is an edited version of her reports. It's important to note that her observations don't directly address the question of whether the treatment works or not, but the conditions she describes are surely a very bad sign.

> I went down to Dr. Hulda Clark's clinic in Tijuana yesterday... She's the lady who wrote *The Cure for All Diseases* and *The Cure for All Cancers*. She believes that all diseases are caused by parasites in the body and if you kill all the parasites and rid yourself of all chemicals in your environment and prevent all metals from getting into your system then you will be cured. I did notice, however, that she did say that if you do not rid yourself of every single little pollutant than it will not work...hmmmm sounds like a loophole in her theory if it doesn't work for you...

The clinic itself was... well... sketchy. There was chaos everywhere and people strolling in and out. There was a weird looking guy walking around stalking all the flies with a swatter... some very sick people were there getting treatments and they were lying on plastic lawn chairs with cushions covered in plastic garbage bags... they were getting IV treatments and their tubes were nailed up on the wall... the whole place didn't look very sanitary and the device they used to test me if I had any parasites was obviously pure quackery. It was this audio thing that if you held one end of a conductor and they pressed the other on your other hand and they placed jars of the stuff they were testing on this metal plate... then when they connected the electric current through your body it made sounds... supposedly the woman doing the testing, also the receptionist, could tell the difference between positive and negative (I heard no obvious differentiating sounds).

I saw an elderly couple from Tenn. there and it was so sad. The husband was so sick and he was just lying there trying to ignore the flies landing on him in the hot, hot, hot clinic care room, just adjacent to the waiting room with no door for privacy. His wife was running around trying to track down anyone who could possibly find her some ice to cool her husband down and no one would help her. I feel like if they could have had a resource to hear about the conditions of the clinic before they traveled there they never would have come...

I was supposed to go back today and pay $150 to hear what her treatment plan would be, but I did suspect it meant staying at the clinic, to make sure that I maintained a "non-toxic environment" (but also I guess pick up a couple of Mexican bugs while I was at it). That didn't seem like something I wanted to do, so I decided to keep the $150 and go out to dinner with friends, which in my opinion would do better for my health than Dr. Hulda Clark could provide.

Anyway, I think I'll stick to more mainstream holistic healers...

Please note that the CancerGuide.org site is a fine project, with no axe to grind.

# The End

In February 2001, Mexican authorities inspected Clark's center and ordered it to shut down. According to a report in the San Diego Union Tribune, the clinic had never registered and was operating without a license. In June, the authorities announced that the clinic would be permitted to reopen but could offer only conventional care.

If anyone has any information that Clark's team are still tolerating such squalid and insulting conditions for their patients, I should like to know about it. Her fees are not as high as some but way too high for this deplorable standard of hygiene and care.

The important point to get across is you have choices. There is no need to feel desperate. I have explained to you many ways on which you can beat cancer, without the need to go to a dirty flea pit like Clark's operation and be charged $10,000s, to be told (without proof) that you are "cured".

I'm sure this section will be seen as a hatchet job by Clark's many admirers. But I would not be serving the community if I minced words and didn't make the facts as plain as I see them.

In any case, Ms. Clark is no longer with us. Hopefully her ridiculous ideas will follow her rapidly to the grave.

**I repeat" whatever results she and her helpers got was from well-known and proven therapies, like diet and lifestyle change. The ridiculous "cures" she touted were irrelevant.**

# 17.2 The Protocel Hoax

Protocel® is one of the names given to a mixture of chemical compounds developed in the 1930's by a chemist named James Sheridan who claimed that that the formula came to him from God in a dream and would cure cancer and other diseases.

Sheridan claimed his formula contains a substance called "croconic acid". There is no such substance anywhere in the universe. It's a scam, even though he did not charge. The fact that Sheridan (supposedly) did not monetize his fantasy does mean therefore it really works!

I advize you to avoid this treatment like the plague. Unfortunately, it is being promoted from the rooftops by foolish, ignorant or downright crooked marketers, making outrageous false claims.

One website trumpets it as "... a safe alternative cancer treatment which has successfully treated people and animals for a wide array of diseases for more than thirty years without dangerous side effects."

I tell you it is a lie. I know people KILLED by this folly. Of course those grubbing up dollars (who are worse than greedy oncologists in my view) will never tell you that. The important point is whether you can kill cancer cells without killing the patient. If not, it's too toxic. Sheridan's formula has never passed any safety tests. He tells a long whining story about how it's all somebody else's fault that these tests were not done.

But the NCI says he never delivered the data they asked for. All they could ever get out of Sheridan and his bunch were testimonials.

You must condition yourself to ignore testimonials. **Testimonials are not science.** In fact many of them are not honest. Those where the story happens to be true, have always got better for some other reason. Same problem with the Laetrile story: it has never been proven and someone who got better *while* taking it did not necessarily get better *because* of taking it.

If you want testimonials, go for chemotherapy! There are literally millions of people who will happily proclaim they were cured by chemo. Testimonials cannot be the benchmark of what's right in medicine.

That's marketing trickery.

Meanwhile, remember what I told you in section 2: many cancers go away if you just leave well alone. So recovery while taking a treatment is not proof it works; only data, statistics, can prove you did better than Nature herself.

The worst and most despicable part of this Protocel story is that promoters commonly state that the NCI actually approved Sheridan's formula and stated it was effective. It's a lie that is easy to beat; just go to the NCI website here and find the truth:

http://www.cancer.gov/cancertopics/pdq/cam/cancell/HealthProfessional/page2

Part of the danger and reckless stupidity is that patients are asked to avoid many key nutrients, such as vitamin C and Vitamin E, glutathione, lipoic acid, carnitine and L-cysteine. If you avoid those enough, you'll die for sure.

What you won't hear said often is that Protocel contains highly toxic substances, like nitric acid, sodium sulfite, potassium hydroxide (also known as caustic potash) and sulfuric acid. I wouldn't allow any patient to put this filth in their body. It's no better than chemotherapy and, I repeat, claims that it is safe and harmless are mere commercial lies.

So here is an unproven formula, with nothing to commend it but myth and opinion, based on phoney compounds, supported only by "testimonials", that is supposedly superior to Mother Nature's nutrients, which have thousands of years of proven anti-cancer effectiveness?

Not tenable.

The following section also has the same fundamental flaw as "Jim's Juice" (another name for Sheridan's formula): the idea of a "magic bullet" that removes the need for the patient to do anything corrective to help him or herself.

I call it the chemo mentality: the idea that you find some magic bullet, swallow it and you'll be saved from cancer. It's one of the stupidest and most dangerous attitudes of mind I can think of. Nature has been kind enough to tell you that your health is in ruins. You should not ignore this message.

Change what you are doing, change your lifestyle, change everything. Work your way honestly and carefully back to health. But to believe that any formula, juice or junk, will save you is a folly that could cost you your life.

# 17.3 Dichloroacetate (DCA)

**Magic bullets don't work! This story illustrates a useful medical/healing principle:**

You may have heard of DCA or dichloroacetate and its supposed benefits for cancer patients. The science isn't 100% but in rats at least DCA caused tumors to shrink. The hope is it will do the same thing in humans. The trouble is no clinical trials have been carried out. Some desperate cancer sufferers are taking it anyway, saying if they might die what difference does it make if they take a potentially toxic compound.

Unfortunately, it isn't so simple. If it really does work it could be a valuable therapy. But if patients take it without expert supervision and someone dies, the substance might become discredited before it even has a chance. It might even be banned.

You see this compound is a simple readily-available substance. There is no patent on it so drug companies, in their usual way, would love to see DCA buried. It threatens their profits. They don't care about saving lives. They pretend to but it's all about profit. That comes before patient care.

DCA is a small molecule that blocks the enzyme pyruvate dehydrogenase kinase in mitochondria — the energy-production centers in cells — causing more glucose to be metabolized in the mitochondria rather than by a different pathway. It shifts the metabolism of pyruvate from *glycolysis* towards oxidation in the mitochondria. To boil it down even further, DCA shifts the cell's metabolism from anaerobic to aerobic metabolism. Remember that cancer cells deal with glucose by glycolisis (section 3.0.

When DCA was given to rats that were growing human lung tumors, the tumors stopped growing within a week, and three months later were half the size of those in untreated animals. Other experimental drugs have had similar effects. But DCA stands out because it can be taken by mouth and easily penetrates tissues.

Because DCA has been around for years, its structure can't be patented and pharmaceutical companies are not interested in developing the drug. That has left patients to try it for themselves.

Evangelos Michelakis at the University of Alberta in Edmonton, Canada and other DCA research scientists are worried by the development. Although DCA seems safe overall, they point to a clinical trial that was stopped early because those taking the drug developed damage to their peripheral nerves (P. Kaufmann et al. Neurology 66, 324–330; 2006). Without a control group, they point out, it will be impossible to tell whether any improvement in the patients' condition is caused by the drug. Patients could also be taking DCA that is not of pharmaceutical grade and might contain harmful impurities.

Michelakis says the patients could end up undermining efforts to do a controlled clinical trial. The battle between dying patients who want immediate access to unapproved drugs and doctors who urge trials and caution is a perennial one. Some patients argue that they cannot wait for trials and should have the right to take unapproved drugs, regardless of the risks.

But there are key arguments against this. An estimated 95% of cancer drugs that enter clinical trials do not get approval, many because they are ineffective or unsafe, so patients risk shortening their life or making their last days more uncomfortable.

Also, if patients can access DCA — or other unapproved drugs — there is no incentive for them to enter a clinical trial. There is no question that more people will be helped if access to unapproved drugs is restricted and proper trials performed.

## The Latest

Now orthodox pharma is on the case. Researchers at the University of Georgia have discovered a new way to deliver this drug that may one day make it a viable treatment for numerous forms of cancer. They published their findings in the American Chemical Society's journal *ACS Chemical Biology*.

Shanta Dhar, an assistant professor of chemistry in the UGA Franklin College of Arts and Sciences, says, "We have developed a new compound based on DCA that is three orders of magnitude more potent than standard treatments."

Dhar's technology, which she calls Mito-DCA, destroys the cancer by focusing on a part of the cell called mitochondria, hence the name (mitochondria-DCA, get it?)

In their experiments, Dhar and her research team exposed cancer cells to Mito-DCA. The results showed that the engineered chemical substance was able to switch the glycolysis-based metabolism of cancer cells to glucose oxidation, meaning that the cancer cells can once again die via apoptosis.

Mito-DCA also suppressed the production of lactic acid in cancerous cells, which allows them to avoid detection by the body's immune system. With this cloaking device damaged, the body's own T-cells are better able to recognize tumors and eliminate them. In fact one could question whether that might have been the real reason the souped-up DCA was effective!

While the UGA researchers' model focused specifically on prostate cancer, Dhar is hopeful that their technique may prove useful for other forms of cancer.

"This is only the beginning of this project," she said. "We will continue to test Mito-DCA and find new avenues for treatment."

[*ACS Chem. Biol.* 2014, 9, 1178-1187]

# 17.4 Beware The Marshall Protocol

You will have read my clear support for extensive and adequate vitamin D supplementation in section 2.8. Everyone knows that vitamin D is one of the most cancer-protective nutrients knwon to man. So imagine some self-stylcd cancer expert telling you "vitamin D causes cancer".

This is the so-called "Marshall protocol", which directly contradicts this advice. It may come down to just who you want to believe, a professor of nutrition, medically qualified, or some misguided engineer claiming medical status and surrounded by fans who have suspended all judgment and connection with the rest of current medical research.

Trevor Marshall is an Australian electrical engineer who developed an interest in biomedical engineering out of a desire to cure his own sarcoidosis, which he developed in the 1970s (a non-malignant but potentially fatal condition). He calls himself doctor but has no medical degree. His PhD is not even in biology but electrical engineering. Marshall's theories come from mathematical molecular models, not clinical studies.

You must not be distracted by the raving testimonials from his ardent fans. Look at the facts, PLEASE, otherwise you risk killing yourself. I'm not kidding.

Marshall believes, with no evidence, that vitamin D is immunosuppressive—in other words it shuts down your body's immune system. Therefore, he states, the lower your vitamin D is, the better, because vitamin D from any source (food, supplements, or sunlight) in any amount accelerates the disease process.

This is wildly off the rails and very dangerous indeed. There are now thousands of good scientific studies showing vitamin D is one of the main vitamins which empowers the immune system, helps block cancer and will help heal it when present.

According to Marshall's addled view, the low vitamin D levels [measured as serum 25(OH)D] found in many people with chronic diseases such as cancer are a result of the disease, rather than the cause.

If he was right, then of course low levels of vitamin D would be attractive. But it's it a complete fiction, based on no clinical evidence or trials. It's just a fancy notion, stuck in place with pseudo-scientific rhetoric. I repeat, Marshall has not produced a single shred of clinical evidence; just theories.

## Fear of Vitamin D

Devotees of the Marshal protocol avoid sunlight and vitamin D as if they were harbinger's of the plague. They won't eat foods high in vitamin D and live like troglodytes in holes. When they venture into the open air, they walk around with dark glasses and wrapped in blankets, to avoid the sunlight.

Patients are advised to take a medication called Benicar (olmesartan), which is an angiotensin II receptor blocker (ARB). This is supposed to reactivate the immune system. But Benicar is dangerous for people who have weak adrenal function (namely low cortisol and aldosterone production). Cancer patients, especially undergoing chemo and radiation, are likely to have such compromised adrenal function.

If that's not dangerous enough, his clients take pulsed, low-dose antibiotics to further combat the infection that is believed to be lurking. This is continued for 3-5 years. Yet we know from decades of experience that long-term antibiotics will wreck the microbiome and this has recently been shown to be one of the number one protectors against cancer.

Marshall is just totally off the scientific rails.

## Herxeimer Reaction

The most insidious and dangerous aspect of all Marshall's teachings are that if you feel really ill, it's doing you good.

This is supposed to be what's called a Herxeimer reaction, named for German dermatologist Karl Herxeimer, who first noticed it when treating syphilitic patients with mercury. The assumption has always been that it is caused by the metabolism being upset but the breakdown of dying toxic cells and their debris.

It's a real reaction. We may encounter it in other situations than the one first described. For example I noticed it often when treating Candida patients with anti-fungal powder.

But today I often see it quoted as a justification for mismanagement of patients and making them sick with harmful procedures.

**Even worse, in Marshall's teaching, if you don't get the reaction, the therapy is doing you no good at all.** That shows his appalling ignorance of Nature and the healing process. Remember he is an engineer with no clinical experience.

This guy is not just a loose cannon, he and his devotees are a menace to public good.

I urge you to avoid any aspect of his theories and methods. You could get yourself killed—literally.

# Absurd Claim That Vitamin D Does Not Benefit Cancer

One of the myth peddlers Amy Proal (www.bacteriality.com), claims there are studies that demonstrate that vitamin D does not decrease cancer risk. This is the "science of convenience", meaning she omits the torrents of great studies which prove unequivocally it does.

Previous theories linking vitamin D to lower risk of certain cancers have been tested and confirmed in more than 200 epidemiological studies, and understanding of its physiological basis stems from more than 2,500 laboratory studies.

On the other hand, the studies Proal relies on are worthless. This is not nit-picking; several of those studies involve people supplementing with absurdly low doses of vitamin D, 600-800 IU per day, which is too little to be effective. She and Marshall are way out of touch. Recent studies and the modern consensus among knowledgeable nutritionists and physicians (I'm not talking about the hospital dinosaurs) indicate that levels of over 1500 units are needed. 2,000 is even better. I take 4,000.

Just how important is vitamin D? In a brand new paper (*Annals of Epidemiology*, May 22, 2009) epidemiologist Cedric Garland, DrPH, professor of family and preventive medicine at the UC San Diego School of Medicine has proposed a whole new model.

He has produced evidence that vitamin D and calcium levels are critical for healthy cell signaling. Without enough vitamin D, cells may lose their identity as differentiated cells, and revert to a stem cell-like state. That's a dangerous pro-cancerous condition.

For a soundly scientific independent view, consult http://www.vitaminDsociety.org

You can read about Marshall and his oddball theories here (but don't! waste your time):

Wikipedia, http://en.wikipedia.org/wiki/Trevor_Marshall

Joe Mercola does a good deconstruct, using his considerable knowledge of all aspects of alternative protocols:

http://articles.mercola.com/sites/articles/archive/2009/03/14/Clearing-Up-Confusion-on-Vitamin-D--Why-I-Dont-Recommend-the-Marshall-Protocol.aspx

# 17.5 Bicarbonate, Candida and "Professor" Simoncini

Alternative treatments for cancer seem ripe for myth and legend. As I keep saying, many people want to believe that they can be treated quickly and easily by some kind of "magic bullet". They hope, perhaps, that they don't have to do anything different, even though their lifestyle has showed up as something toxic and dangerous.

I can't think of any other reason the ridiculous claims of Italian ex-doctor, Tullio Simoncini would be taken seriously by anybody. Currently living in Rome, he has been using unsubstantiated cancer treatments for 15 years.

On some websites it says that he once was a prominent oncologist. In reality he was never working as a regularly employee of the medical staff at the oncology department, but he worked as a volunteer. He didn't receive any salary. And he only administered treatment to cancer patients under supervision of senior doctors. His main occupation at the time was as a doctor in the Italian Social Security Service, assessing whether disabled people were eligible for pension or not!

In 2003, his license to practice medicine was withdrawn, and in 2006 he was convicted by an Italian judge for wrongful death and swindling. This has not stopped him from continuing to provide his controversial treatments, not only in Italy, but apparently also in foreign countries, such as the Netherlands.

Simoncini claims all you have to do it give the patient IV baking soda (sodium bicarbonate) and the cancer goes away.

Only a fool would think that; but if you are still not sure he might be right: he goes on to claim that ALL cancers are a *Candida albicans* or fungus infection. So all you have to do (he says) is administer bicarbonate, that will kill the Candida and you're done. It's too absurd.

It is easy to find testimonials on the internet, praising Tullio Simoncinis approach. But reports of actual harm caused by acceptance of his ideas are also surfacing. You just won't find them on Tullio Simoncini's or his proponents web sites, as they wish to give you the impression, that their treatment is harmless and cheap in contrast to chemotherapy. One should understand, that these reports are only the "tip of the ice berg". Dead people don't talk, and only seldom do relatives step forward.

Far from cheap, this shyster can easily relieve you of $30,000 or more!

Simoncini does not give any proof for his crank ideas and has never published any supporting data in a scientific journal. He also claims that the treatment is not dangerous, because sodium bicarbonate is also used in standard medical procedures. He fails to mention that this treatment is applied in hospital only to patients with definite disturbances of water and mineral metabolism and under meticulous clinical supervision. The highly concentrated solutions that he administers within a short period can disturb the mineral balance in the body and lead to serious and even fatal complications.

In fact Simoncini's approach is not merely a misguided but harmless notion. Simoncini kills! Stay away from this therapy.

In October 2007, a charge was brought against the Clinic for Preventive Medicine (CPM) in Bilthoven, the Netherlands. This clinic houses a mixture of small enterprises, where physicians and non-physicians offer a great variety of "alternative" treatments.

A 50-year-old patient with breast cancer who had been treated at this clinic was admitted to the emergency department of the University Medical Center of the Free University of Amsterdam, where she died within a few days. The attending physician refused to sign a death certificate, because the patient had died from a non-natural cause.

It appeared that Simoncini had treated her at the Bilthoven clinic, with injections and infusions of sodium bicarbonate.

The clinic medical director denied any involvement, but two tenacious journalists of the Dutch newspaper de Volkskrant succeeded in finding out what had happened.

If you are interested in reading more about Simoncini's misunderstandings/manipulations of science, try this web page:

http://anaxImperator.wordpress.com/2009/06/09/tullio-simoncini-and-the-research-that-wasnt/

You will be shocked to find that in animals studies, bicarbonate is capable of causing and enhancing the growth of cancer. But if you remember Emanuel Revici's discovery that a large proportion of patients get worse by alkalizing and you will readily so why this can happen.

Do NOT try and use alkalis or bicarbonate without knowing whether you have Revici's "alakaline pattern" or "acid pattern". You could kill yourself by ignorance. (see section 10.1)

Just ignore the ignorant fools on the Internet (like Marc Sircus, who attacked me and called me a madman, feeling smug and safe from a libel suit). These jokers all copy each other's pet theories and mistakes just go on and on and on...

# 17.6 Chapparal

You will see this listed in some compilations of holistic cancer therapies. Whether it deserves to be there is another matter. There is some concern over taking such a toxic substance.

This common shrub of the American South-West, is usually prepared in the form of a tea. As expected, the pharmaceutical industry is again trying to out-do nature by exploring the anti-cancer properties of what they refer to as the "active ingredient," nordihydroguaiaretic acid (NDGA).

Chaparral is commonly referred to as the creosote bush. NDGA was shown by S. Birkenfeld to reduce the occurrence of colon cancer in rats, fed a chemical that induced that cancer.

D.K. Shalini demonstrated NDGA's ability to protect genes against carcinogens and published this experiment in Molecular Cell Biochemistry, 1990.

The breast cancer preventive effect of NDGA was demonstrated by D.L. McCormick and A.M. Spicer (Cancer Left, 1987).

Leukemia cell cultures were inhibited by NDGA (A.M. Miller, Journal of Laboratory Clinical Medicine, 1989) Human brain cancer cell growth was likewise inhibited by NDGA (DE. Wilson, Journal of Neurosurgery, 1989.)

Cancer cell inhibition was intensively explored in the doctorate thesis of J Zemora (Auburn University, 1984) Regression of the deadly melanoma and treatment of choriocarcinoma and lymphosarcoma have been sited by CR. Smart in Cancer Chemotherapy Reports, 1969, and echoed by the American Cancer Society, 1971.

D. Vanden Berghe demonstrated the anti-cancer and anti-viral activity of other chaparral extracts and P. Train wrote of use as an anti-bacterial.

Because of a rare case in which signs of liver damage showed up after several months of taking chaparral leaf, M. Katz in the Journal of Clinical Gastroenterology, 1990, warned that "the public and the medical profession must be wary of all 'harmless' non-prescription medications, whether purchased in pharmacies or elsewhere."

All in all, it's better to avoid this option. It's too risky and there are far better methods available.

# 17.7 Cannabis (Marijauna, Hash)!

You've probably heard that marijuana has been used by cancer patients to counteract the nausea and vomiting caused by chemotherapy.[1] [see references at the end of this section]

Gradually this has grown to the tale the marijuana "cures cancer". It's nonsense. What may be true is that derivatives of this herb have potential. But that's far from drug-taking. As you've just read in the previous section, we use yew and periwinkle plant derivatives in chemo; but that doesn't mean we smoke or chew them! We are talking extracts only.

The notion of marijuana used as an anti-neoplastic started with a paper in the *Journal of the National Cancer* Institute in 1975, demonstrating the supposed activity of marijuana derivatives, as I said. It described the retarding effect on the growth of lung cancer in mice in as little as ten days and even more pronounced beneficial effects, with continued use.[2]

Proponents of legal marijauna have been quick to sieze this snippet of science and turn government regulations into a conspiracy to keep a natural wonder herb from the deserving public. I DON'T BUY INTO THIS.

Hash is junk and dangerous junk at that. I'll give you some guidelines here but I'm not recommending it.

# 17.7a THC vs. Brain Tumors

Gliomas (tumors in the brain) are especially aggressive malignant forms of cancer. These tumors are notoriously difficult to treat and often result in rapid death.

Surprisingly, therefore, cannabinoids such as THC (tetra-hydro-cannabinol) seem to act as antineoplastic agents, particularly on glioma cell lines which "induced a considerable regression of malignant gliomas" in animals. [3,4,5]

Italian investigators at the University of Milan, Department of Pharmacology, Chemotherapy and Toxicology, also reported that cannabidiol (CBD, which is non-psychoactive), inhibited the growth of various human glioma cell lines in vivo and in vitro in a dose dependent manner.[6]

In 2004, Guzman and colleagues reported that cannabinoids inhibited glioma tumor growth in animals and in human glioblastoma multiforme (GBM) and showed this was by the mechanism of inhibiting vascular-endothelial growth factor (VEGF), the signaler that generates more blood supply for tumors.[7]

It is claimed that natural cannabinoids have little effect on normal cells.[8]

# 17.7b Skin Cancers and Leukemia

Cannabinoids may help control non-melanoma skin cancers.[9] Again, it seems to do

this by inhibiting VEGF and thus blood supply to the tumor.

Cannabinoids have a positive effect on leukemia cells. THC is a potent inducer of apoptosis, even in low doses and as early as 6 hours after exposure to the drug (NOT smoking pot). These effects were seen in leukemic cell lines as well as in peripheral blood mononuclear cells.[10]

## 17.7c Synergy with Chemo

Studies also suggest that the administration of cannabinoids, in conjunction with conventional anti-cancer therapies, could enhance the effectiveness of standard cancer treatments. Moreover, investigators at the University of California, Pacific Medical Center, reported that the administration of a combination of the plant's constituents is superior to the administration of isolated compounds alone.[11] All holistic doctors know that the "active compound" idea is a myth used to leverage something to patent and make profits from. The many constituents of a pharmacological source act together in ways we cannot really know.

# 17.7d Cannabis May Cause Cancer

Don't think this is a 100% done deal. A new study has shown that smoking marijuana as often as weekly over an extended period of time appears to greatly boost a young man's risk for developing a particularly aggressive form of testicular cancer, the nonseminoma, which accounts for about 40% of all cases.

Across North America, Europe, Australia and New Zealand, testicular cancer rates have doubled in the past half-century. That has led some researchers to suggest that the upward trend might be due to a simultaneous and comparable rise in the use of marijuana.[12]

The BBC quotes the British Lung Foundation in stating that cannabis is 20 times more likely to cause lung cancer than tobacco.[13]

## Marijuana Synthetics are Dangerous

Finally, I feel obliged to add this important warning:

Modern day synthetic (manufactured) cannabinoids are NOT the old folk herb you have been reading about. They are extremely toxic and cannot be given any kind of safety clearance.

Tests suggest that synthetic cannabinoids might be up to 100 times more toxic than the natural plant herbal equivalent dose.

# The Last Word

Finally, I feel obliged to add this important warning:

Modern day synthetic (manufactured) cannabinoids are NOT the old folk herb you have been reading about. They are extremely toxic and cannot be given any kind of safety clearance.

Tests suggest that synthetic cannabinoids might be up to 100 times more toxic than the natural plant herbal equivalent dose.

"People have the mind-set that this is just pot," says Dr. Lewis Nelson, a medical toxicologist at NYU Langone and Bellevue hospitals and director of training at the city's poison control center. "But it's not."

"Synthetic marijuana is really a misnomer. It's really quite different, and the effects are much more unpredictable. It's dangerous, and there is no quality control in what you are getting."

So read the data with this in mind. Don't be naive and fall for the druggie lobby's propaganda.

Leave well alone is my advice.

"People have the mind-set that this is just pot," says Dr. Lewis Nelson, a medical toxicologist at NYU Langone and Bellevue hospitals and director of training at the city's poison control center. "But it's not."

"Synthetic marijuana is really a misnomer. It's really quite different, and the effects are much more unpredictable. It's dangerous, and there is no quality control in what you are getting."

So read the data with this in mind. Don't be naive and fall for the druggie lobby's propaganda.

Leave well alone is my advice.

## Sources:

1. P. V. Tortorice, Pharmacotherapy, 1990; H.J. Eyre, Cancer, 1984.

2. Journal of the National Cancer Institute, Vol. 55, No. 3, September 1975

3. Guzman et al. 1998. Delta-9-tetrahydrocannabinol induces apoptosis in C6 glioma cells. FEBS Letters 436: 6-10.

4. Guzman et al. 2000. Anti-tumoral action of cannabinoids: involvement of sustained ceramide accumulation and extracellular signal-regulated kinase activation. Nature Medicine 6: 313-319.

5. Guzman et al. 2003. Inhibition of tumor angiogenesis by cannabinoids. The FASEB Journal 17: 529-531.

6. Massi et al. 2004. Antitumor effects of cannabidiol, a non-psychotropic cannabinoid, on human glioma cell lines. Journal of Pharmacology and Experimental Therapeutics Fast Forward 308: 838-845.

7. Guzman et al. 2004. Cannabinoids inhibit the vascular endothelial growth factor pathways in gliomas (PDF). Cancer Research 64: 5617-5623.

8. Allister et al. 2005. Cannabinoids selectively inhibit proliferation and induce death of cultured human glioblastoma multiforme cells. Journal of Neurooncology 74: 31-40.

9. Casanova et al. Inhibition of skin tumor growth and angiogenesis in vivo by activation of cannabinoid receptors. 2003. Journal of Clinical Investigation 111: 43-50.

10. Powles et al. 2005. Cannabis-induced cytotoxicity in leukemic cell lines. Blood 105: 1214-1221

11. Marcu et al. 2010. Cannabidiol enhances the inhibitory effects of delta9-tetrahydrocannabinol on human glioblastoma cell proliferation and survival. Molecular Cancer Therapeutics 9: 180-189.

12. Feb. 9th 2009 online issue of the journal Cancer.

13. http://www.bbc.co.uk/news/health-18283689

**This territory is so controversial, I have given full references.**

Made in the USA
San Bernardino, CA
22 December 2016